# Computed Tomography for Technologists

## EXAM REVIEW

SECOND
EDITION

# Computed Tomography for Technologists

## EXAM REVIEW

**Lois E. Romans, RT, (R)(CT)**

Wolters Kluwer

Philadelphia • Baltimore • New York • London
Buenos Aires • Hong Kong • Sydney • Tokyo

*Acquisitions Editor*: Sharon Zinner
*Development Editor*: Amy Millholen
*Editorial Coordinator*: Caroline Define/Tim Rinehart
*Editorial Assistant*: Virginia Podgurski
*Marketing Manager*: Shauna Kelley
*Production Project Manager*: Kim Cox
*Design Coordinator*: Stephen Druding
*Manufacturing Coordinator*: Margie Orzech
*Prepress Vendor*: SPi Global

Second Edition

**Cataloging-in-Publication Data available on request from the Publisher**

ISBN: 978-1-4963-7726-5

# Preface

Never has the field of CT been more exciting. Technological developments, such as 256-slice MDCT and dual-source systems, have opened the door to new CT applications. To stay abreast of new advances, technologists must oftentimes relearn information from their original training programs that, until recently, was little used and all but forgotten. One example is seen in the explosion in cardiac CT applications. Although cardiac anatomy and physiology is included in the basic RT curriculum, until recently, CT technologists had little opportunity to put that knowledge to use. Now, to effectively perform cardiac protocols, technologists must reacquaint themselves with the basics of ECG tracings and the intricacies of cardiac anatomy.

Many CT technologists find themselves in an unenviable position. They are expected to possess a wide range of knowledge relating to their science, but few are provided a comprehensive source for that information. The quest for information most often means sifting through a variety of texts written for other audiences, in an attempt to glean pertinent data. Technologists must sort through physics texts geared toward other physicists and patient care texts written for nursing students with only a few paragraphs relevant to CT practice. Perhaps most problematic is finding a reliable source for relevant information about newer applications and techniques. Information on new protocols is primarily found in journal articles and texts written by radiologists. While providing valuable information, these sources tend to be scarce in the background information a typical CT technologist needs to fully understand the intricacies of a new exam procedure. Instead, these sources often provide specific diagnostic criteria, useful to the radiologist, but not as relevant to the technologist.

My goal was to make the data more accessible to CT technologists. To that end, I've reviewed a wide variety of resources and attempted to extract the information most pertinent to the practicing CT technologist. My efforts resulted in the companion to this text, *Computed Tomography for Technologists: A Comprehensive Text.*

*Computed Tomography for Technologists: Exam Review* is intended to be used in a fashion similar to CliffsNotes, to help readers by providing a bulleted list of key aspects of the *Comprehensive Text,* and to provide questions that test their understanding of the material. This *Exam Review* text can stand alone if the reader has already been exposed to the more comprehensive material at some time in the past and is simply looking for a quick review.

Students preparing for the ARRT's advanced level certification exam will find the practice exam in the text and the exam simulator offered as an ancillary resource particularly helpful. They were created to serve three main purposes. One is to allow the reader to evaluate their current level of CT understanding and assess possible weak areas for further study. Second, brief explanations are provided to bring to the surface knowledge that the technologists may have known cognitively. The explanations are purposefully brief, although I have included references to the *Comprehensive Text,* should the reader wish to pursue a more in-depth study of specific topics. Finally, practice exams help to refamiliarize the reader with the process of taking multiple choice examinations. In many cases, test-taking skills can be improved with practice, and too often, technologists, with their original Registry exam many years in the past, have become rusty at such skills.

I have made every effort to include questions from the entire spectrum of CT procedures. I have placed an emphasis on deductive reasoning, because it is essential that the technologist be aware of how one adjustment may have myriad consequences.

The questions in the practice exams reflect the content categories included on the ARRT certification exam. They have been roughly broken down into four main types: (1) questions that concern patient care (13%); (2) questions regarding safety, primarily concerning radiation safety and dose (12%); (3) those concerning the physical properties in the production of x-ray and the corresponding generation of the CT image (34%); and (4) those that refer to actual imaging procedures, including the identification of cross-sectional anatomy (41%).

This text can also be an excellent resource to technologists new to radiography. In recognition of the ever-expanding role of general radiographers, program graduates are now expected to possess a basic understanding of CT. Therefore, curriculum for general radiography incorporates many aspects of CT. An exam simulator found on the companion student site on thePoint is customizable so that users can practice taking the CT exam or the CT portion of the radiography exam.

Finally, radiation therapists and nuclear medicine technologists may also find this to be a valuable resource. CT simulation is a core skill in radiation therapy, there-fore therapists benefit from basic education in many aspects of CT. Similarly, with the advent of PET-CT and SPECT-CT fusion imaging, nuclear medicine technologists may find that they need to learn CT skills, particularly those that relate to CT radiation dose, cross-sectional anatomy, and radiographic contrast media.

*Lois E. Romans, RT, (R)(CT)*
*University of Michigan Health Systems*
*Ann Arbor, Michigan*

# User's Guide

This User's Guide shows you how to put the helpful features of *Computed Tomography for Technologists: Exam Review*, second edition, to work for you.

Content is presented in a **user-friendly bulleted format**.

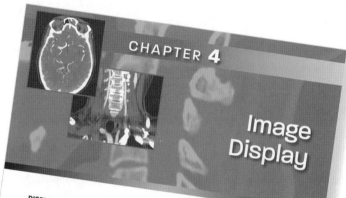

**Review Questions** at the end of each chapter are registry-style multiple choice questions.

### Endoluminal Imaging

■ Endoluminal imaging is a form of VR that is specifically designed to look inside the lumen of a structure.

■ Because the technique aims to simulate the view of an endoscopist, it is commonly referred to as virtual endoscopy.

■ Endoluminal imaging visualizes a structure as if it were hollow and the viewer were inside of it. Once inside, the viewer can "fly through" the structure; that is, the viewer can move forward or backward at will.

### Three-Dimensional Modeling

■ VR data sets can be used to create 3D models using 3D printers.

■ Three-dimensional printing is the common name for the additive manufacturing technique that creates 3D solid objects from a digital file. Models are produced by laying down successive layers of material until the object is created.

### Region-of-Interest Editing

■ The process of selectively removing or isolating information from the data set is referred to as region-of-interest editing or segmentation. The purpose is to better demonstrate the areas of interest by removing obscuring structures from the display.

■ Manual segmentation refers to the process by which a user identifies and selects data to be saved or removed.

■ Fully automated segmentation is a software feature that attempts to remove unwanted data automatically. However, in many situations, the source images are too complex and the software cannot readily identify the unwanted data.

■ Semiautomatic segmentation methods combine many of the benefits of manual and automatic segmentation techniques. The user guides the otherwise automatic process by providing initial information about the region of interest.

### Factors That Degrade Reformatted Images

■ Segmentation errors occur when important vessels or other structures are inadvertently edited out of the data set.

■ Excessive image noise in the source images will significantly limit the quality and utility of 3D rendered images.

■ Artifacts on the source data will also degrade the reformatted images. The most common artifacts are a result of motion or from metallic objects that produce streaks.

● Stair-step artifacts can occur when voxels are not isotropic.

## REVIEW QUESTIONS

1. Raw data that result from an MDCT scan acquisition are used so that the 1-mm slices are combined to produce thicker slices for viewing. This is called
   a. 3D reformation.
   b. image reconstruction.
   c. segmentation.
   d. multiplanar reformation.

2. In what situation would overlapping reconstructions for subsequent image rendering not be indicated?
   a. Slice thickness = 0.5 mm, DFOV = 25
   b. Slice thickness = 2 mm, DFOV = 35
   c. Slice thickness = 5 mm, DFOV = 45
   d. Slice thickness = 7 mm, DFOV = 45

3. Assume the raw data are still available. In what scenario would it be impossible to create an MPR?
   a. Source images vary in slice thickness.
   b. Source images vary in gantry tilt.
   c. Source images vary in image center.
   d. Source images vary in DFOV.

4. What plane is the MPR depicted by Figure 8-1?
   a. Sagittal
   b. Coronal
   c. Oblique
   d. Curved

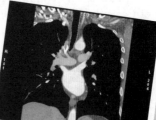

**FIGURE 8-1**

5. Which of the following is a TRUE statement regarding MPRs?
   a. They are created from raw data.
   b. They are 3D in nature.
   c. All MPR images have the same image quality as the source image.
   d. They can be created either at the operator's console or at a separate workstation.

6. A limitation of scanner-created MPRs is that
   a. only one examination protocol per scanner can be programmed to automatically create MPRs.
   b. they take more time to create than manually produced MPRs.

**Anatomical images** in the cross-sectional anatomy chapters have important structures identified.

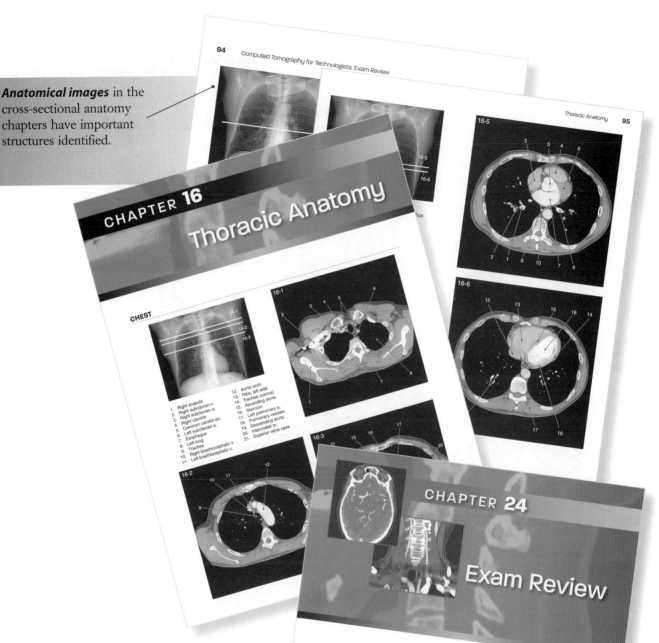

**Mock exam chapter** is a practice test for the ARRT certification exam, with the same number of questions and same breakdown of questions for each content area (patient care, safety, image production, and procedures).

**Answers to review questions** are printed at the back of the book as an appendix. Answer rationales and chapter/heading references to the *Comprehensive Text* are provided.

## Appendix

### Answers to Review Questions

#### CHAPTER 1: BASIC PRINCIPLES OF CT

1. Answer–d. Manufacturers use different names to describe features in a CT system. Names that have been used to describe the preliminary image include Topogram (Siemens), Scout (GE Healthcare), Scanogram (Toshiba), Pilot (Picker), and CR Image (Shimadzu). The term "spiral scan" is used to describe the method of scanning that includes a continuously rotating x-ray tube and constant table that travel throughout the scan acquisition. (Comprehensive Text Chapter 1; Heading: Terminology)

2. Answer–b. Low-contrast resolution is the ability of the system to display small density differences, such as when an image of the brain clearly shows the difference between the white and gray matter. Choices (a) and (c) are synonyms for a system's ability to define small objects distinctly. Temporal resolution, choice (d), refers to acquisition speed. (Comprehensive Text Chapter 1; Heading: Terminology)

3. Answer–a. (Comprehensive Text Chapter 1; Heading: Computed Tomography Defined)

4. Answer–d. A 1,024 matrix contains 1,024 rows of pixels down and 1,024 columns of pixels across. The total number of pixels in a matrix is the product of the number of rows and the number of columns. (Comprehensive Text Chapter 1; Heading: Computed Tomography Defined)

5. Answer–d. Beam attenuation is a basic radiation principle in which higher-density objects absorb more of the x-ray beam; subsequently fewer photons reach the detectors. The alteration in the beam varies with the density of the structure it passes through. This phenomenon is essential to produce images in which varying shades of gray reflect varying densities within the object. (Comprehensive Text Chapter 1; Heading: Beam Attenuation)

6. Answer–c. A low-attenuation object is one that allows x-rays to pass through relatively unimpeded. Because the trachea contains air, which does not attenuate much of the x-ray beam, it will be repre-

sented by a black area on the image. (Comprehensive Text Chapter 1; Heading: Beam Attenuation)

7. Answer–b. In the Hounsfield system, the attenuation capacity of water is assigned 0, that of air −1,000, and that of bone 1,000. Objects with a beam attenuation less than that of water have an associated negative number. If an object is slightly less dense than water, an HU of slightly less than 0 can be expected. (Comprehensive Text Chapter 1; Heading: Hounsfield Units)

8. Answer–a. Oral or intravenous iodinated agents fill certain structures with a higher-density material, subsequently raising the structure's ability to attenuate the x-ray beam. It is important to note that the contrast agent does not change the body tissues but only resides in them. (Comprehensive Text Chapter 1; Heading: Beam Attenuation)

9. Answer–d. The x-ray beam used in CT contains a variety of x-ray photons, ranging from those that are weak to those that are relatively strong. (Comprehensive Text Chapter 1; Heading: Polychromatic X-ray Beams)

10. Answer–a. Artifacts can be attributed to many different reasons, but they always degrade the image. (Comprehensive Text Chapter 1; Heading: Polychromatic X-ray Beams)

11. Answer–d. Filtering the x-ray beam removes long-wavelength, or "soft," x-rays that do not contribute to the CT image but increase the patient's radiation dose. A second purpose of filtration is to reduce beam-hardening artifacts by creating a more uniform beam intensity. An x-ray beam can only be filtered after it is generated (i.e., leaves the anode); therefore, neither choices (a) nor (c) are possible. (Comprehensive Text Chapter 1; Heading: Polychromatic X-ray Beams)

12. Answer–d. Thinner slices reduce volume averaging by decreasing the amount of patient information included in each voxel. (Comprehensive Text Chapter 1; Heading: Volume Averaging)

13. Answer–a. To accurately image the many small structures of the inner ear, a thin slice is required. It is true that there is a trade-off when it comes to

151

## Student Resources

The online student resource center at **http://thePoint.lww.com/RomansER2e** features an online **exam simulator** that allows for additional practice and mastery of the material.

See the inside front cover for details on how to access the student resource center.

**thePoint®**

# Reviewers

The publisher, author, and editors gratefully acknowledge the valuable contributions made by the following professionals who reviewed this text:

**Matthew G. Aagesen, MD**
*Musculoskeletal Fellow*
University of Michigan Health System
Ann Arbor, Michigan

**Jeff L. Berry, MS, RT (R) (CT)**
*Radiography Program Director*
Department of Medical Imaging and Radiation Sciences
University of Oklahoma Health Sciences Center
Oklahoma City, Oklahoma

**Jonathan R. Dillman, MD**
*Abdominal Radiology Fellow*
University of Michigan Health System
Ann Arbor, Michigan

**James H. Ellis, MD, FACR**
*Professor of Radiology*
University of Michigan Health System
Ann Arbor, Michigan

**Frances Gilman, MS, RT, R, CT, MR, CV, ARRT**
*Assistant Professor and Chair*
Department of Radiologic Sciences
Thomas Jefferson University
Philadelphia, Pennsylvania

**Ella A. Kazerooni, MD, FACR**
*Professor of Radiology*
*Director, Cardiothoracic Radiology*
University of Michigan Health System
Ann Arbor, Michigan

**William Nelson, MA, RT(R)**
*Faculty*
Radiography Program
Washtenaw Community College
Ann Arbor, Michigan

**Leanna B. Neubrander, BS, RT (R) (CT)**
*Instructor, Department of Radiologic Sciences*
Florida Hospital College of Health Sciences
Orlando, Florida

**Dr. Saabry Osmany, MD**
*Department of Nuclear Medicine and PET*
Singapore General Hospital
Singapore

**Deena Slockett, MBA, RT (R), (M)**
*Associate Professor, FHCHS*
*Program Coordinator*
Department of Radiologic Sciences
Orlando, Florida

**Suzette Thomas-Rodriguez, BS (Medical Imaging), ARRT(R) (CT) (MRI)**
*Senior Lecturer*
Department of Radiological Sciences
College of Science Technology and Applied Arts of Trinidad & Tobago
Port-of-Spain, Trinidad

**Amit Vyas, MD**
*Neuroradiology Fellow*
University of Michigan Health System
Ann Arbor, Michigan

# Table of Contents

## SECTION IV: Imaging Procedures and Protocols

# SECTION I

# Physics and Instrumentation

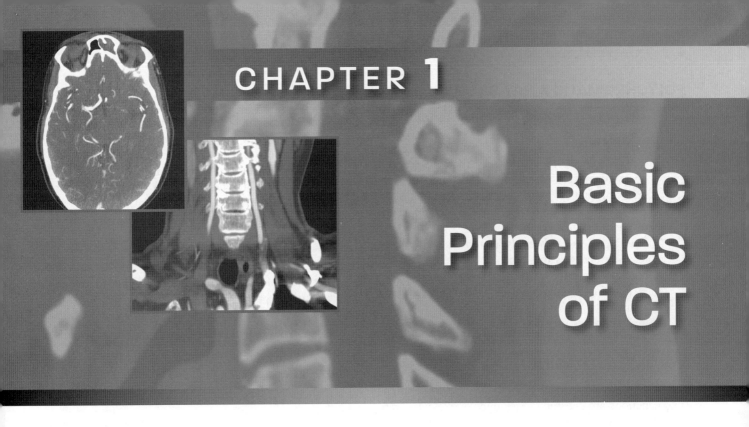

# CHAPTER **1**

# Basic Principles of CT

## BACKGROUND AND TERMINOLOGY

- The main advantages of CT over conventional radiography are in the elimination of superimposed structures, the ability to differentiate small differences in density of anatomic structures and abnormalities, and the superior quality of the images.
- CT image quality is evaluated using a number of criteria including spatial resolution, low-contrast resolution, and temporal resolution.
- The CT process creates cross-sectional images with information collected when an x-ray beam passes through an area of anatomy.
- Each CT slice represents a specific plane in the patient's body, referred to as the $z$ axis. The $z$ axis determines the thickness of the cross-sectional slice.
- Data that form the CT slice are further sectioned into elements. Each two-dimensional square is a pixel in which the width is indicated by $x$, and the height by $y$. If the $z$ axis is taken into account, the result is a cube, referred to as a voxel.
- A matrix is the grid formed from the rows and columns of pixels.

## BEAM ATTENUATION

- X-ray photons pass through or are absorbed or scattered by structures in varying amounts, depending on the average photon energy of the x-ray beam and the characteristics of the structure in its path.
- The degree to which an x-ray beam is reduced is referred to as attenuation.

- Objects that have little ability to attenuate the beam are said to have low attenuation. Objects that have the ability to absorb much, or all, of the beam are said to have high attenuation.
- Historically, lower attenuation structures are represented by a black or dark gray area on the image. Higher attenuation structures are represented by a white or light gray area on the image.
- The number of photons that interact with an object depends on the thickness, density, and atomic number of the object.
- The amount of the x-ray beam that is scattered or absorbed per unit thickness of the absorber is expressed by the linear attenuation coefficient ($\mu$).
- Differences in linear attenuation coefficients among tissues are responsible for x-ray image contrast. To differentiate an object on a CT image from adjacent objects, there must be a sufficient density difference between the two objects.
  - Oral or intravenous administration of a contrast agent is often used to create a temporary artificial density difference between objects.
- Hounsfield units quantify the degree that a structure attenuates an x-ray beam.
- There are 2,000 HU for naturally occurring anatomic structures, ranging from −1,000 for air to 1,000 for dense bone.
- HU measurements are not absolute. A number of factors can contribute to inaccurate values including poor equipment calibration, image artifacts, and volume averaging.

3

## POLYCHROMATIC X-RAY BEAM

- The x-ray beam used in CT is polychromatic. That is, the beam comprises photons with varying energies.
- The CT detectors cannot differentiate and adjust for differences in attenuation that are caused by low-energy x-ray photons. This can produce image artifacts.
- An artifact is an object seen on the image but not present in the object scanned.
- Filtering the x-ray beam helps to reduce the range of x-ray energies that reach the patient by eliminating the photons with weaker energies.
  - Filtering improves image quality by reducing artifacts.
  - Filtering reduces the radiation dose to the patient.

## VOLUME AVERAGING

- The process in CT by which different tissue attenuations are averaged to produce one less accurate pixel reading is called volume averaging or the partial volume effect.
- Thicker CT slices increase the likelihood of missing very small objects.
- Thinner slices result in a higher radiation dose to the patient, and if the area to be scanned is large, will produce a huge number of slices.
- Scanning procedures are designed to provide the image quality necessary for diagnosis at an acceptable radiation dose.
- The process of using raw data to create an image is called image reconstruction.
  - The reconstruction that is automatically produced during scanning is often called prospective reconstruction.
  - Reusing raw data to generate new images is called retrospective reconstruction.

## SCAN MODES

- Older CT systems operated exclusively in a "step-and-shoot" fashion.
- In the 1990s, technical developments resulted in helical scanning, which allows for uninterrupted imaging.
- Helical scanners were further improved to incorporate multiple rows of detectors that allowed data for many slices to be acquired with each gantry rotation.

## IMAGE PLANES

- Directional terms used in medicine are based on the body being viewed in the anatomic position. This position is characterized by an individual standing erect, with the palms of the hands facing forward.
  - Anterior and ventral refer to movement forward (toward the face).
  - Posterior and dorsal describe movement toward the back surface of the body.
  - Inferior and caudal refer to movement toward the feet (down).
  - Superior, cranial, and cephalic define movement toward the head (up).
  - Lateral refers to movement toward the sides of the body.
  - Medial refers to movement toward the midline of the body.
  - Distal (away from) refers to movement toward the end of an extremity.
  - Proximal is defined as situated near the point of attachment.
- Body planes can be imagined by thinking of large sheets of glass cutting through the body in various ways.
  - All planes that are parallel to the floor are called horizontal, or transverse, planes.
  - Planes that stand perpendicular to the floor are called vertical, or longitudinal, planes.
  - A coronal plane divides the body into anterior and posterior sections.
  - A sagittal plane divides the body into right and left sections.
  - The sagittal plane that is located directly in the center, making left and right sections of equal size, is called the median, or midsagittal, plane.
    - A parasagittal plane is located to either the left or the right of midline.
  - Oblique planes are analogous to sheets of glass that are slanted and lie at an angle to one of the three standard planes.
- Changing the imaging plane in CT may provide additional information. The imaging plane may be adjusted to accommodate specific anatomy or to reduce artifacts created by surrounding structures.

## OVERVIEW OF CT OPERATION

- X-ray photons are created when a substance is bombarded by fast-moving electrons.
- To make the electrons move quickly, high voltage, or kV, is used. This propels the electrons from the x-ray tube filament to the anode.
- The area of the anode where the electrons strike and the x-ray beam is produced is the focal spot.
- The quantity of electrons propelled is controlled by the tube current and is measured in milliamperes (mA).
- The intensity of the x-ray beam is controlled by the kilovolt peak (kVp) setting.

- The vast majority of the kinetic energy of the projectile electrons is converted to thermal energy. Less than 1% is converted to x-ray energy.
- Increasing the voltage increases the energy with which the electrons strike the target and, therefore, increases the intensity of the x-ray beam.
- The ability of the tube to withstand heat is called its heat capacity.
- The ability of the tube to rid itself of heat is its heat dissipation.
- Detectors record the number of x-ray photons that pass through the patient.
- Each detector cell is sampled many times per second by the data acquisition system (DAS).
- The digital data from the DAS are then transmitted to the central processing unit (CPU).
- The reconstruction process takes the individual views and reconstructs the densities within the slice.
- Digitized data are then sent to a display processor that converts them into shades of gray that can be displayed on a monitor.
- The CT process can be broken down into three phases:
  - Phase 1 is data acquisition (get data).
  - Phase 2 is image reconstruction (use data).
  - Phase 3 is image display (show data).

## REVIEW QUESTIONS

1. Which is NOT a synonym for the preliminary (or localizer) image taken at the start of a CT examination?
   a. Topogram
   b. Scout
   c. Scanogram
   d. Spiral
2. The ability of a system to differentiate, on the image, objects with similar densities is known as
   a. high-contrast resolution.
   b. low-contrast resolution.
   c. spatial resolution.
   d. temporal resolution.
3. Each two-dimensional square of data that make up the CT image is called a
   a. pixel.
   b. voxel.
   c. matrix.
   d. fragment.
4. How many pixels are contained in a 1,024 matrix image?
   a. 1,024
   b. 2,048
   c. 262,144
   d. 1,048,576
5. Beam attenuation can be defined as
   a. the phenomenon by which artifacts result when lower-energy photons are preferentially absorbed, leaving only higher-intensity photons to strike the detector array.
   b. x-ray energy that is produced from bombarding a substance with fast-moving electrons.
   c. the ability of the detector to capture transmitted photons and change them to electronic signals.
   d. the phenomenon by which an x-ray beam passing through a structure is decreased in intensity or amount because of absorption and interaction with matter.
6. Which of the following is a low-attenuation structure?
   a. Iodine-filled aorta
   b. Rib
   c. Trachea
   d. Calcified arteries
7. An object is slightly less dense than water. What is the expected Hounsfield measurement?
   a. −940
   b. −10
   c. 50
   d. 850
8. Why does the administration of iodinated contrast media result in an enhanced image?
   a. Iodinated contrast material increases the ability of the enhanced structure to attenuate the x-ray beam.
   b. Iodinated contrast material decreases the average photon energy of the x-ray beam; therefore, more photons are absorbed by the patient.
   c. The administration of iodinated contrast material results in a smaller pixel, thereby increasing spatial resolution, which results in an enhanced image.
   d. Iodinated contrast material alters the atomic number of body tissues. In the case of blood vessels, it temporarily changes their color from red to blue, hence the name "x-ray dye."
9. The x-ray beam sources for CT produce x-ray energy that is polychromatic. This means that
   a. when viewed by the naked eye, the beam exhibits many different colors.
   b. it produces, as a by-product, a substance known as poly-chlorinated biphenyl.
   c. photons contained in the beam are all of the same wavelength.
   d. the beam comprises photons with varying energies.
10. An object that appears on the image but is not present in the object scanned is called a (an)
    a. artifact.
    b. anomaly.
    c. shadow.
    d. ghost.
11. Which is an advantage of filtering the x-ray beam?
    a. Filtering reduces the anode heat load.
    b. A filtered beam produces images with substantially less quantum mottle.
    c. Filtering the beam prevents energy from being converted to heat; therefore, 100% of the energy is converted to x-rays.
    d. Filtering reduces the radiation dose to the patient.
12. Scan thickness is *primarily* important for the part it plays in
    a. noise reduction.
    b. the contrast scale.
    c. detector aperture opening.
    d. volume averaging.

13. You are working with the radiologists to establish examination protocols for your department. Which of the following is a logical consideration when determining an appropriate slice thickness for studies of the internal auditory canal?
    a. Because the auditory ossicles are quite small, a thin slice will be necessary to reduce the chance that volume averaging will obscure their appearance on the image.
    b. The appropriate slice thickness will vary considerably from patient to patient. Therefore, each technologist should be free to adjust the slice thickness as he or she deems necessary for the particular patient.
    c. A slice thickness of 5 to 7 mm is adequate because the structures of interest are not particularly small, and the examination is most often ordered as a screening study for asymptomatic patients.
    d. The thickest slice available should be used to reduce the radiation dose to the corneas.
14. How many CT numbers are assigned to each pixel in the image matrix?
    a. One-half the number of all values recorded from the detector array
    b. One
    c. The number of HU per pixel is one-tenth the display field of view
    d. Two values for a 256-matrix; 4 values for a 512-matrix
15. Which is another name for raw data?
    a. Image data
    b. Scan data
    c. Reconstructed data
    d. Displayed data

16. When in the anatomic position, the arms are
    a. raised above the head, palms facing backward.
    b. crossed over the chest, palms on opposite shoulders.
    c. down by the sides, palms facing forward.
    d. by the sides, with elbows bent, palms facing backward and resting on the hips.
17. In Figure 1-1, arrow #1 depicts a (an)
    a. coronal plane.
    b. transverse plane.
    c. sagittal plane.
    d. axial plane.

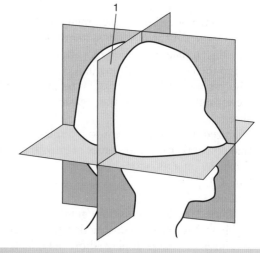

**FIGURE 1-1**

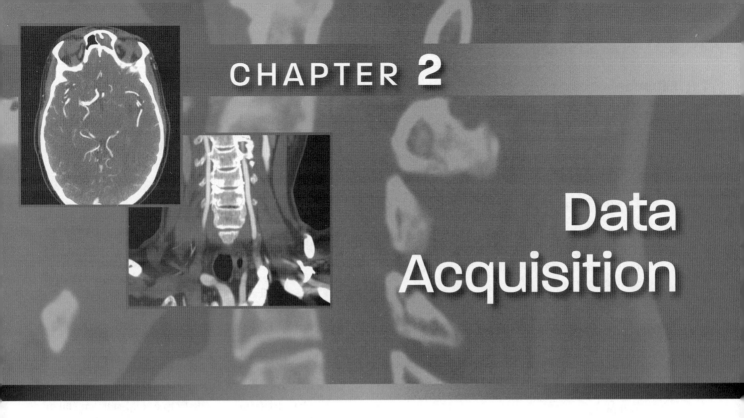

# CHAPTER 2

# Data Acquisition

## DATA ACQUISITION

- Data are acquired when x-rays pass through a patient to strike a detector and are recorded.
- The major components used for data acquisition are those contained in the gantry and the patient table.

## GANTRY

- Components are mounted in the gantry on a rotating scan frame.
- Gantries vary in total size as well as in the diameter of the aperture. Typical aperture size ranges from 70 to 90 cm.
- The gantry can be tilted to adjust the scan plane.
- Early scanners used cables to rotate the gantry frame. This required the gantry to rotate in one direction and then stop to change direction and rotate in the opposite direction.
- The development of slip rings permits the gantry frame to rotate continuously, making helical scan methods possible.

### Generator

- High-frequency generators are used in CT. They are located within the gantry.
- Generators produce high voltage and transmit it to the x-ray tube. The power capacity of the generator is listed in kilowatts (kW). The power capacity of the generator determines the range of exposure techniques available.
- Generators produce high kV to increase the intensity of the resulting x-ray beam. This increases the penetrating ability of the beam and reduces the patient dose. A high kV setting also allows a lower mA setting, which helps to reduce the heat load on the x-ray tube.
- Cooling mechanisms housed within the gantry help to reduce temperature fluctuations that could affect system performance.

### X-ray Source

- The x-ray tubes used in CT are a modification of a standard rotating anode tube.
- CT tubes often contain more than one size focal spot. Small focal spots improve spatial resolution, but, because they concentrate heat onto a smaller portion of the anode, they cannot tolerate as much heat.
- To increase the number of simultaneously acquired slices, some multislice systems employ the periodic motion of the focal spot in the longitudinal direction ($z$ axis). This is called a flying focal spot or $z$-flying focal spot.
- Anode heat capacity is measured in million heat units (MHU).
- Anode heat dissipation rate is measured in thousand heat units (KHU).

## Filtration

- Filters are used to shape the x-ray beam. They reduce the radiation dose to the patient and help to reduce image artifact. Filtering the x-ray beam helps to reduce the range of x-ray energies that reach the patient by removing the lower energy x-rays.
- Different filters are used when scanning the body than when scanning the head.
- Bowtie filters are often used to scan the body. These reduce the beam intensity at the periphery of the beam, corresponding to the thinner areas of a patient's anatomy.
- Collimators restrict the x-ray beam and reduce scatter radiation. Reducing the scatter improves contrast resolution and decreases patient dose.
- Source collimators affect slice thickness by narrowing or widening the x-ray beam. Because they act on the x-ray before it passes through the patient, they are also called prepatient collimators.
- Some CT systems also use predetector collimation. These act on the x-ray after it has emerged from the patient and before it strikes the detector. These are sometimes referred to as postpatient collimators. Their purpose is to prevent scattered radiation from reaching the detectors.

## Detectors

- Detectors collect information regarding the degree to which each anatomic structure attenuates the x-ray beam. A detector array comprises detector elements situated in an arc or a ring, each of which measures the intensity of transmitted x-ray radiation along a beam projected from the x-ray source to that particular detector element.
- The number of detector cells that collect data is controlled by the selection of scan field size.
- Detectors can be made from different substances, each with their own advantages and disadvantages.
- The optimal characteristics of a detector are as follows:
  - High detector efficiency–defined as the ability of the detector to capture transmitted photons and change them to electronic signals
  - Low, or no, afterglow–defined as a brief, persistent flash of scintillation that must be taken into account and subtracted before image reconstruction
  - High scatter suppression
  - High stability

- Detector efficiency is dependent on the stopping power of the detector material, scintillator (solid-state types) or charge collection (xenon types) efficiency, geometric efficiency, and scatter rejection.
- The geometric efficiency of a detector refers to the amount of space occupied by the detector collimator plates relative to the surface area of the detector.
- Capture efficiency refers to the ability with which the detector obtains x-ray beams that have passed through the patient.
- Absorption efficiency refers to the number of photons absorbed by the detector and is dependent on the physical properties of the detector face.
- Response time is the time required for the signal from the detector to return to zero so that it is ready to detect another x-ray event.
- The dynamic range is the ratio of the maximum signal measured to the minimum signal the detectors can measure.
- Detectors can be made from a solid-state crystal or from xenon gas-filled chambers. All new detectors are of the solid-state crystal variety.
- Xenon gas detectors are much less efficient than solid-state detectors. However, they are less expensive to produce, somewhat easier to calibrate, and are highly stable.
- Solid-state detectors are also called scintillation detectors because they use a crystal that fluoresces when struck by an x-ray photon.
  - A photodiode transforms the light energy into electrical energy.
- Solid-state detectors are very efficient, absorbing nearly 100% of the photons that reach them.
- Older solid-state detectors produced a brief afterglow.
- Solid-state detectors are more sensitive to fluctuation in temperature and moisture than the gas variety.
- The size, shape, and placement of the detector elements affect the amount of scatter radiation that is recorded.
  - Detector spacing is measured from the middle of one detector to the middle of the neighboring detector. It accounts for the spacing bar placed between each detector element.
  - The size of the detector opening is called the aperture.
  - A small detector is important for good spatial resolution and scatter rejection.

## Scanner Generation

- The configuration of the x-ray tube to the detectors determines scanner generation.

- First- and second-generation scanners are no longer used.
- The third-generation design consists of an x-ray tube that produces a fan-shaped beam that covers the entire field of view and a detector array.
  - An advantage of this configuration is that the tube is directly focused on the detector array. This fixed relationship allows the beam to be highly collimated, which greatly reduces scatter radiation.
  - A disadvantage of this configuration is the more frequent occurrence of ring artifact (as compared with the fourth-generation design).
  - The third-generation design is the most widely used configuration in the industry today.
- Fourth-generation scanners use a detector array that is fixed in a 360° circle within the gantry. The tube rotates within the fixed detector array and produces a fan-shaped beam.
  - Because the emerging beam does not strike the detectors at exactly the same time, motion artifacts are more of a problem.
  - Overscans are used to reduce the motion artifacts.
  - Because the tube is closer to the patient, the same technique will produce a higher dose, as compared with a third-generation system.
- Fifth-generation scanners are referred to as electron beam (EBCT) or ultrafast CT. The design of these systems varies considerably from that of other generations in that neither the x-ray beam nor the detectors move.
- Sixth-generation, or dual-source scanners use two side-by-side tube and detector arrays. The two systems may be energized using the same or different kVp's.
  - The use of two different kVp settings, often referred to as spectral scanning, provides the potential to analyze material composition to aid in tissue characterization.

## Detector Electronics

- The data-acquisition system (DAS) measures the number of photons that strike the detector, converts the information to a digital signal, and sends the signal to the computer.
- The DAS is positioned in the gantry, near the detectors.
- To be useful for the CT system computer, the analog signals from the detector must be converted into a digital format. This task is accomplished by the analog-to-digital converter (ADC).
- Detectors are sampled many times, as many as 1,000 times per second by the DAS.

- The number of samples taken per second is known as the sampling rate, sample rate, or sampling frequency.
- Image artifacts can occur if the sampling rate is too low.

## PATIENT TABLE

- The process of moving the table by a specified measure is called incrementation, feed, step, or index. Helical CT table incrementation is measured in millimeters per second because the table moves continuously throughout the data acquisition.
- The degree to which the table can move horizontally is called the scannable range.
- An anatomic landmark is chosen when a patient is first positioned within the gantry and the table position is manually set to zero. This is referred to as referencing the table.

### REVIEW QUESTIONS

1. Which of the following components is NOT housed within the gantry?
   a. Three-phase generator
   b. High-frequency generator
   c. Slip rings
   d. Xenon gas detectors
2. The power capacity of the generator is listed in
   a. milliamperes (mA).
   b. thousand heat units (KHU).
   c. million heat units (MHU).
   d. kilowatts (kW).
3. Which of the following describes a slip ring device?
   a. A recoiling system cable used to rotate the gantry frame
   b. A brushlike apparatus that provides continuous electrical power and electronic communication across a rotating surface
   c. A device used to shape the x-ray beam, thereby reducing the radiation dose to the patient and reducing image artifact
   d. A device that restricts the x-ray beam emerging from the gantry to thin ribbons
4. Which is a disadvantage of a small focal spot size?
   a. Reduced spatial resolution
   b. Reduced detector efficiency
   c. Increased penumbra
   d. Reduced heat capacity
5. The ability of the tube to withstand by-product heat is called
   a. heat capacity.
   b. heat dissipation.
   c. thermal potential.
   d. thermal transference.
6. In Figure 2-1, what is the object marked X called?
   a. Collimator
   b. Bowtie filter
   c. Focal spot
   d. Detector

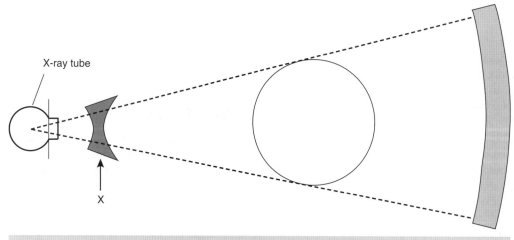

**FIGURE 2-1**

7. Regarding the detectors in the CT system, geometric efficiency is controlled primarily by
   a. detector material (solid-state crystals or xenon gas chambers).
   b. type of photodiode used.
   c. filtration.
   d. detector spacing and aperture.
8. Which of the following is a characteristic of xenon gas detectors?
   a. Low efficiency
   b. Sensitive to temperature and moisture
   c. May exhibit afterglow
   d. Also called scintillators
9. Figure 2-2 illustrates a scanner with a
   a. second-generation design.
   b. third-generation design.
   c. fourth-generation design.
   d. fifth-generation design.
10. Which component of the CT system converts the electric signal supplied by the detectors into a digital format?
   a. Photodiode
   b. Array processor
   c. Display processor
   d. Analog-to-digital converter

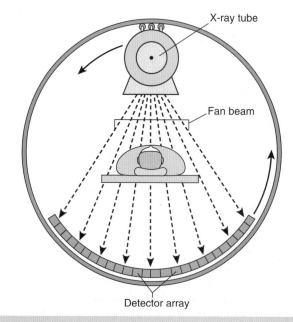

**FIGURE 2-2**

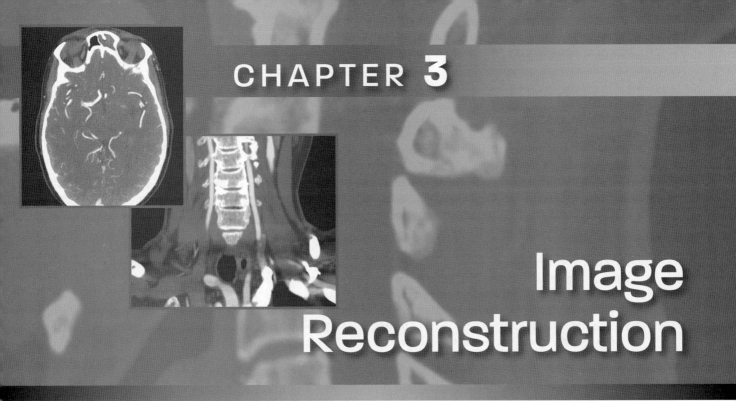

# CHAPTER 3

# Image Reconstruction

## IMAGE RECONSTRUCTION TERMINOLOGY

- To create a CT image, the system uses all of the information collected from the detectors during the data-acquisition process, and through a series of steps, it manipulates the data so as to produce a useful image that can be sent to a display device. This process of manipulating data is called image reconstruction.
- Image reconstruction functions are performed using a computer; therefore, an understanding of basic computer science concepts is helpful.
- An algorithm is a precise set of steps to be performed in a specific order to solve a problem. Algorithms are the basis for most computer programming.
- Reconstruction algorithms are used in CT to convert information obtained from the detector array into information suitable for image display.
- Fast Fourier transform (FFT) is an efficient algorithm that is used in image analysis and many other applications.
- Interpolation is a mathematical method of estimating the value of an unknown value using the known values on either side of the unknown value.
- Many forms of interpolation exist, although linear interpolation is the simplest type. Linear interpolation assumes that an unknown point falls along a straight line between two known points.

## EQUIPMENT COMPONENTS USED FOR IMAGE RECONSTRUCTION

- Hardware is the portion of the computer that can be physically touched.
- Software is instructions that tell the computer what to do and when to do it.
- Thousands of bits of data from each scan are saved on the computer's hard disk. These stored data can be retrieved and manipulated to form an image.
- An enormous amount of information is collected for each image. Advances in computer technology have played a key role in the evolution of CT technology.
- Saving data on auxiliary devices for possible future viewing is referred to as archiving.
- The principal components of a computer are an input device, an output device, a central processing unit, and memory.
- Input devices feed data into the computer. Examples are keyboard, mouse, touch-sensitive plasma screen, and CT detector mechanisms.
- Output devices accept processed data from the computer. Examples include monitor, laser camera, printer, and archiving equipment such as servers, optical disks, or magnetic tape.
- The central processing unit (CPU) interprets computer program instructions and sequences tasks. The CPU is made up of a microprocessor, a control unit, and primary memory.

- A CPU design referred to as an array processor was the standard in CT systems. Advances in computer technology have reduced the prevalence of array processors.
- There are three principal types of computer memory:
  - Read-only memory (ROM)–primary memory that is imprinted at the factory and is used to store frequently used instructions such as those required for starting the system.
  - Random access memory (RAM)–primary memory includes instructions that are frequently changed, such as the data used to reconstruct images. RAM is so named because all parts of it can be reached easily at random.
    - ◆ The opposite of RAM is serial access memory (SAM), which stores data that can only be accessed sequentially.
  - Write-once, read-many (WORM) memory does not allow saved information to be rewritten, reformatted, or erased.

## DATA TYPES

- Raw data include all measurements obtained from the detector array. Raw data require much more computer storage than that of image data.
- The terms scan data and raw data are used interchangeably to refer to the data sitting in the computer waiting to be made into an image.
- Image reconstruction that is automatically produced during scanning is called prospective reconstruction.
- It is called retrospective reconstruction when the same raw data are used later to generate a new image.
- To form an image, the computer assigns one HU value to each pixel. This value is the average of all attenuation measurements for that pixel.
- Image data are those that result once the computer has processed the raw data and displayed an image.

## OVERVIEW OF IMAGE RECONSTRUCTION

- The path that the x-ray beam takes from the tube to the detector is referred to as a ray.
- The detector reads each arriving ray and measures how much of the beam is attenuated. This measurement is called a ray sum.
- A complete set of ray sums is known as a view. Many views are needed to create an image.
- The system accounts for the attenuation properties of each ray sum and correlates them with the position of the ray. The result of this correlation is called an attenuation profile. An attenuation profile is created for each view in the scan.

- The information from all of the profiles is projected onto a matrix. The process of converting the data from the attenuation profile to a matrix is known as back projection.
- Filtering is done to minimize artifacts that can occur during the back projection process.
- The process of applying a filter function to an attenuation profile is called convolution.
- Many different filters are available that use different algorithms depending on which parts of the data must be enhanced or suppressed.
- Scan field of view (SFOV) determines the area, within the gantry, from which the raw data are acquired.
- Regardless of what size SFOV is selected, or where the patient is positioned within the gantry, scan data are always collected around the isocenter.
- SFOV selection determines the number of detector cells collecting data.
- Out-of-field artifacts can occur if any part of the patient lies outside the SFOV.
- Selecting the display field of view (DFOV) determines how much of the raw data is used to create an image.
- Changing the DFOV will affect image quality by changing the amount of raw data that is averaged together for each pixel.

### REVIEW QUESTIONS

1. "A precise set of steps to be performed in a specific order to solve a problem" describes
   a. an algorithm.
   b. beam attenuation.
   c. the mean of a random variable.
   d. the binomial probability formula.
2. What is interpolation?
   a. A technique for expressing waveform as a weighted sum of sines and cosines
   b. An efficient algorithm used to compute DFT and its inverse
   c. The difference between the first quartile and the third quartile. This is one way to describe the spread of a set of data.
   d. A mathematical method of estimating an unknown value using the known values on either side of the unknown
3. Which is an example of a computer input device?
   a. Microprocessor
   b. Primary memory
   c. CT detector mechanisms
   d. Laser camera
4. The central processing unit (CPU) performs what function?
   a. Dissipates excessive heat that builds up on the target material
   b. Interprets computer program instructions and sequences tasks
   c. Samples the detectors
   d. Restricts the x-ray beam to thin ribbons

5. All the thousands of bits of data acquired by the CT system with each scan are called
   a. image data.
   b. calibration vectors.
   c. raw data.
   d. ray sums.

6. The DAS reads each arriving ray and measures how much of the beam has been attenuated. This is
   a. a ray sum.
   b. a view.
   c. back projection.
   d. a sample.

7. In CT image creation using a third-generation design, a complete set of ray sums is known as a (an)
   a. convolution equation.
   b. algorithm.
   c. spatial frequency filter.
   d. view.

8. The process of converting the data from the attenuation profile to a matrix is known as
   a. reformation.
   b. archiving.
   c. back projection.
   d. referencing.

9. The process of applying a filter function to an attenuation profile is known as
   a. data processing.
   b. convolution.
   c. archiving.
   d. reformation.

10. Increasing the scan field of view
    a. increases the number of detector cells collecting data.
    b. increases the range of HU displayed on the image.
    c. decreases the pixel size.
    d. decreases the display field of view.

11. Figure 3-1 was taken of the abdomen using a 25-cm display field of view. What is necessary to reconstruct the image with a larger display field of view?
    a. The scanner must have an image magnification function.
    b. The scan field must be larger than 25 cm and raw data must be available.
    c. Image data must be available and the scanner must have reformation software.
    d. Scan data must be acquired in a spiral mode.

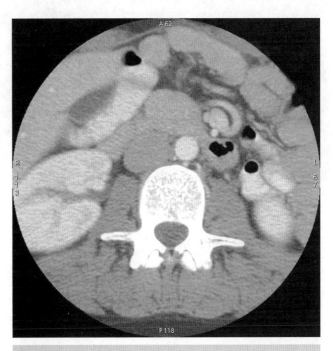

**FIGURE 3-1**

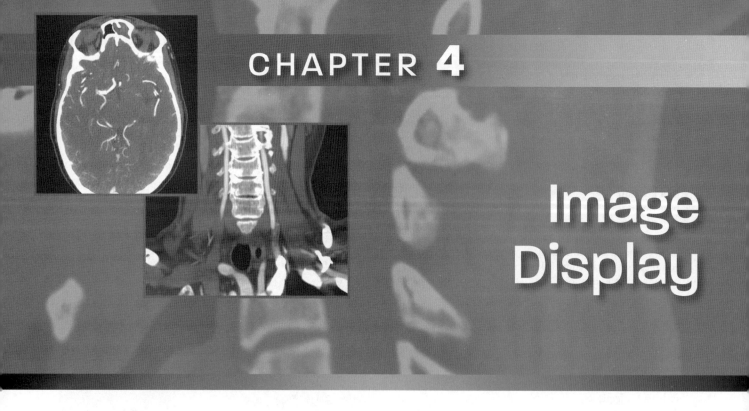

# CHAPTER 4

# Image Display

## DISPLAY MONITORS

- Black-and-white or color monitors display the CT image.
- The display device within the monitor can be either a cathode-ray tube or some form of flat panel.
- The monitors used in CT require analog signals. Therefore, it is necessary to convert the digital signal from the computer's memory back to an analog format. Digital-to-analog converters (DACs) accomplish this task.
- The way an image is viewed on the monitor can be adjusted by changing the window setting.

## WINDOW SETTINGS

- Window settings are largely subjective. They are also influenced by factors such as the patient's size and body composition.
- Ideally, images would be displayed so that a different shade of gray was used for each Hounsfield value represented.
- However, although there are more than 2,000 Hounsfield units, not all values can be appreciated; newer medical monitors can display up to 1,024 shades of gray. Furthermore, the human eye can differentiate only a fraction of those shades.
- To solve the problem of more Hounsfield units than discernible shades of gray, a gray scale is used.
- Applying the gray scale, the display processor assigns a certain number of HU to each level of gray.

- The number of HU assigned to each level of gray is determined by the window width.
- If a wide window width is selected, for example 700, then 700 values must be distributed over the available shades of gray. Therefore, many HU are included in each shade of gray. This can make it difficult to discern subtle density differences on the image.
- The window width selects the quantity of HU to be displayed as shades of gray.
- By selecting the center value, the window level selects the range of HU that will be displayed.
- All values higher than those in the selected range will appear white on the image.
- All values lower than those in the selected range will appear black on the image.
- The window level should be set at a point that is roughly the same value as the average attenuation number of the tissue of interest.
- Wide window widths (500–2,000 HU) are best for imaging tissue types that vary greatly, when the goal is to see the various tissues on one image.
- Because wider window settings decrease image contrast, they suppress the appearance of noise.
- Tissue types with similar densities should be displayed in a narrow window width (50–500 HU). This will provide greater density discrimination and contrast.

## IMAGE DISPLAY OPTIONS

- A region of interest, or ROI, is an area on the image defined by the operator.

- Placing an ROI is the first step in a number of image display and measurement functions.
- The Hounsfield measurement of an object can provide valuable diagnostic information. However, because measurement may be negatively affected by volume averaging or image noise, caution should be used when Hounsfield values are used in the diagnosis of disease.
- If a cursor is placed on the image, the system will display the value for the pixel that is covered by the cursor.
- If an ROI is placed over an area, the reading is an average of the HU within the area.
- An HU reading derived from a single pixel can be useful in some instances, particularly when a quick check of a density is needed.
- ROI measurement should be used whenever the values will be considered in formulating a diagnosis. When an area is used, the standard deviation reading is also provided.
- The standard deviation indicates the amount of CT number variance within the ROI.
- A standard deviation of 0 indicates that every pixel within the ROI has the same HU. A standard deviation cannot be less than 0.
- The higher the standard deviation, the greater the variation among pixels within the region.
- Factors that produce a high standard deviation are as follows:
  - Mixed attenuation tissue
  - ROI that includes streak artifact
  - Incorrectly placed ROI
- Distance measurements are helpful in reporting the size of an abnormality or when placing a biopsy needle. The software can also calculate the degree of angulation of the measurement line from the horizontal or vertical plane.
- The CT distance scale that often appears along the margins of an image can be used in the same way as a scale of miles is used in a map key.
- It is important to annotate images with any information that may not be immediately apparent.
- It is standard practice to include a reference image with lines posted to indicate the locations of each slice.
- Image magnification is not the same as decreasing the display field of view. Magnifying the image does not improve its image quality. It simply makes the image larger.
- Image magnification is often useful when acquiring distance measurements or placing an ROI. A larger image can make precise placement easier.
- Image magnification uses only image data (not raw data). Magnification is a useful tool that should be used on isolated images within a study.

- Magnification has inherent limitations and should not be used as an alternative to correct display field selection.

## REVIEW QUESTIONS

1. What is the function of the digital-to-analog converters?
   a. Converts the data into shades of gray to be displayed
   b. Converts the digital signal from the computer into an analog signal for the display monitor
   c. Converts the light emitted from crystal detectors into an electric current
   d. Converts the analog signal from the detectors to a digital signal for the computers
2. The window settings for Figure 4-1 are intended for evaluating
   a. bone.
   b. mediastinum.
   c. lung.
   d. the contrast-enhanced heart.

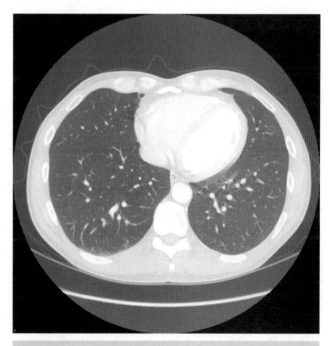

**FIGURE 4-1**

3. Why is it necessary to convert the digitized data from the reconstruction processor to shades of gray?
   a. To allow an HU to be assigned to each structure
   b. To remove streak artifacts from the final image
   c. To enhance the desirable aspects of the image and suppress the undesirable aspects
   d. So that an image can be displayed on the monitor
4. What Hounsfield values are in the naturally occurring range (i.e., not man-made objects like surgical clips)?
   a. −1,000 to 1,000
   b. −600 to 0
   c. 0 to 1,200
   d. −2,000 to 4,000

5. Decreasing the window width in a CT image decreases
   a. slice thickness.
   b. mAs.
   c. the appearance of quantum mottle (image noise).
   d. the anatomic diversity displayed.
6. The window width of a specific CT image is set at 300, and the level (or center) is set at 100. How is a structure with a measurement of 280 HU displayed?
   a. It is white.
   b. It is a light shade of gray.
   c. It is a dark shade of gray.
   d. It is black.
7. If the main tissue of interest is liver, which of the following is the best approximate window level setting?
   a. −600
   b. 0
   c. 50
   d. 600
8. On a CT image, an ROI is placed within a structure and measured. Its standard deviation is 0. What can be determined about this structure?

   a. It is composed of water or something with the same density as water.
   b. It is composed of fat.
   c. It is very homogeneous.
   d. It is very heterogeneous.
9. For which application are the raw data necessary?
   a. To magnify the image
   b. To decrease the display field size
   c. To create a histogram
   d. To obtain a Hounsfield measurement of a specific structure
10. A magnification factor of 1.5 is used to enlarge the image data, resulting in
   a. a decrease in the pixel size.
   b. an increase in the pixel size.
   c. an inaccuracy in any subsequent distance measurement.
   d. an image that is larger and may allow a more accurate cursor placement for measurements.

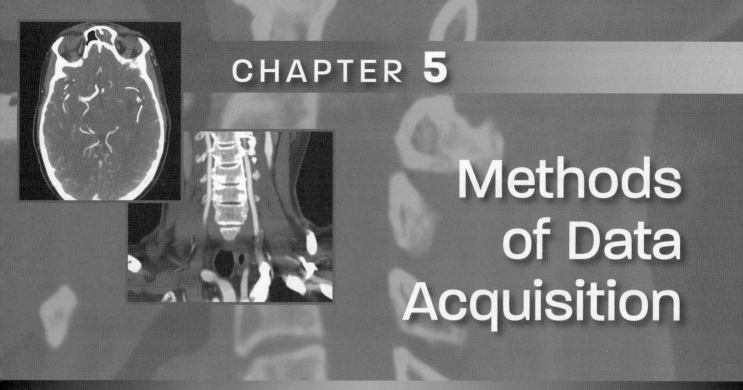

# CHAPTER 5

# Methods of Data Acquisition

There are three general methods in which scanners acquire data: 1) preliminary, or localizer, scanning; 2) axial, or step-and-shoot, scanning; and 3) helical, or spiral, scanning.

## LOCALIZER SCANS

- Localizer scans are digital image acquisitions that are created while the tube is stationary and the table moves through the scan field. They are not cross-sectional; rather the single projection causes anatomic structures to appear superimposed, like those depicted by conventional radiography.
- The position of the x-ray tube determines the orientation of the image.
  - If the tube is positioned above the patient, the localizer scan will be an anteroposterior (AP) view.
  - If the tube is positioned on either side of the patient, the localizer scan will be a lateral view.
- Localizer images are called by various names, depending on the manufacturer. The terms scout, surview, topogram, scanogram, preview, and pilot have all been used.
- In all routine studies, at least one localizer scan is acquired.
  - An AP view allows the technologist to ensure appropriate image centering in the $x$ direction.
  - A lateral view allows the technologist to ensure appropriate image centering in the $y$ direction.
  - Including all the areas to be scanned on the localizer image ensures that they lie within the scannable range or $z$ direction. The extent of the anatomic area included on the localizer image is controlled by the technologist and is dependent on the type of study.
- Miscentering a patient in either $x$ or $y$ direction can result in out-of-field artifacts.
- Proper patient centering is also important when automatic exposure control techniques are used.
- It is imperative that the operator input the correct directional instructions into the CT system before data acquisition is initiated. Failure to do so can result in incorrect image annotation and result in serious medical errors.
- Localizer images allow the technologist to prescribe the location of cross-sectional slices.
- Most scan procedures rely on beginning and ending landmarks that can be readily identified on the scout image.
  - With some protocols (e.g., adrenal glands) it is impossible to use readily identifiable landmarks to accurately predict the cross-sectional location of the organ of interest. In these cases the technologist must make an educated guess. Two different approaches can be used in these situations:
    1. One cross-sectional slice is taken and checked for accuracy before proceeding with the examination.
    2. Additional cross-sectional slices are included to both superior and inferior margins of the estimated location. This approach will increase the radiation dose to the patient but

is necessary when the delay that results from the first approach is not feasible.

- Localizer images allow the technologist to prospectively select the optimal display field of view (DFOV) and the correct image center.

## STEP-AND-SHOOT SCANNING

- Key aspects of the step-and-shoot method are that the CT table moves to the desired location and remains stationary while the x-ray tube rotates within the gantry, collecting data.
- This method is also referred to as axial scanning, conventional scanning, serial scanning, or sequence scanning.
- In this method of scanning there is a slight pause in scanning between data acquisitions, as the table advances to the next location. This is referred to as the interscan delay.
- The practice of grouping more than one axial scan in a single breath-hold is called "clustering."
- Scans produced with the step-and-shoot method result in images that are perpendicular to the $z$ axis (or tabletop) and parallel to every other slice, like slices of sausage.
- When evaluating image quality using phantoms (that do not breathe or move), step-and-shoot methods result in the highest image quality, superior to that of helical methods.
- Axial scans can be programmed to acquire data for contiguous slices (in which one slice abuts the next) or in a noncontiguous fashion in which some areas of the patient are skipped between slices or slice data overlap.
  - Gapped images are taken when a survey of an area is needed. Because some areas are not exposed, studies made up of gapped slices will reduce the radiation dose to the patient. High-resolution chest studies are often performed with gapped slices.
  - Axial protocols that use overlapping slices are rare because they increase the radiation dose to the patient but typically do not provide additional diagnostic information.
- All scanners offer the option of axial scanning. Although helical scanning has replaced many axial protocols, there are still some procedures in which axial methods are preferred.
- The primary disadvantage to the axial method is that the cumulative effect of the interscan delay adds to the total examination time. Even seemingly short delays (<30 seconds) can be significant when examining blood vessels, which remain contrast-filled for very short periods.
- Another disadvantage is that axial data have more limitations regarding reconstruction options than do data acquired with helical methods.

- Slice misregistration occurs when a patient breathes differently with each data acquisition. Valuable information may be missed because of this effect. Therefore, it is preferable to obtain images (particularly of the chest) in a single breath-hold.

### Single-Detector Row Systems

- Until the 1990s, all commercial scanners contained many detector elements aligned in a single row.
- In SDCT, opening or closing the collimator controls the slice thickness by controlling the portion of the detector's width that is exposed to the incoming x-rays.
- In SDCT, the largest allowable slice thickness is less than the detector width, typically 10 mm.
- The radiation emitted from the collimated x-ray source in these systems is commonly referred to as a fan beam.
- Each gantry rotation produces data for a single slice.
- In SDCT, the area of patient anatomy to be covered during an examination is found by multiplying the slice increment selected by the number of slices acquired.
  - For example, 25 contiguous slices, each 5 mm in width, will cover 125 mm of patient anatomy (lengthwise).

### Multidetector Row Systems

- Newer CT systems continue to use many detector elements situated in a row. However, they may contain from 4 to 320 parallel rows.
- In MDCT scanners, a single rotation can produce multiple slices. Therefore, MDCT provides longer and faster $z$ axis coverage per gantry rotation.
- In addition, many MDCT systems have increased the speed of gantry rotation, which further increases volume coverage per unit time.
- In MDCT slice thickness is determined by a combination of the x-ray beam width (controlled by the collimators) and the detector configuration.
- The radiation emitted from the collimated x-ray source is commonly referred to as a cone beam.
- MDCT can be used for either axial or helical data acquisitions.
- In some MDCT systems, the parallel rows are of equal size, referred to as a uniform array.
- In some MDCT systems, the center rows of detectors are thinner than those at the periphery. These variable-width detector rows are also called adaptive arrays, nonuniform arrays, or hybrid arrays.
- In MDCT, data from multiple parallel rows of detector elements can be combined in various ways, a process known as binning. These different combinations result in a different slice thickness.

- For example, a four-slice scanner that contained 16 detector rows, each 1.25 mm wide, can be programmed so that a single gantry rotation can yield any of the following:
  - ◆ 4 slices, each 1.25 mm
  - ◆ 4 slices, each 2.5 mm (grouping two detector rows for each slice)
  - ◆ 4 slices, each 3.75 mm (grouping three detector rows for each slice)
  - ◆ 4 slices, each 5 mm (using all the available detectors in groups of four).

## Dual-Source CT

- ▪ The design uses two sets of x-ray tubes and two corresponding detector arrays in a single CT gantry.
  - This design is known as dual-source or dual focal spot CT.
- ▪ A primary goal of the dual-source design is increased scan speed. This is particularly important in cardiac CT studies.
  - The radiation dose to the patient is no higher when dual-source CT is used.
- ▪ The advent of dual-source CT scanners have necessitated a change in nomenclature of MDCT regarding z-axis coverage.
  - The number of detector rows in the z-axis and the number of slices acquired in a single rotation are no longer interchangeable terms.
  - Systems with two alternating focal spots allow the same number of detector rows to be sampled twice. Thus, the number of image slices generated is double the number of detector rows. However, the volume coverage (i.e., z axis coverage) remains the same.
  - Hence, a 128-detector row scanner with two alternating focal spots can be referred to as 256-slice CT.
- ▪ A second potential advantage stems from the fact that the two x-ray tubes, while working simultaneously, can be programmed by the operator to use different kVp settings. This produces x-ray photons possessing different energies. The beam attenuation of an object is dependent both on the density of the object and on the energy of the x-ray beam. Therefore, additional information can be learned about the object scanned when two x-ray energies are used and the difference in attenuation is analyzed. For example, this strategy can be used to differentiate iodine from other dense materials.

### Dual-Energy CT

- ▪ Dual-source and dual-energy CT are not the same.
  - Dual-source refers to the simultaneous use of two x-ray tubes that can be operated at the same or different kVp settings.

- Dual-energy CT, also called spectral imaging, refers to any acquisition of CT data at two different kVp settings.
- Dual-energy scans can be studies that simultaneously acquire data a two different kVp settings (when performed on a dual-source scanners). Dual-energy scans can also be performed on single-source CT systems. Different approaches can be used.
  - ◆ Sequential helical scans can be done with different kVp settings.
  - ◆ A single helical scan can be performed with rapid switching of the x-ray tube kVp setting between two settings.

## HELICAL SCANNING

- ▪ Three basic ingredients define a helical scan process: a continually rotating x-ray tube, constant x-ray output, and uninterrupted table movement.
- ▪ Helical scanning is also called spiral, volumetric, or continuous acquisition scanning.
- ▪ Helical scanning offers many advantages, including the ability to optimize iodinated contrast agent administration, the reduction of respiratory misregistration, and the reduction of motion artifacts from organs such as the heart.
- ▪ The end result of helical scan methods is a block of data, not separate slices as occurs with axial methods. Acquiring information in a volume allows data manipulation possibilities not available with the older axial methods. However, it is important to remember that although the end result is a block of data, in most cases the information is acquired in a ribbon—and not a block at a time, thus placing certain limitations on data manipulation.
- ▪ Newer 256 and 320 detector systems do allow for 160 mm of coverage in a single axial rotation, which is generally enough to cover the heart and some other organs. In this scenario, information is acquired in a block and allows extensive options for data manipulation.
- ▪ The major improvements that led to the development of helical scan methods are
  - Gantries with a slip ring design
  - More efficient tube cooling
  - Higher x-ray output (i.e., increased mA capability)
  - Smoother table movement
  - Software that adjusts for table motion
  - Improved raw data management
  - More efficient detectors
- ▪ There are fundamental differences between traditional axial images and those acquired in a helical scan process. An axial image is taken so that each slice is parallel to every other slice. In contrast,

with helical scanning the beginning point of the slice is not in the same plane as the end point of the slice. Hence, helical CT creates slices that are at a slight tilt, similar to the rungs in a spring.

- Helical interpolation methods create images that closely resemble those acquired in a traditional axial mode. They, in effect, "unslant" the helical slice.
- Different helical interpolation techniques exist. Two of the most common schemes are the 360° and the 180° linear interpolations. These are abbreviated 360LI and 180LI.
- Any method of interpolation is associated with some, although often quite minimal, loss of image resolution.
- In general, the more the interpolation required to process an image, the more pronounced these disadvantages become. As the angle of the slice becomes steeper, the interpolation required to adjust the data increases.
- Interpolation methods can result in a slice that is wider than that selected by the operator. The actual width of the slice (as opposed to the one selected) is referred to as the effective slice thickness or the slice-sensitivity profile (SSP).
- Early helical interpolation methods resulted in considerable slice thickness blooming (in which the effective slice thickness was wider than the selected slice thickness). However, interpolation methods quickly improved, and this disadvantage is not nearly as pronounced on current scanners.

## Pitch

- Pitch is a parameter that is commonly used to describe the CT table movement during a helical scan acquisition.
- It is most commonly defined as the travel distance of the CT scan table per 360° rotation of the x-ray tube, divided by the x-ray beam collimation width.
- When the table feed and beam collimation are identical, pitch is 1. When the table feed is less than the beam collimation, pitch is less than 1 and scan overlap occurs.
- The concept of pitch is more complicated when discussing MDCT than in SDCT.
- To understand pitch in an SDCT system, consider what happens to the table speed when the pitch is set at 1.
  - If pitch is 1, and a 5-mm slice thickness is selected, the table will move 5 mm for each 360° rotation of the x-ray tube. However, if a 10-mm slice thickness is selected, the table will move 10 mm for each gantry rotation.
- Now consider what happens when the pitch is set at 2.
  - If the pitch is 2, and a 5-mm slice thickness is selected, the table will move 10 mm for each 360° rotation of the x-ray tube.

- To understand how pitch affects the image, imagine what happens to the data if the spiral is stretched out, like pulling the ends of a spring. The slant becomes more pronounced.
- As pitch increases, so does the slice angle. More interpolation is required to straighten the image. Consequently, as pitch increases, the effects of interpolation become more pronounced.
- It may seem that increasing the pitch would result in data for some anatomic areas being skipped. This is not true. Information is collected for each table position regardless of pitch. However, as pitch increases, fewer data are acquired for each table position.
- Pitch is sometimes expressed as a ratio of table speed to slice thickness. Hence, a pitch of 2:1 indicates that the table will move twice the distance of the slice thickness for each rotation of the gantry. This is the same statement as saying the pitch is 2.
- Increasing the pitch will result in a scan covering more anatomy lengthwise for a given total acquisition time. It will also reduce the radiation dose to the patient.
- A decrease in pitch slows down the table speed. A pitch of less than 1 will result in overlapping slices. Therefore, decreasing the pitch will decrease the amount of anatomy covered per unit time and increase the radiation dose to the patient.
- A compromise is necessary when the pitch is extended beyond 1. In exchange for the shortened examination time and the reduced patient radiation dose comes the loss of image sharpness and a decrease in the SSP.
- The operator may select the pitch on a helical scan. Like mA setting, available pitch settings vary, depending on the manufacturer. These sacrifices are not linear. In fact, these disadvantages are minimal when the pitch does not exceed 1.5. The impact on the image is more significant when pitch is extended beyond this point.
- Pitch is often increased slightly to allow an entire area to be covered in a single breath-hold. It is also an appropriate option when the tube heat limits the length of a helical scan acquisition.
- In MDCT, the simultaneous data acquisition from parallel rows of detectors requires rapid table movement during scanning. MDCT stretches our earlier concept of pitch.
- Pitch is still defined as the relationship between slice thickness and table travel per rotation. But in MDCT, the terms collimation and slice thickness are no longer synonymous. This detail has given rise to more than one definition of pitch as it relates to MDCT systems.
- The most common definition of pitch (and the one favored by physicists) is referred to as beam

pitch and relates more closely to the definition established in SDCT.

- Beam pitch is defined as table movement per rotation divided by beam width.
  - The beam width can be determined by multiplying the number of slices by the slice thickness.
  - For example, with a 64-slice MDCT at 64 × 0.5 mm slice thickness and a table-feed of 48 mm per rotation, the pitch is 1.5. The equation is:

$$48/(64 \times 0.5) = 48/32 = 1.5$$

- The less common definition of pitch uses the detector aperture (rather than the x-ray beam width). This is termed detector pitch and is defined as table movement per rotation time divided by the selected slice thickness.
- The distance covered in an MDCT helical scan sequence can be calculated using the following equation:

Pitch × total acquisition time × 1/rotation time
× (slice thickness × slices per rotation)
= amount of (lengthwise) anatomy covered

- For example, in a scan sequence in which the pitch is 1.5, acquisition time is 20 seconds, 1 mm slice thickness, 4 slices per rotation, gantry rotation is 0.5 seconds, then 240 mm anatomy is covered. The equation is:

$$1.5 \times 20\,s \times 1\,mm/0.5\,s \times (1 \times 4) = 240\,mm$$

- Because helical scans result in a block of data, a choice can be made as to where, within that block, an image is created. This flexibility allows the creation of overlapping slices retrospectively. It does this without increasing the radiation dose to the patient, as is the case when axial images are scanned in an overlapping fashion.
- In some situations changing the slice incrementation retrospectively can reduce the partial volume effect.
- Overlapping images are also an asset to multiplanar and three-dimensional image reformation. Using overlapping images helps reduce the stairstep appearance often seen along the edges of a reformatted image.
- Data incrementation can be changed on SDCT, but slice thickness cannot be retrospectively altered using SDCT data.
- MDCT systems offer opportunities for retrospectively changing slice thickness that are not available on SDCT systems.
- MDCT images acquired with a thin slice can be added together to create a thicker slice for viewing.

For example, four slices of 0.5 mm each could be combined to create a 2-mm slice for viewing.

- However, the reverse is not always true. That is, on many systems if the data are acquired with a slice thickness of 2 mm, the data cannot retrospectively be divided to produce four 0.5-mm slices.
- Therefore, in MDCT, there can be a difference between how the images are acquired and how they are viewed. This difference has resulted in the necessity to differentiate between slice thickness (how the data were acquired) and image thickness (how the data are reconstructed).
- In MDCT, image thickness may be greater than the slice thickness, but in most cases the image thickness may not be less than slice thickness.

## REVIEW QUESTIONS

1. Compared with conventional radiographic images, CT localizer images
   a. do not superimpose anatomic structures.
   b. are of slightly poorer image quality.
   c. result in a much higher radiation dose to the patient.
   d. result in a much lower radiation dose to the patient.
2. Refer to Figure 5-1. What view will result when a localizer image is taken with the x-ray tube in this position?
   a. Anteroposterior (AP) view
   b. Posteroanterior (PA) view
   c. Lateral view
   d. Decubitus view

Localizer scan

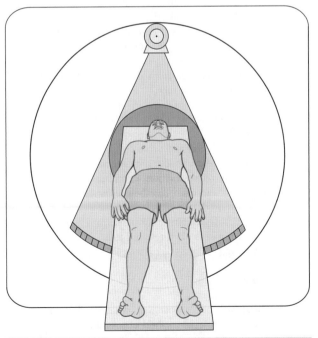

**FIGURE 5-1**

3. Examine the localizer image in Figure 5-2. What is the likely outcome; should the technologist proceed with the examination?
   a. The images will be noisy, from too low an mA setting.
   b. The images will contain streaks, from metallic objects in the scannable range.
   c. The images will be mislabeled, with the right side labeled as left, and anterior will be labeled posterior.
   d. The images will contain ring artifacts, from a misaligned detector element.

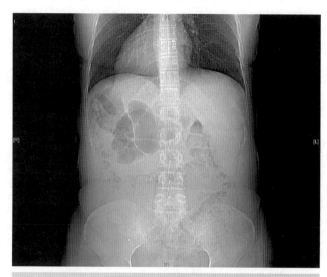

**FIGURE 5-2**

4. Which are key aspects of the axial method of data acquisition?
   a. The table remains stationary while the x-ray tube rotates within the gantry, collecting data.
   b. Multiple parallel rows of detectors are needed.
   c. The table moves continuously throughout the data acquisition.
   d. Each slice is created from data acquired during a 180° rotation of the x-ray tube.
5. The interscan delay inherent in an axial scan method is caused by which factor?
   a. Tube cooling
   b. Detector realignment
   c. Table movement between data acquisitions
   d. Serial image reconstruction algorithms that must reconstruct data from each slice before data for the next slice can be acquired
6. The practice of grouping more than one axial scan in a single breath-hold is often referred to as
   a. reformatting.
   b. clustering.
   c. dynamic scanning.
   d. volumetric scanning.
7. Compared with helical scanning, what are the primary disadvantages to the axial method of scanning?
   a. Low-contrast resolution is inferior.
   b. Spatial resolution is inferior.

c. Radiation dose is much higher; noise is more pronounced.
   d. Total examination time is longer; data reconstruction is more limited.
8. What is it called when a patient breathes differently with each data acquisition and areas of anatomy seem to be misplaced in the $z$ axis?
   a. Misregistration
   b. Retrospective reconstruction
   c. Slice thickness blooming
   d. Slice-sensitivity profile degradation
9. Basic ingredients defining a helical scan include all of the following EXCEPT:
   a. a continually rotating x-ray tube.
   b. multiple parallel rows of detectors.
   c. constant x-ray output.
   d. uninterrupted table movement.
10. All of the following are synonyms for helical scanning EXCEPT:
    a. volumetric scanning.
    b. spiral scanning.
    c. continuous acquisition scanning.
    d. dynamic scanning.
11. All of the following were improvements necessary to make helical scanning possible EXCEPT:
    a. fourth-generation scanner design.
    b. gantries with slip ring designs.
    c. software that adjusts for table motion.
    d. improved raw data management.
12. The goal of helical interpolation methods is to
    a. calculate the appropriate mAs for a given patient size.
    b. take the slant and the blur out of the helical image so that they closely resemble images taken from axial methods.
    c. automatically assign the optimal window width and level to each reconstructed image.
    d. eliminate artifacts from voluntary and involuntary patient motion.
13. What is the pitch in the following scenario: 16-slice scanner, 0.5-mm slice thickness, table movement of 12 mm per rotation?
    a. 1
    b. 1.25
    c. 1.5
    d. 2
14. How much anatomy (lengthwise) will be covered in a helical scan when the following parameters are selected: 15 seconds total acquisition time, 0.5 seconds gantry rotation time, 2 mm slice thickness, 4 slices per rotation, pitch of 1.5?
    a. 40 mm
    b. 90 mm
    c. 160 mm
    d. 360 mm
15. Which of the following is NOT a reconstruction possibility when an MDCT system produces four 1-mm slices with each gantry rotation?
    a. Slices can be combined to create two 2-mm slices.
    b. Slices can be combined to create one 4-mm slice.
    c. Slices can be divided to produce sixteen 0.25-mm slices.
    d. Slices can be reconstructed to create images that overlap by 0.5 mm.

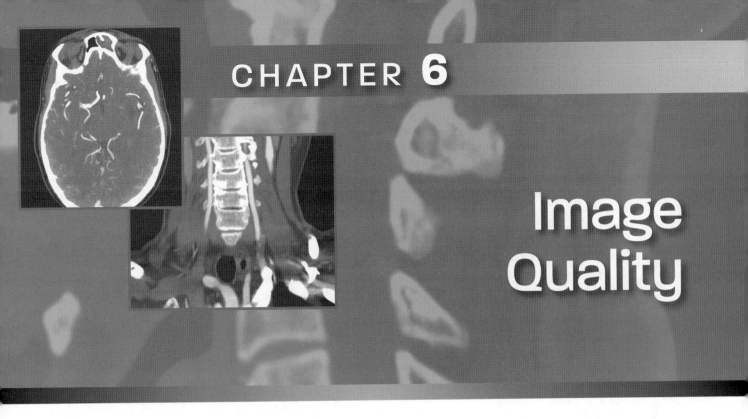

CHAPTER **6**

# Image Quality

## SCANNING PARAMETERS DEFINED

- Many factors affect the quality of the image produced. Those factors that can be controlled by the operator are collectively called scan parameters. Scan parameters include milliampere (mA) level, scan time (in seconds), slice thickness, field of view, scan algorithm, and kilovolt peak (kVp). For helical scan methods, pitch is also a selectable parameter.
- As in standard radiography, the total x-ray beam exposure in CT is dependent on a combination of mA setting, scan time, and kVp setting.

### Milliampere Second

- Milliampere level and scan time together define the quantity of the x-ray energy. The product of these two parameters is known as milliampere seconds (mAs).
- The current of electrons that flow from the x-ray tube's filament to strike the anode is measured in mA. Increasing the mA increases the number of electrons that will produce x-ray photons.
- The use of a small filament size concentrates the focal spot, reducing the penumbra (i.e., geometric unsharpness), which in turn, positively affects image quality. Unfortunately, small filaments cannot tolerate high mA. Therefore, systems typically provide two separate filaments. A small filament is provided for lower mA settings (typically < 350 mA) and a large filament for higher settings.

- Scan time, for SDCT, is the time the x-ray beam is on for the collection of data for each slice.
- Most often, scan time is the time it takes for the gantry to make a complete 360° rotation, although with overscanning and partial scanning options, there may be some mild variation.
- In most situations, a full scan (360°) is also used in MDCT. Therefore, in most cases, the scan time in MDCT is the time it takes for the x-ray tube to make a 360° rotation, even though many slices may be produced.
- In MDCT cardiac applications, images may be created from data acquired from less than a 360° rotation; hence the scan time for these protocols are shorter.
- The quantity of x-ray produced is a product of mA and scan time. A specific mAs setting can be obtained from a variety of combinations, based on the mA setting and scan times available with a specific system.
- Higher mA settings allow shorter scan times to be used. A short scan time is critical in reducing image degradation as a result of patient motion.
  - Even with a cooperative patient who remains still and suspends respiration on command, motion can be a factor because of involuntary movement such as peristalsis and cardiac motion.
  - The degree to which involuntary motion affects an image is largely dependent on the area scanned.

- Improvements in scanner design in recent years have allowed scans to be performed with higher mA setting and much shorter scan times.
- The factors that influence the mAs selection in CT are basically the same as in conventional radiography. Specifically, the thicker and denser the part being examined, the more the mAs required to produce an adequate image.
  - For example, a CT study of the lungs will require less mAs than that of the abdomen because the chest is composed primarily of the lungs, which contain air and are less dense than the organs of the abdomen.
- mAs can be obtained from various combinations of mA and scan time settings.
- Reducing the mAs while holding the kVp constant reduces the radiation dose to the patient.
- Automatic tube current modulation (ATCM) is software that automatically adjusts the tube current based on the estimated attenuation of the patient at a specific location.
  - This software adjusts mAs during each gantry rotation to compensate for large variation in x-ray attenuation, such as when scans move from the shoulders to the rest of the thorax.
  - The design of automatic tube current modulation software varies by manufacturer. In one method, the estimates are derived from scout views done in both anteroposterior and lateral projections. From these views, the mA is programmed to vary by location along the length of the patient.
  - Centering the patient in the gantry is vital with this design.
  - Automatic exposure control techniques can significantly reduce the patient's radiation dose; 35% to 60% reductions have been reported.

## Tube Voltage (kVp)

- The kVp setting defines the quality (or average energy) of the beam.
- Compared with mA selection, choices of kVp are more limited. On some systems, the kVp setting is fixed, typically at 120 kVp.
- Increasing the kVp setting increases the intensity of the x-ray beam and the beam's ability to penetrate a thick, dense anatomic part.
- Routine body CT for adult patients is performed with 120 to 140 kVp. Pediatric patients are often scanned with 80 kVp.
- Dose is reduced if the kVp is reduced while the mAs is held constant. However, excessively lowering the kVp may result in a dramatic increase in the amount of x-ray attenuated by patient tissue, because the x-ray beam will be too weak to penetrate the patient.

- It is more common practice to manipulate the mAs, rather than the kVp, when modifying the radiation dose. This is because the choice of mA is more flexible, and its effect on image quality is more straightforward and predictable than is a change in kVp.

## Uncoupling Effect

- CT physics is somewhat different from that of film-screen radiography, in which the relationship between dose and image quality is clear and well understood by technologists.
- In film-screen radiography, when the radiation dose is too high, the film is overexposed and the image obtained is too dark. It can be said that the image is "coupled" with the dose.
- In CT (and other digital technology), the image quality is uncoupled from the dose, so even when an mA or kVp setting that is too high is used, a good image results.
  - The uncoupling effect can make it difficult to identify when a dose that is higher than necessary is used.

## Slice Thickness

- Slice thickness has a significant impact on image quality. When discussing image quality, we are primarily interested in the slice thickness (how the data were acquired) rather than image thickness (how the data are reconstructed for display).

## Field of View

- Scan field of view (SFOV) determines the area, within the gantry, for which raw data are acquired. Scan data are always acquired around the gantry's isocenter.
- Display field of view (DFOV) determines how much, and what section, of the collected raw data are used to create an image.

## Reconstruction Algorithm

- Reconstruction algorithms determine how data are filtered in the reconstruction process.
- Many different filters are available that use different algorithms depending on which parts of the data must be enhanced or suppressed.
- Some algorithms help to reduce the appearance of artifacts by reducing the difference between adjacent pixels, but must sacrifice spatial resolution. These are often called smoothing algorithms.
- Some filters accentuate the difference between neighboring pixels to optimize spatial resolution, but make sacrifices in low-contrast resolution. These are often called bone or detail filters.

### *Iterative Reconstruction*

- Iterative reconstruction (IR) techniques refer to image reconstruction algorithms that begin with an assumption and then improve the image by continually analyzing scan data and making adjustments until the assumption and real time data are in agreement.
- IR techniques require considerably more computing power than do filter back projection (FBP). Historically, computer speeds were much slower, making IR techniques impractical. Hence, despite significant drawbacks, FBP has been the standard in CT.
- As computing power and speeds rose exponentially in the 1990s and 2000s, IR methods made a comeback. IR is particularly valuable in its ability to enhance image quality for lower dose scans.
  - Even with modern computers, the algorithms are still very time-consuming. Full IR methods also result in images that have a different appearance; acceptance of the new look by technologists and radiologists can be a barrier to its use.
- IR software programs used a blend of FBP and IR techniques to reduce the reconstruction time, create images more in keeping with viewers' expectations, and reduce artifacts.
- Each vendor offers its own version of software. While each vendor's software does basically the same thing, there is variation in the methodologies. Each software approach is associated with slightly different strengths and limitations.

## Pitch

- Pitch is the relationship between slice thickness and table travel per rotation during a helical scan acquisition. Pitch settings vary depending on manufacturer and detector row number and configuration.

## Scan Geometry

- In most situations, an image is created from the data acquired from one 360° rotation of the x-ray tube. This is referred to as a full scan.
- A partial scan is when images are created from less than a 360° rotation. A partial scan is typically 180° plus the degree of arc of the fan angle. They are also referred to as half-scans. Because they possess only half of the otherwise available data, they are inferior to standard full scans.
- An overscan uses information from more than a 360° rotation. The overscan adds approximately the width of the FOV to the full scan, resulting in a 400° rotation.
  - Overscans were most commonly used in fourth-generation scanner designs.

## IMAGE QUALITY DEFINED

- At the most fundamental level, image quality is a comparison of the image to the actual object. However, the true test of the quality of a specific image is whether it serves the purpose for which it was acquired.
- In CT, image quality is directly related to its usefulness in providing an accurate diagnosis. The usefulness of an image can only be assessed on a case-by-case basis.
- There are other, more objective measures of CT image quality. These tools help make possible comparisons of one imaging system to another, or the same system over time.
- Many factors influence how well a CT image represents the actual object scanned.
- Image accuracy is also referred to as image fidelity.
- The two main features of image quality (that can be measured) are
  - Detail (or high-contrast) resolution—the ability to resolve (as separate objects) small, high-contrast objects.
  - Contrast resolution—the ability to differentiate between objects with very similar densities as their background.

## Spatial Resolution

- Detail resolution is also called spatial resolution. It is the system's ability to resolve, as separate forms, small objects placed very close together.
  - An example of an imaging scenario that depends on spatial resolution is small bone fragments in a crushed ankle.
- There are two methods of measuring spatial resolution:
  - It can be measured directly using a line pairs phantom.
  - It can be calculated from analyzing the spread of information within the system. This is known as the modulation transfer function, or MTF.
  - By using one of these methods, it is possible to compare a system's performance with another CT system or the same system on a different day.
- A line pairs phantom contains closely spaced metal strips imbedded in acrylic. The phantom is scanned, and the number of strips that are visible is counted.
  - A line pair is not a set of two lines, but rather, a line and the space between lines. Therefore, if 20 lines can be seen in a 1-cm section in an image of the phantom, the spatial resolution is reported as 20 line pairs per centimeter (lp/cm).
- The number of line pairs visible per unit length is also called spatial frequency.

- How frequently an object will fit into a given space is its spatial frequency.
- Therefore, large objects will have a low spatial frequency, and small objects will have a high spatial frequency.

■ The MTF is the most commonly used method of describing spatial resolution ability, not only in CT but also in conventional radiography.

■ The MTF is the ratio of the accuracy of the image compared with the actual object scanned.
- The MTF scale is from 0 to 1. If the image reproduced the object exactly, the MTF of the system would have a value of 1. If the image were blank and contained no information about the object, the MTF would be 0.
- MTF graphs chart spatial frequency on the *x* axis and MTF along the *y* axis. An MTF curve that extends farther to the right indicates higher spatial resolution, which means the imaging system is better able to reproduce small objects.

■ Compared with conventional radiography, CT has significantly worse spatial resolution. (It is the contrast resolution that distinguishes CT from other clinical modalities.)

■ The spatial resolution of a CT image can be described in two dimensions.
- Resolution in the *xy* direction is called in-plane resolution.
- Resolution in the *z* direction is called longitudinal resolution.

## Factors Affecting Spatial Resolution

### Matrix, DFOV, Pixel Size

■ Matrix size and display field of view (DFOV) selection determine pixel size. This relationship is represented by the equation: Pixel Size = DFOV/Matrix Size
- Pixel size plays an important role in the in-plane spatial resolution of an image.
- Each pixel has a width *x*, and a length *y*. In CT, pixels are square, so $x = y$.
- Matrix size refers to how many pixels are present in the grid. Because the perimeter of the square matrix is held constant, the greater the total pixels present in the image, the smaller each individual pixel.
- DFOV determines how much raw data will be used to reconstruct the image.
- Changing the DFOV will also alter the size of the image on the screen.
- Increasing the DFOV increases the size of each pixel in the image. The pixel size reflects how much patient data are contained within each square. A larger pixel will include more patient data. A larger pixel results in poorer spatial resolution.

### Slice Thickness

■ Raw data are segmented in the longitudinal (head/foot) direction by the slice thickness. Each segmented portion of data is called a voxel.

■ Voxel size plays a role in volume averaging, and therefore affects longitudinal resolution.

■ Historically, the impact of slice thickness on image quality is substantially more pronounced than is pixel size.

■ New scanners offer the choice of very thin slices (between 0.5 and 1 mm). These thin slices can result in isotropic (or near-isotropic) voxels.

■ An isotropic voxel is a cube, measuring the same in the *x*, *y*, and *z* directions.

■ Sampling theorem: because an object may not lie entirely within a pixel, the pixel dimension should be half the size of the object to increase the likelihood of that object being resolved.

### Reconstruction Algorithm

■ All CT systems offer a choice of different reconstruction algorithms. The appropriate reconstruction algorithm depends on which parts of the data should be enhanced or suppressed to optimize the image for diagnosis.
- Some will "smooth" the data more heavily, by reducing the difference between adjacent pixels.
- This can reduce the appearance of metal artifacts, but does so at the cost of reduced spatial resolution.
- Some filters accentuate the difference between neighboring pixels to optimize spatial resolution. But these make sacrifices in low-contrast resolution. These filters are often called bone or detail filters.

### Focal Spot Size

■ Focal spot size affects image quality, but the effect is minimal.

■ Larger focal spots cause more geometric unsharpness in the image and reduce spatial resolution.

### Pitch

■ The pitch used in helical scanning can affect spatial resolution.

■ In general, increasing the pitch reduces the resolution. This effect is more pronounced in SDCT than in MDCT systems.

### Motion

■ Motion creates blurring in the image and degrades spatial resolution.

■ Shortened scan times may improve spatial resolution to the extent that they may reduce the effects of both involuntary motion (e.g., peristalsis) and overt patient motion.

# CONTRAST RESOLUTION

- Contrast resolution (or low-contrast resolution) is the ability to differentiate a structure that varies only slightly in density from its surrounding.
  - An example of an imaging scenario that depends on contrast resolution is that of a liver lesion surrounded by healthy liver tissue.
- Contrast resolution may also be referred to as the sensitivity of the system; hence, the term low-contrast sensitivity is also used.
- CT is superior to all other clinical modalities in its contrast resolution. CT can differentiate an object with a 0.5% contrast variation. This translates to just a 5-HU difference.
- Contrast resolution is measured using phantoms that contain objects, typically cylindrical, of varying sizes and with a small difference in density (typically from 4 to 10 HU) from the background. An observer must detect objects as distinct.
- Because the difference between an object and the background can be small, noise plays an important role in low-contrast resolution.

## Noise

- Image noise is the undesirable fluctuation of pixel values in an image of a homogeneous material, such as a water phantom.
- We can recognize noise as the grainy appearance or "salt-and-pepper" look on an underexposed image.
- A major cause of noise is quantum mottle. Quantum mottle occurs when there are an insufficient number of photons detected. It is inversely related to the number of photons used to form the image.
- In CT, the number of x-ray photons detected per pixel may also be referred to as signal-to-noise ratio (SNR).
- The presence of noise on an image degrades its quality, particularly its contrast resolution.

## Factors Affecting Contrast Resolution

- The mAs selected for a scan directly influences the number of photons used to produce the CT image, thereby affecting the SNR and the contrast resolution.
- Doubling the mAs of the study increases the SNR by 40%.
- The radiation dose to the patient increases linearly with mAs. Therefore, mAs will improve contrast resolution, but at the cost of a higher radiation dose to the patient.
- Determining the appropriate mAs for a scan must be made in the context of the clinical task at hand. A relatively high amount of noise may be tolerable if the clinical task is primarily dependent on the image's spatial resolution, such as the identification of emphysema in the lung. Conversely, a study to detect a kidney lesion depends on the images' low-contrast resolution, and therefore requires that mAs be set to a level that reduces noise.

### Slice Thickness

- Slice thickness has a linear effect on the number of x-ray photons available to produce the image. Because thicker slices allow more photons to reach the detectors, they have a better SNR and appear less noisy. However, this improvement comes at the cost of spatial resolution in the $z$ axis.

### Reconstruction Algorithm

- Bone algorithms produce lower contrast resolution.
- Soft tissue algorithms improve contrast resolution.

### Other Contrast Resolution Considerations

- Subject contrast relates to the inherent properties of the object scanned.
  - If everything else is held constant, small objects are more difficult to see than are larger objects.
  - The relationship between object size and visibility is called the contrast-detail response. Measuring and charting this relationship results in what is known as a contrast-detail curve.
- The inherent contrast of an organ relates to its physical properties, particularly when compared with that of its surrounding organs. For example, the lung is said to possess high inherent contrast because it is primarily air filled. The low-attenuation lungs provide a background that makes nearly any other object easily discernible.
- The displayed contrast of an image is dependent on the window settings used for its display. Low-contrast objects must be displayed at optimal window settings to be discernible from their background.

# TEMPORAL RESOLUTION

- In discussions of image quality, temporal (from the root "tempo") refers to the characteristic of being limited by time.
- The temporal resolution of a system refers to how rapidly data are acquired.
- Temporal resolution is controlled by gantry rotation speed, the number of detector channels in the system, and the speed with which the system can record changing signals.
- Temporal resolution of a CT system is typically reported in milliseconds (ms), which are thousandths of a second.
- High temporal resolution is of particular importance when imaging moving structures and for studies dependent on the dynamic flow of iodinated contrast media.

## REVIEW QUESTIONS

1. All of the following are scan parameters EXCEPT
   a. mAs.
   b. slice thickness.
   c. matrix.
   d. pitch.
2. Which of the following combinations of mA and scan time will result in 350 mAs and be the best choice for a cardiac scan?
   a. mA = 300, scan time = 0.50 seconds
   b. mA = 200, scan time = 2 seconds
   c. mA = 350, scan time = 1 second
   d. mA = 700, scan time = 0.5 seconds
3. Which can be attributed to the uncoupling effect?
   a. Even when the mAs or kVp setting is too high, a good image results.
   b. When mAs or kVp settings are either too high or too low, quantum mottle results.
   c. mA and scan time have no relationship to the quantity of x-ray produced.
   d. Normal x-ray physics are reversed; mAs controls the quality of the x-ray beam, whereas the kVp controls the quantity of the x-ray beam.
4. Which is a disadvantage of a bone algorithm?
   a. It reduces spatial resolution.
   b. It smooths data, reducing the difference between adjacent pixels.
   c. It accentuates the difference between neighboring pixels.
   d. It reduces the visibility of soft tissue structures.
5. What is a partial scan?
   a. A scan that collects two matching samples, taken 180° apart
   b. A scan that collects data from a 360° tube arc
   c. A scan that collects data from a 360° tube arc, plus the width of the field of view
   d. A scan that collects data from 180° tube arc, plus the degree of arc of the fan angle
6. What is the true test of the quality of a specific image?
   a. Whether it serves the purpose for which it was acquired
   b. Whether it has a limiting resolution of 7 lp/mm or greater
   c. Whether it has an MTF of greater than 1
   d. Whether pixel size is 0.5 mm or smaller
7. What two main features are assessed to measure image quality?
   a. mAs and kVp
   b. Spatial resolution and contrast resolution
   c. Temporal resolution and the degree of motion artifact
   d. Focal spot size and DFOV
8. Which of the following is an imaging challenge that depends on contrast resolution?
   a. A calcified nodule in the lung
   b. Tiny, contrast-filled arteries that are just 1 mm apart
   c. Bony erosion in the ossicles of the internal auditory canal
   d. Distinguishing between the white matter and gray matter of the brain
9. What is spatial frequency?
   a. The number of line pairs visible per unit length
   b. The ratio of the accuracy of the image compared with the actual object scanned
   c. The ratio of pixel size to slice thickness
   d. The number of x-ray photons detected per pixel
10. A graphical representation of the CT systems' capability of passing information through it to the observer is called
    a. interpolation.
    b. modulation transfer function (MTF).
    c. receiver operator characteristics.
    d. contrast-detail response.
11. Using a standard 512 matrix for all studies, which contains the smallest pixels?
    a. A scan of the internal auditory canals, in which DFOV is 16 cm
    b. A scan of the brain, in which DFOV is 25 cm
    c. A scan of the chest, in which DFOV is 35 cm
    d. A scan of the abdomen, in which DFOV is 42
12. Which term describes an isotropic voxel?
    a. A rectangular solid
    b. A square
    c. A cube
    d. A slab
13. The ability to differentiate a structure that varies only slightly in density from its surrounding is referred to as
    a. spatial resolution.
    b. high-contrast resolution.
    c. detail resolution.
    d. low-contrast resolution.
14. An image of a water phantom displays a range of pixel values. What can be said about this image?
    a. It was reconstructed with a "soft" algorithm.
    b. It is "noisy."
    c. The mAs setting used to produce the image was too high.
    d. A thick slice was used.
15. When discussing the quality of a CT image, what is meant by temporal resolution?
    a. The internal auditory canal is often used to evaluate a system's overall quality. Because the internal auditory canals are located in the temporal bone, this is called its temporal resolution.
    b. The ability of a system to display an object that has a density that is very similar to its background.
    c. How rapidly data are acquired; it is controlled by gantry rotation speed, the number of detector channels in the system, and the speed with which the system can record changing signals.
    d. The ability to resolve, as separate objects, small, high-contrast objects.

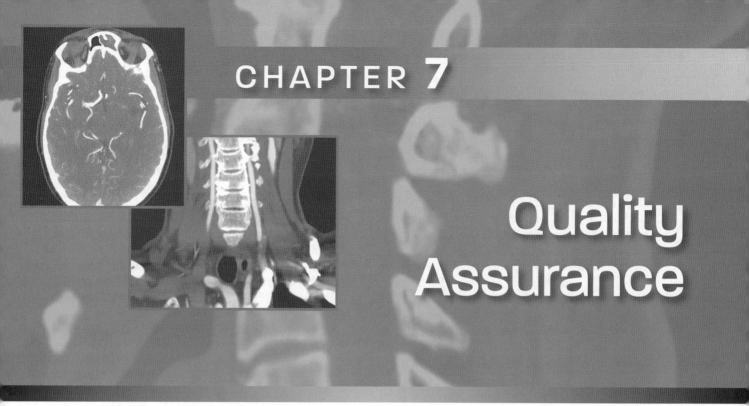

CHAPTER **7**

# Quality Assurance

## QUALITY ASSURANCE METHODS

- Quality control programs are designed to ensure that the CT system is producing the best possible image quality while delivering the minimal radiation dose to the patient.
- Responsibility for quality control programs is often shared between technologists and medical physicists.
  - Technologists typically perform and record routine quality control tests.
  - A medical physicist is required to obtain dosimetric data. Testing done by a physicist is typically performed annually or semiannually.
- Quality assurance programs should be designed around three basic concepts:
  - The tests that make up the program must be performed on a regular basis.
  - The results from all tests must be recorded using a consistent format.
  - Documentation should indicate whether the tested parameter is within specified guidelines.

### Quality Control Phantoms

- Many phantoms are designed with multiple components so that they can be used to examine a broad range of scanner parameters.
- A line pairs phantom can be used to measure spatial resolution directly. This test is usually performed monthly.
- A phantom that contains objects of varying size that have only a small density difference from their background is used to evaluate contrast resolution. Because low-contrast resolution is affected by image noise, and image noise is primarily a result of inadequate mAs, the phantoms are scanned at different mAs settings. This test is usually performed monthly.
- The slice thickness accuracy of a scanner can be evaluated using a phantom that includes a ramp, spiral, or step wedge. This test is usually performed semiannually.
- Scanner manufacturers often provide a phantom that is designed specifically for verifying the accuracy of the laser lights. This test is usually performed semiannually.
- Image noise is assessed with scans of a water phantom (or any phantom known to be of uniform density). Variations between pixels as indicated by the standard deviation indicate noise. This test is usually performed weekly.
- Cross-field uniformity refers to the ability of the scanner to yield the same CT number in a homogeneous object (i.e., water phantom) regardless of the location of the region of interest (ROI). When several ROIs are placed in a phantom, it is expected that each will possess the same measurement. If fluctuations exist, a problem with the system's uniformity can be diagnosed. This test is usually performed weekly.
- Linearity refers to the relationship between CT numbers and the linear attenuation values of the scanned object at a designated kVp value. Daily calibrations help to avoid fluctuation in linearity.

To assess linearity, a phantom containing a variety of objects with known densities is scanned and the objects measured. The values are graphed and should result in a straight line between the average CT number and the linear attenuation coefficients. Linearity is typically measured semiannually.

- Technologists must understand the factors that affect the radiation dose to the patient. Technologists should advise anyone who must remain in the scan room of radiation protection strategies.
- Medical physicists must obtain dose measurements for each of a facility's CT scanners. Measurements are made using standard head and body CTDI phantoms and a pencil ionization chamber. Values are compared with reference doses. Values that are higher than the reference doses must be documented, including the reason for the higher dose level.

## Image Artifacts

- Artifacts are anything appearing on the image that is not present in the object scanned. Artifacts have many different presentations and can be attributed to many causes.
- They can be broadly classified as
  - Physics based (resulting from the physical processes associated with data acquisition)
  - Patient based
  - Equipment induced
- Artifacts can seriously degrade the quality of CT images, sometimes to the extent that the images are nondiagnostic.
- Prompt and accurate identification of artifacts can sometimes permit them to be corrected without a service call; or, if the severity of the artifact requires a service engineer, the call can be placed promptly.
- Beam-hardening artifacts result when lower-energy photons are preferentially absorbed, leaving only the higher-energy beams to strike the detector. The degree of beam hardening is dependent on the composition of the part examined and the extent the beam must travel through various tissues.
  - The x-ray beam is hardened more by dense objects.
  - Beam hardening can result in cupping or streak artifacts.
- CT systems use filtration, calibration correction, and beam-hardening correction to minimize beam-hardening artifacts.
- The best strategy available to the operator to avoid beam hardening is to select the appropriate scan field of view. This ensures that the correction filtration, calibration, and beam-hardening correction software are used.

- A partial volume artifact can occur when a dense object lies to the edge of the FOV. This can result in the object showing up in only a small number of views collected from the tube's 360° path. The inconsistencies between the views cause shading artifacts to appear in the image. Partial volume artifacts can be reduced by using thinner slices.
- Undersampling occurs when there is not enough information collected during an acquisition. Undersampling causes inaccuracies related to reproducing sharp edges and small objects. The result is known as aliasing artifacts, which is when fine stripes appear to be radiating from a dense structure. Aliasing artifacts can be reduced by increasing scan time or by reducing the helical pitch.
- The edge gradient effect results in streak artifacts arising from irregularly shaped objects that have a pronounced difference in density from surrounding structures. Edge gradient artifacts are largely unavoidable, but are somewhat reduced by thinner slices. Using low HU value oral contrast, such as water, in place of a barium suspension can eliminate the streak artifacts from the gastrointestinal tract.
- Artifacts from patient motion typically appear as shading, streaking, blurring, or ghosting. Voluntary motion can be reduced by adequately preparing patients for the examination. This includes clearly explaining to patients what is expected of them, the use of position aids, and, in some situations, the use of immobilization devices such as straps.
- The chest and abdomen should be scanned using the shortest possible scan time to minimize artifact from involuntary motion.
- Cardiac protocols often include pharmacologic methods to lower the patient's heart rate in an effort to reduce motion artifacts from heart palpitations.
- Metallic objects in the SFOV will create streak artifacts. They occur, in part, because the density of the metal is beyond the range of HU values that the system is designed to handle. The dynamic range on new scanners has been expanded, reducing the impact of metallic streak artifacts. However, beam hardening, partial volume, edge gradient, and aliasing all contribute to the streaks that result from metal in the SFOV.
  - Patients should be asked to take off any removable metal objects before scanning begins.
  - For nonremovable items, it is sometimes possible to angle the gantry to avoid the metal objects.
  - When it is impossible to avoid the metal objects, increasing the technique, especially kVp, may help penetrate some objects, and using thin slices will reduce the contribution owing to partial volume artifacts.

- Out-of-field artifacts are caused by anatomy that extends outside the selected SFOV. When an SFOV is selected that is larger than the patient, and the patient is appropriately centered within the gantry, out-of-field artifacts are avoided. Encouraging patients to raise their arms out of the way of the SFOV will also avoid artifact. For exceptionally large patients who exceed even the largest SFOV, out-of-field artifacts are inevitable.
- Ring artifacts occur primarily with third-generation scanners and appear on the image as a ring or concentric rings. They are caused by faulty or miscalibrated detector elements. In some instances, technologists may eliminate circular artifacts by recalibrating the scanner.
- An electrical current surge within the x-ray tube can result in tube arcing (also called high-voltage arcing). There is no specific pattern in the appearance of tube arc artifacts: they can be slight streaks that are nearly undetectable or they can be so severe that they render the image useless. A service engineer should be called when tube arcing occurs. In addition to the error message, the technologist should describe the arcing pattern and the frequency of the error.
- Helical interpolation artifacts can occur in spiral scans when higher pitches are used. Helical interpolation artifacts result in subtle inaccuracies in CT number and can lead to interpretation errors. These artifacts can be avoided by using a low pitch when possible.
- Windmill artifacts appear only on MDCT helical systems. They are attributed to the wider collimation that is required to accommodate the larger number of detector channels. Because of the wide collimation, the x-ray beam becomes cone shaped rather than fan shaped. This can result in artifacts from the so-called cone beam effect. They appear as either streaks or bright and dark shading near areas of large density differences. Cone beam artifacts are more pronounced for the outer detector rows. Manufacturers are addressing the problem with innovative cone beam reconstruction algorithms.

## REVIEW QUESTIONS

1. All of the following are key aspects of a quality assurance program EXCEPT
   a. the tests that make up the program must be performed on a regular basis.
   b. all tests must be completed by a medical physicist.
   c. the results from all tests must be recorded using a consistent format.
   d. documentation should indicate whether the tested parameter is within specified guidelines.

2. Figure 7-1 is that of a
   a. line pairs phantom.
   b. phantom used to assess slice thickness.
   c. water phantom.
   d. phantom used to assess the accuracy of the laser light.

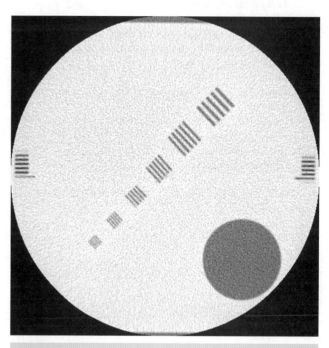

**FIGURE 7-1**

3. How often is the accuracy of a scanner's slice thickness tested?
   a. Daily
   b. Weekly
   c. Monthly
   d. Semiannually

4. A water phantom is scanned and several ROIs are placed in the resulting image. The ROIs placed at the perimeter of the image measure differently from the ROIs near the center. This indicates a problem with
   a. linearity.
   b. cross-field uniformity.
   c. noise.
   d. low-contrast resolution.

5. A water phantom is scanned and several ROIs are placed in the resulting image. The standard deviation measurements from the ROIs range from 15 to 25. What can be said about the image?
   a. It is noisy.
   b. The spatial resolution is 15 to 25 lp/cm.
   c. The low-contrast resolution is within normal limits.
   d. The radiation dose is unnecessarily high.

6. What can be done to improve the linearity of a CT system?
   a. Daily calibrations
   b. Increasing mAs
   c. Decreasing kVp
   d. Widening the window width when viewing the images

7. What quality control test must be performed by a medical physicist?
   a. Cross-field uniformity
   b. Spatial resolution
   c. Radiation dose measurements
   d. Laser light accuracy
8. Which is a TRUE statement regarding beam hardening?
   a. The beam is hardened more by bone and less by fat.
   b. The beam is hardened more by air and less by bone.
   c. Nothing can be done to minimize beam-hardening artifacts.
   d. Lowering the kVp is the best method of reducing beam-hardening artifacts.
9. Artifacts that result from undersampling are called
   a. out-of-field artifacts.
   b. metallic artifacts.
   c. cone beam artifacts.
   d. aliasing artifacts.
10. Identify the type of artifact indicated by the arrows in Figure 7-2.
    a. Aliasing
    b. Edge gradient
    c. Motion
    d. Tube arc

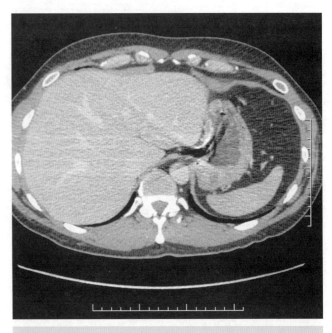

**FIGURE 7-2**

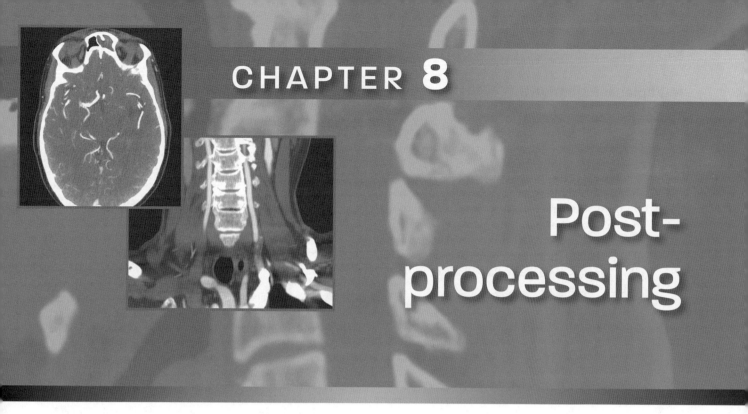

# Post-processing

Techniques that manipulate either raw data or image data after scanning has taken place and result in the creation of new images are called postprocessing.

Although the terms are frequently used interchangeably, in this text the term "reconstruction" is used when raw data are manipulated to create pixels that are then used to create an image. The term "reformation" is used when image data are assembled to produce images in different planes, or to produce 3D images.

## RETROSPECTIVE RECONSTRUCTION

- Reconstructing raw data to create new images can only be done from the operator's console.
- Although many parameters can be changed retrospectively, the images that result are always in the same plane and the same orientation as were the original images.
- Display field of view (DFOV), image center, and reconstruction algorithm can be changed retrospectively on both axial and helical data.
- On helical data, image incrementation can be changed retrospectively. This is often done to produce overlapping images, which are then used in multiplanar or 3D reformations.
- A 50% overlap is common. For example, a case scanned with a slice thickness of 5 mm would be reconstructed every 2.5 mm.
- Overlapping reconstructions of data for use as source images in MPR or 3D reformation are particularly useful when the slice thickness

substantially exceeds pixel size. It is less beneficial when the voxel size is isotropic.
  - To determine whether a voxel is isotropic, compare the pixel size to the slice thickness. A voxel is isotropic when the *xy* direction is equal to the slice thickness.
- On MDCT systems, data from parallel rows of detectors can be combined in different ways to create thicker slices for viewing or storing.
- The goal of using a thin slice for scanning and reconstructing thicker slices for viewing and storing is to maintain the advantage of high-resolution imaging but also create image files that are manageable and more easily reviewed by radiologists.

## IMAGE REFORMATION

- The terms image reformation and image rendering are synonyms.
- To reformat a CT examination, all of the source images must have an identical DFOV, image center, and gantry tilt, and they must be contiguous. Because lining up the images exactly is vital, even a small amount of motion will seriously degrade the reformatted image.
- Image reformation uses only image data (not raw data) to generate images in a plane or orientation different from the prospective image.
- Reformatted images can be of either a 2D or 3D nature.
- In general, the thinner the original slice, the better the reformatted image.

33

## Multiplanar Reformation

- Reformation that is done to show anatomy in various planes is referred to as multiplanar reformation (MPR).
- MPRs are two-dimensional in nature.
  - Unlike 3D displays, 2D image displays always represent the original CT attenuation values.
- On most scanners, MPRs can be created either at the operator's console or at a separate workstation.
- MPRs can be created in coronal, sagittal, or oblique planes. Curved planar reformation (CPR) allows images to be created along the centerline of tubular organs.
- MDCT has made MPR more useful because the volumetric data sets that result from MDCT methods produce very high quality MPR images. Current software allows the reformats to be generated quickly and easily.
  - When voxels are isotropic in the source data, MPRs created in any plane will have the same image quality as the original axial reconstruction.
  - When voxels are not isotropic in the source data, image quality can be improved by using overlapping source images.
- Manual methods of MPR require the operator to input criteria, such as the thickness and plane of the desired reformatted image.
  - Real-time (or interactive) reformation refers to the feature that allows the operator to manually change the image plane while the software continually updates the image.
- Scanner-created MPRs are programmed in the system to be generated automatically. They can save time for the technologists and ensure that the MPRs are always done. Typically, only straight sagittal and coronal planes can be programmed to be automatically generated.
- Most picture archive and communication systems (PACS) allow MPRs to be created on the PACS workstation. This allows the radiologist to create the images that are the most suitable for a specific diagnosis. However, if high-quality MPRs are to be created from PACS workstations, then the thinnest possible slices must be available. This means that all of the slices must be sent to the PACS workstation, rather than just the thicker slices often reconstructed for viewing purposes.

## Three-Dimensional Reformation

- Three-dimensional reformation attempts to represent the scan volume in a single image.
- Unlike 2D displays, 3D techniques manipulate CT values to display an image; the original CT value is not included.

- Because 3D rendering can be time consuming, the software is generally available on independent consoles so the operator's console remains available for scanning patients.
- Three-dimensional techniques draw an imaginary line from the viewer through the data volume. Displays are generated by taking into account some or all (depending on the technique used) of the CT values along each line.
- The principles of MPR apply to 3D reformats, especially the axiom that the thinner the original slices, the better the final 3D image.
- A variety of 3D techniques exist that display data from the scan volume in different ways.

### Surface Rendering

- Surface rendering (SR) is also called shaded surface display (SSD). This technique creates images that display the outline or outside shell of the structure.
- In most forms of SR, a threshold CT value must be selected. The software will then include or exclude the voxel depending on whether its CT number is above or below the threshold. It uses this information to create an image of the surface of an object.
  - Selecting the appropriate threshold CT values of the voxels that will be displayed is critical.
- SR is useful for examining tubular structures, such as the inside surfaces of airways, the colon, and blood vessels.
- Maximum intensity projection (MIP) and minimum intensity projection (MinIP) are examples of a technique known as projection displays.
  - The MIP selects only the highest-value voxels from the data set for display.
  - The MinIP selects the minimum value voxels for display.
- It is frequently useful to limit the data set before creating the projection displays. This technique can remove structures that may obscure the area of interest.

### Volume Rendering

- Volume rendering (VR) has become the favored 3D imaging technique. VR is a 3D transparent representation of the imaged structure.
- An advantage of the VR technique is that all voxels contribute to the image. This allows VR images to display multiple tissues and show their relationship to one another.
- VR allows the user a high degree of interactivity. The user can change the look of the VR by changing variables such as the color scale, applied lighting, opacity values, and window settings.

### Endoluminal Imaging

- Endoluminal imaging is a form of VR that is specifically designed to look inside the lumen of a structure.
- Because the technique aims to simulate the view of an endoscopist, it is commonly referred to as virtual endoscopy.
- Endoluminal imaging visualizes a structure as if it were hollow and the viewer were inside of it. Once inside, the viewer can "fly through" the structure; that is, the viewer can move forward or backward at will.

### Three-Dimensional Modeling

- VR data sets can be used to create 3D models using 3D printers.
- Three-dimensional printing is the common name for the additive manufacturing technique that creates 3D solid objects from a digital file. Models are produced by laying down successive layers of material until the object is created.

## Region-of-Interest Editing

- The process of selectively removing or isolating information from the data set is referred to as region-of-interest editing or segmentation. The purpose is to better demonstrate the areas of interest by removing obscuring structures from the display.
- Manual segmentation refers to the process by which a user identifies and selects data to be saved or removed.
- Fully automated segmentation is a software feature that attempts to remove unwanted data automatically. However, in many situations, the source images are too complex and the software cannot readily identify the unwanted data.
- Semiautomatic segmentation methods combine many of the benefits of manual and automatic segmentation techniques. The user guides the otherwise automatic process by providing initial information about the region of interest.

## Factors That Degrade Reformatted Images

- Segmentation errors occur when important vessels or other structures are inadvertently edited out of the data set.
- Excessive image noise in the source images will significantly limit the quality and utility of 3D rendered images.
- Artifacts on the source data will also degrade the reformatted images. The most common artifacts are a result of motion or from metallic objects that produce streaks.
  - Stair-step artifacts can occur when voxels are not isotropic.

## REVIEW QUESTIONS

1. Raw data that result from an MDCT scan acquisition are used so that the 1-mm slices are combined to produce thicker slices for viewing. This is called
   a. 3D reformation.
   b. image reconstruction.
   c. segmentation.
   d. multiplanar reformation.
2. In what situation would overlapping reconstructions for subsequent image rendering not be indicated?
   a. Slice thickness = 0.5 mm, DFOV = 25
   b. Slice thickness = 2 mm, DFOV = 35
   c. Slice thickness = 5 mm, DFOV = 42
   d. Slice thickness = 7 mm, DFOV = 45
3. Assume the raw data are still available. In what scenario would it be impossible to create an MPR?
   a. Source images vary in slice thickness.
   b. Source images vary in gantry tilt.
   c. Source images vary in image center.
   d. Source images vary in DFOV.
4. What plane is the MPR depicted by Figure 8-1?
   a. Sagittal
   b. Coronal
   c. Oblique
   d. Curved

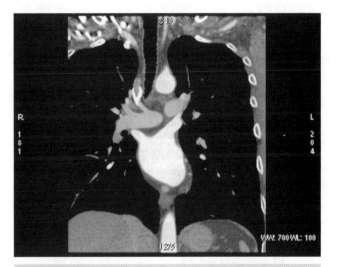

**FIGURE 8-1**

5. Which of the following is a TRUE statement regarding MPRs?
   a. They are created from raw data.
   b. They are 3D in nature.
   c. All MPR images have the same image quality as the source image.
   d. They can be created either at the operator's console or at a separate workstation.
6. A limitation of scanner-created MPRs is that
   a. only one examination protocol per scanner can be programmed to automatically create MPRs.
   b. they take more time to create than manually produced MPRs.

c. in most cases, only straight sagittal and coronal planes can be automatically generated.

d. they are not consistently produced, so technologists must remember to check to see whether they were created.

7. Which is a disadvantage to workstation-created MPRs?

a. They require that the raw data be sent to the workstation, which is difficult to transmit via the PACS.

b. To produce the highest quality MPRs, the thinnest slices must be sent to the workstation. This amount of data can slow down the PACS.

c. Most radiologists have not been trained to create MPRs.

d. Workstations are only able to create MPRs in the sagittal and coronal planes.

8. Another name for surface rendering is

a. volume rendering.

b. segmentation.

c. projection display.

d. shaded surface display.

9. In creating a surface-rendered image, what can happen if the threshold set is too narrow?

a. Actual protruding structures can be imperceptible.

b. Nontissue materials, such as fluids, can be displayed as if they were tissue and can obscure protruding structures.

c. Too much data are included so that less powerful computers may not be able to generate a display.

d. The SR image generated cannot be rotated.

10. An MIP is a good method to display all of the following EXCEPT

a. pulmonary nodules.

b. fracture extent.

c. contrast-filled coronary arteries.

d. bronchial tree.

11. What type of 3D display is depicted in Figure 8-2?

a. Volume rendering

b. Surface rendering

c. MIP

d. MinIP

12. Which has become the favored 3D imaging technique in CT?

a. Volume rendering

b. Surface rendering

c. MIP

d. MinIP

13. VR techniques assign each voxel an opacity value based on its ___. This value determines the degree the voxel will contribute to the final image.

a. location

b. Hounsfield units

c. depth

d. width

14. The process of selectively removing or isolating information from the 3D data set is referred to as

a. clipping.

b. cutting.

c. segmentation.

d. dissociation.

15. In Figure 8-3, what is the most likely cause of the artifact indicated by the arrows on this reformatted image?

a. Motion

b. Noise

c. Metallic objects

d. Windmill artifacts

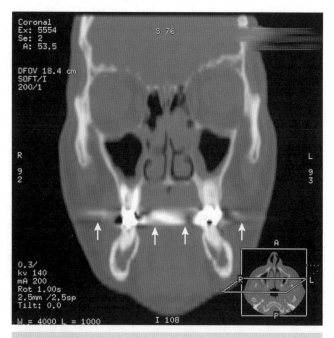

**FIGURE 8-3**

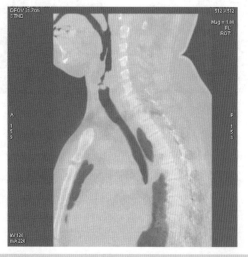

**FIGURE 8-2**

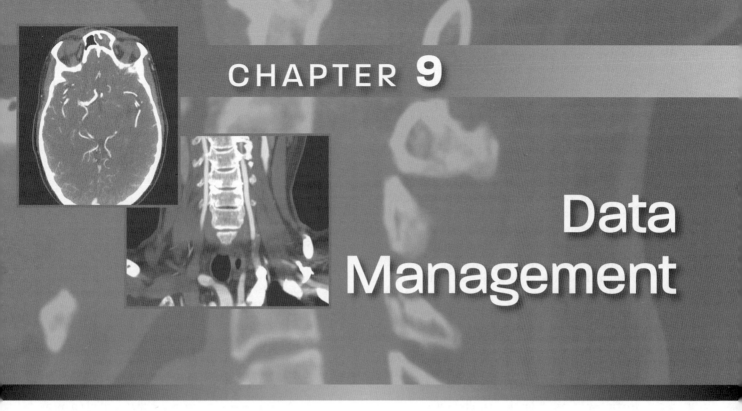

# CHAPTER 9

# Data Management

## INTRODUCTION

Digital connectivity is becoming as mainstream in health care as in every other aspect of life. Healthcare consumers increasingly expect the convenience that technology brings to other businesses. Healthcare organizations are responding by offering digital, consumer-based services such as online scheduling, online bill paying, and digital communication with clinicians.

- Patient portals are secure online applications that provide patients with 24-hour access to their personal health information from anywhere with an Internet connection. Using a secure username and password, patients can view health information such as recent appointments, medications, allergies, and test results.
- Clinical decision support (CDS) software aims to provide clinicians and medical staff with knowledge and situation-specific information, intelligently filtered and presented at the appropriate time to help healthcare providers make clinical decisions.
  - In regards to radiology, a key use of CDS is to help ordering clinicians to quickly determine what type of imaging exam is needed for a patient with specific symptoms. In the future, such software may be mandated by the Centers for Medicare and Medicaid Services (CMS). The goal is to reduce the number of inappropriate exams, thereby improving the quality of health care by reducing unnecessary exposure to radiation and also reducing cost.

- Electronic Health Information Exchange (HIE) allows healthcare providers and patients to appropriately access and securely share a patient's vital medical information—improving the speed, quality, safety, and cost of patient care.

## INTRODUCTION TO IMAGING INFORMATICS

- The collection, classification, storage, retrieval, and dissemination of recorded information is known as informatics.
- Imaging informatics is a subspecialty that is vital to radiology as it is devoted to how information about medical images is exchanged within the radiology department and throughout the medical enterprise.
  - Although it is often thought of as how images get from one place to another, imaging informatics is actually much broader in scope.
- Imaging professionals must work with many different electronic information systems from both outside the radiology department and within it.
  - Hospital information systems (HIS) focus on administrative issues, such as patient demographic data, financial data, and patient locations within the hospital.
  - Clinical information systems (CIS) may be integrated into the HIS, but are often separate systems that keep track of clinical data.
  - Computerized physician (or provider) order entry (CPOE) systems electronically transmit clinician orders to radiology and other departments.

- A generic term for a digital patient record is an electronic health record, or EHR. These are often composed of electronic medical records (EMR) from a variety of sources, including radiology. However, in general usage, EHR and EMR are used synonymously.
- In the radiology department, two key components form the information infrastructure: the radiology information system (RIS) and the picture archive and communication system (PACS).
- The RIS is most often used for scheduling patients, storing reports, patient tracking, protocoling examinations, and billing. Ideally, the RIS ties together all the computer systems within the radiology department. Such connectivity is commonly referred to as intraoperability.
- The term PACS encompasses a broad range of technologies necessary for the storage, retrieval, distribution, and display of images.
- Film-based systems are being replaced by electronic systems. Film is usually referred to as "hardcopy," whereas electronic images are often referred to as "softcopy."
  - Film-based systems are being replaced by PACS for both financial and quality reasons.
- In some departments, the conversion from a primarily film-based system to a PACS is gradual, starting with a select set of modalities, or with just a small set of functions. Other departments completely convert to an entirely digital department that includes image acquisition, transfer, interpretation, storage, and transmission.
- In addition to the RIS and PACS, radiology departments often use a variety of other software to meet their specialized needs. Examples are software systems that keep a record of the radiation dose to patients, keep track of exams performed or interpreted by radiology learners (e.g., residents and student technologists), to facilitate the download and viewing of images that were created externally, to track revenue or insurance payouts, or for radiologists use when dictating results.

## PACS FUNDAMENTALS

- A PACS uses a computer network to integrate image acquisition devices, display workstations, and storage systems. The PACS technology has a huge influence on the workflow of radiologists and technologists. It can also have an impact on referring physicians, allowing them easy remote access to the images of their patients.
- To be included in a PACS system, images must be in a digital form. CT is intrinsically digital. Modalities such as conventional radiography have been modified to allow direct digital capture.

- A skilled team of information technology (IT) personnel is necessary to keep the PACS running smoothly.
- Although IT staff troubleshoot most problems, to ensure optimal workflow and image quality, technologists should be familiar with the basic elements of the PACS.

## Networking

- A network is a group of two or more computers linked together.
- Although the network and the PACS are two distinct environments, they are interdependent.
- Computer networks can be configured in many different ways.
  - Those that are close together (in the same building) are called local area networks (LAN).
  - Those that are farther apart and connected by telephone lines, cables, or radio waves are called wide area networks (WAN).
  - "Wired" networks are those that are linked by a physical connection.
  - "Wireless" networks are those that use radio waves to transmit data between computers.
- PACS use the client-server network architecture.
  - Server computers are passive, waiting for requests from other networked computers. They facilitate communication between and deliver information to other computers. A server typically accepts connections from a large number of clients.
  - End users interact directly with client computers to send data requests to one or more connected servers. Clients usually connect to a small number of servers.
  - Each client or server in the network may also be referred to as a node.
- PACS may have one or more servers. The server computers that are integral to the functioning of the PACS are referred to as core servers.
- Bandwidth is a term used to describe the amount of data that can be transmitted between two points in the network in a set period of time.
  - Bandwidth represents the capacity of the network connection. It is primarily dependent on the transmission medium but also depends on factors such as the number of computers sharing the same bandwidth.
- Image data can be compressed to make transmission more efficient.
  - The compression method is said to be lossless if no image data are lost during the process.
  - Lossy compression methods introduce compression artifacts; it is difficult to know for certain the level of lossy compression that can be applied to an image without decreasing the diagnostic accuracy.

- A protocol defines a common set of rules and signals that computers on the network use to communicate.

## Electronic Standards

- The Digital Imaging and Communication in Medicine (DICOM) standard is a universally adopted standard for medical image interchange.
- Vendors publish DICOM Conformance Statements to convey what DICOM standards they adhere to.
- The Health Level Seven (HL7) organization works to develop universal standards for clinical and administrative data throughout the healthcare arena. HL7 is also used to refer to some of the specific standards created by the organization.

## Image Acquisition

- Image acquisition from the CT scanner to the PACS should be done by a direct digital DICOM capture. This provides the same spatial resolution and image manipulation capabilities as exists on the operator's console.
  - A less favorable option for transferring image data from the CT scanner to the PACS is the analog method known as frame grabbing. Similar to a screen capture, converting data using this method loses the pixel measurements of the original image.

## Workstation Monitors

- Until the 1990s, all monitors in the radiology department used cathode-ray tube (CRT) technology. To suit the needs of radiology, the typical color CRT monitors used in televisions were modified. Monochrome CRTs were created with special phosphors that could produce the required brightness, reduce distortion, and display images with higher spatial resolution.
- More recently, liquid crystal display (LCD) and plasma display technologies are options for medical display devices.
- The purchase price of the LCD and plasma monitors is approximately two to three times higher than the price of CRT monitors of equal spatial resolution. However, this cost is offset by the longer life span of the new monitors. In addition, LCD monitors consume less energy than do their CRT counterparts and emit less heat (which lowers room cooling costs).
- Quality assurance is simpler with LCD and plasma technologies–CRT monitors require frequent calibration that is not necessary with the newer designs. In addition, the brightness levels of CRT monitors degrade relatively quickly.

- Brightness (or luminance) is an important characteristic because subtle aspects of an image tend to be more easily seen on brighter displays.
- Historically, monitors used for medical display have been predominately gray scale, rather than color. The main reason for this is that a monochrome display is brighter and sharper than its color counterpart. Color displays require a higher maximum luminance compared with grayscale monitors. However, applications such as PET/CT and Doppler ultrasound require color display, so PACS workstations often include both a monochrome and a color monitor.

## Data Storage

- Radiology departments generate a tremendous amount of data. Innovations, such as 256-slice CT technology, indicate that the growth of digital information will continue.
- The process of saving image data from the originating modality to an electronic medium is called archiving. Archived images can later be retrieved to be displayed on the monitor, copied onto a disk, or filmed.
- Several devices are available for archiving, and can be broadly classified as online (when images are instantly accessible), near-line (when images are automatically retrieved from a storage system), or offline (when image devices must be located and manually loaded into the system).
- A system known as a redundant array of inexpensive disks (or drives; RAID) is a storage solution that capitalizes on the fact that data stored on hard disks can be accessed quickly and reliably.
- Optical devices include compact discs (CD), digital versatile discs (DVD), and Blu-ray discs. Although the technology is similar, the capacity of a DVD is greater than that of a CD; Blu-ray discs have even greater data storage capacity than do DVDs.
- Optical media are often used in a device called an optical jukebox. These are robotic storage systems that automatically load and unload the optical discs.
  - They are also called optical disc libraries, robotic drives, or autochangers.
- Magnetic tape consists of a long narrow strip of plastic with a magnetizable coating. It is most often packaged in cartridges and cassettes. The device that performs the actual writing or reading of data is known as the tape drive. Tapes are also used with autochangers and tape libraries.
- To access data on magnetic tape, it must be rewound to the appropriate location on the tape (sequential access). This is in contrast to optical media that offers random access. Therefore, magnetic tape is somewhat slower.

## Image Distribution

- Image distribution channels can be department-wide, hospital-wide, or more recently, enterprise-wide. Enterprise distribution refers to the ability to deliver images to geographically diverse locations. These can meet the needs of off-campus outpatient clinics or radiologists who wish to review studies from home.
- The Internet is increasingly being used as a key element in meeting image distribution requirements.
- Any image distribution system must have a well-designed security system to keep confidential patient information safe and to meet regulatory requirements.
  - Many security strategies exist, including firewalls, passwords and usernames, and secure socket layers.
  - Virtual private networks, or VPNs, are also being used to make the Internet a safe medium for the secure transmission of clinical data. VPNs in the medical computing world are used to enhance security by encrypting the information at the source and decrypting it at the destination.

## REVIEW QUESTIONS

1. Which electronic system allows clinicians to input an electronic order for a CT examination and transmits that order to the CT department?
   a. RIS
   b. PACS
   c. HIS
   d. CPOE
2. What two electronic elements form the radiology information infrastructure?
   a. RIS and PACS
   b. HIS and CIS
   c. CPOE and EMR
   d. LAN and SSL
3. Which of the following is NOT a true statement regarding PACS?
   a. Vast amounts of data pass through any PACS.
   b. PACS technology has a huge impact on the workflow of radiologists and technologists.
   c. To be included in a PACS system, images must be in a digital form.
   d. Once the hardware for the PACS is installed, the system runs virtually maintenance-free.
4. Computers that act on requests from other networked computers, rather than from a person inputting directly into it, are called
   a. LANS.
   b. star topologies.
   c. servers.
   d. P2P.
5. The computers that are integral to the functioning of the PACS are referred to as
   a. archival devices.
   b. core servers.
   c. routers.
   d. bridges.
6. The amount of data that can be transmitted between two points in the network in a set period of time is known as
   a. bandwidth.
   b. pixel volume.
   c. memory capacity.
   d. frequency.
7. A scheme that compresses an image without any loss of information when the image is decompressed is called
   a. lossy.
   b. fractional coding.
   c. scalar and vector quantization.
   d. lossless.
8. DICOM refers to a
   a. specific geometric arrangement of computers in a network.
   b. universally adopted standard for medical image interchange.
   c. type of magnetic tape used to store data.
   d. peer-to-peer computer network such as the Usenet news server.
9. Which is NOT true of an LCD monitor?
   a. The purchase price of an LCD is approximately half that of a CRT monitor.
   b. LCD monitors have a longer life span compared with CRT monitors.
   c. Assuring the continued quality of the LCD is much simpler than that of the CRT monitor.
   d. LCD monitors maintain their luminosity better than do CRT monitors.
10. A device that is used to automatically load and unload optical discs is called a (an)
    a. ethernet.
    b. tape drive.
    c. media vending machine.
    d. optical jukebox.

# SECTION II

# Patient Care

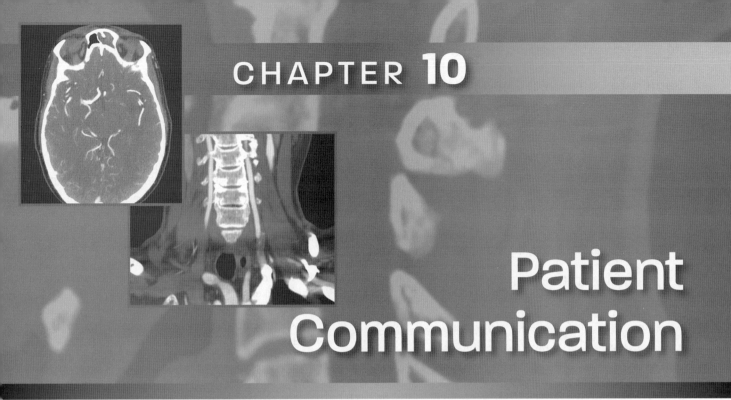

# CHAPTER 10

# Patient Communication

## BENEFITS OF EFFECTIVE COMMUNICATION

■ Effective communication skills are essential and allow technologists to perform safe, diagnostically useful studies. Obtaining an accurate medical history and ensuring that the patient understands what is expected of him or her during a CT examination are critical steps.

■ Research reveals that professionals who communicate effectively spend no more time, per patient, than do those who report feeling "too rushed to spend time talking." In fact, some studies have shown that total examination time actually *decreased* as communication increased.

■ Patients have a right to expect quality service throughout the entire healthcare experience, including the following:
  ● How healthcare workers communicate with patients, from the registration desk to the billing department
  ● How they and their families are treated by the staff
  ● The type of information they are given

■ Providing patients with the quality service they expect not only is worthwhile and important medically but also makes good business sense. There is a clear link between effective communication and a reduction in malpractice claims. Patients feel most satisfied when they feel fully informed. They need to have their questions answered. Patients also express a desire to have interactions that feel personal, caring, and respectful. They want technologists to relate to them as people. Dissatisfied patients have reported feeling that the provider focuses on them only as a disease process (e.g., "the diabetic") or as an organ to be examined (e.g., "the abdomen").

■ The benefits of effective communication include improved patient safety, improved examination quality, improved patient retention, increased referrals, greater profitability, reduced risk of malpractice suits, improved collections, better staff morale, reduced staff turnover, and greater workflow efficiency.

■ There are a number of ways communication can inadvertently go awry. Technologists often feel pressed for time and consequently rush the visit. Sometimes they use excessive medical terminology, or they can underestimate the patient's desire for information.

## THE COMMUNICATION PROCESS

■ Communication can be defined as the "process of creating meaning." Two words in this sentence are critical: *create* and *meaning*. Messages are generated by the speaker, but meanings are generated from within the mind of the receiver. Many times the sender thinks that the message is clear. But the receiver, who must interpret the message through his or her own specific frame of reference, may hear something entirely different. Communication is so difficult because at each step in the process, there is a potential for breakdown. In fact, it is estimated that 40% to 60% of meaning is lost in the transmission of messages from sender to receiver.

## Barriers to Communication

- Language–the choice of words a sender selects will influence the quality of the communication. It is important to remember that no two people will attribute the exact same meaning to the same words.
- Power struggles–defensiveness, distorted perceptions, guilt, transference, past transgression. These issues crop up when either the sender or the receiver suffers from low self-esteem or insecurity.
- Misreading of body language, tone, and other nonverbal forms of communication–it is important to understand that a majority of communication is nonverbal. This means that when we attribute meaning to what someone else is saying, the verbal part of the message actually means less than does the nonverbal part. The nonverbal part includes such aspects as body language and tone.
- Fuzzy transmission–unreliable or inconsistent messages.
- Receiver distortion–selective hearing, ignoring nonverbal cues. This often happens if the receiver doesn't like portions of the sender's message. By simply ignoring pieces of the message, the receiver gets a message more to his or her liking.
- Assumptions–assuming others see situations the same as you or have the same feelings as you. Healthcare workers become so accustomed to the hospital environment that they sometimes forget how frightening and strange it can be to someone with no medical background.
- Preconceptions–in the process of communicating, our prejudices often slip through.
- Past experiences–how we perceive communication is affected by past experiences with the individual.
- Cultural differences–effective communication requires deciphering the basic values, motives, aspiration, and assumptions that operate across geographical lines. Given some dramatic differences across cultures in approaches to such areas as time, space, and privacy, the opportunities for miscommunication while we are in cross-cultural situations are plentiful.

## Nonverbal Communication

- As much as 90% of the meaning we derive from communication comes from the nonverbal cues that the other person gives. Often, a person may say one thing but communicate something totally different through vocal intonation and body language. Mixed messages create tension and distrust because the receiver senses that the communicator is being less than candid.
- Nonverbal communication can be categorized in five ways:
  - Visual–includes facial expression, eye contact, posture, and gestures.
  - Tactile–the use of touch, such as a handshake or pat on the back, to impart meaning.
  - Vocal–the intonation of a person's voice.
  - Use of time, space–this includes keeping people waiting, standing too close to another.
  - Objects or values–the appearance of objects, such as a messy waiting room, can send inadvertent messages to patients and their families.

## PRACTICAL ADVICE

- Communication is a two-way process; therefore, both the speaker and listener have responsibilities.
- The speaker's responsibilities
  - Be audible. Speak loudly enough so that your listener can hear you without undue strain. Be clear.
  - Be aware that your listener may not have understood you.
  - Be willing to ask questions of your listener to see if he or she understands you.
  - Offer the listener an opportunity to ask for clarification.
  - Be willing to restate and clarify your message.
- The listener's responsibilities
  - Let the speaker know whether he or she is inaudible.
  - Let the speaker know that you are attentive. Look at the speaker. Nod or shake your head.
  - If the speaker's message is unclear, let him or her know that you need a point clarified.
  - Be aware that you may not have understood the speaker. Don't be impatient if you occasionally do not understand everything. Try to keep from getting angry. Be willing to paraphrase what you think the speaker means.

## Communication Habits to Avoid

- Don't use false reassurance.
- Don't ignore a patient's wishes.
- Don't speak like you are talking to a child.
- Don't assume that a nonresponsive patient can't hear.
- Don't carry on a separate conversation with a coworker while a patient is present.
- Don't think being professional means being cold.
- Don't blame the patient.
- Don't use abbreviations or medical lingo.

## Communication Habits to Adopt

- Be a good listener.
- Use focused questions.
- Use the patient's name.
- Use touch to comfort and be aware of nonverbal messages.
- Develop a rapport with the patient.

- Explain before acting.
- Give the patient an opportunity to ask questions.
- Use reflective speech.
- Give consistent messages.

## REVIEW QUESTIONS

1. Mr. Jones is scheduled for a CT of the chest. As you review his history, he confides that he is extremely concerned that the study will find cancer, particularly as he has smoked cigarettes for more than 20 years. Your response is which of the following?
   a. "Don't worry, everything will be fine; this test is just a precaution."
   b. "I understand your concern. The U.S. Surgeon General says that cigarette smoking is the major single cause of cancer mortality in the United States."
   c. "I understand your concern, and know that waiting to get an answer can be excruciating. We will get the results to your physician just as soon as we can."
   d. "You may be able to sue the cigarette companies if you do have cancer. You should probably contact a lawyer."

2. You are taking a patient's medical history. You are unsure what he means when he says, "Oh, yeah, I've had lots of times when my kidneys just shut down and they had to give them a kick start." Using reflective speech, you
   a. record on the history sheet exactly what the patient said.
   b. say, "So you've experienced kidney failure in the past that required dialysis?"
   c. ask him to repeat what he just said, so that a coworker can also listen.
   d. say, "Oh, that happens to me sometimes, too. Have you tried drinking a lot of water?"

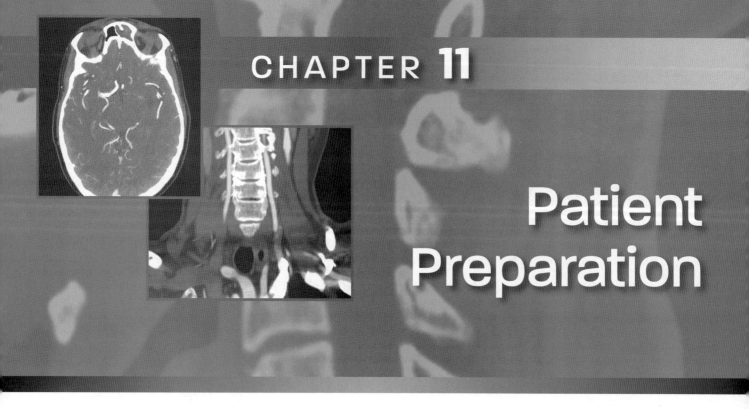

# CHAPTER 11

# Patient Preparation

Many steps must occur before scanning a patient. Often, these tasks are performed in collaboration with other staff members including clerks, radiology nurses, and radiologists. The exact order of the steps and what staff member will perform what task varies widely from facility to facility.

## INITIATING THE EXAMINATION

- All CT examinations must be initiated by a clinician with appropriate credentials. In addition to physicians, clinicians who may order diagnostic tests include nurse practitioners (NP) and physician assistants (PA).
- In situations in which a doctor's order must be relayed by clerks or other staff members, there exists the potential for transcription errors. Therefore, it is recommended that the original requisition written by the ordering clinician be faxed or electronically transmitted to the imaging facility.
- Before any CT examination is performed, a copy of the original order requisition must be reviewed by the technologist so that she can verify that the appropriate examination has been planned.
- Ideally, some patient screening should occur at the time the examination is scheduled. This will help to schedule patients more efficiently by adequately planning for issues such as contrast media allergies and claustrophobia. Electronic scheduling systems often assist with the screening process by prompting clerical staff to ask questions pertinent to the appropriate scheduling of the ordered exam.

- The most accurate method for transmitting orders to the radiology department is via an electronic system in which the ordering clinician places the electronic order herself. Generically called computerized physician order entry (CPOE), these systems eliminate the transcription errors that can arise when an intermediary (e.g., clerk or nurse) must read a handwritten order and translate it into an electronic order.

## Selecting the Appropriate Protocol

- The proper selection of protocol is the purview of the radiologist, often with a technologist's input. In some instances, protocol selection is constrained by a specific scanner's capabilities. The overarching goal is to select the protocol that will answer the clinical question(s) posed with the least risk to the patient. Risks to the patient include those attributed to radiation exposure, contrast media reactions, or complications such as bleeding or infection that may arise from procedures such as biopsies or fluid drainage. The protocol selected must consider the patient's ability to tolerate the examination.
- In some institutions, radiologists review each CT request, consider the patient's medical history, and assign a specific protocol. Technologists will then carry out the selected protocol unless their review of the actual patient (rather than just the paperwork) brings up questions or concerns.
- In other facilities, radiologists set up specific algorithms for technologists to follow. These might include matching specific clinical indications to

specific examination protocols. These algorithms most often require the technologist to review a number of criteria from the patient's medical history (e.g., laboratory values related to renal function, allergies) before selecting the appropriate protocol. Technologists seek the radiologists' advice only when uncertainties arise.

■ Technologists must understand the criteria used to determine when various protocols are appropriate. This is an important patient safeguard in that technologists can identify potential errors before an examination is performed.

## ROOM PREPARATION

■ Scanner calibrations and tube warm-up procedures should be done while the room is free of both patient and CT staff.

■ The room should be checked for cleanliness, items from previous patients discarded, and supplies stocked and in their designated location.

■ The appropriate equipment, such as head holder or foot extension, should be attached. Positioning devices such as angle sponges should be clean and readily accessible. Appropriate safety equipment, such as thyroid or breast shields, should be ready for use. On the infrequent occasion that someone other than the patient will remain in the scan room during the examination, appropriate safety equipment (e.g., lead aprons or a lead screen) must be provided.

## MEDICAL HISTORY

■ An appropriate medical history is a vital aspect of any CT examination. It will help to ensure a patient's safety, guide the selection of examination protocol, and offer the radiologist valuable diagnostic information. Many organizations employ an electronic method for collecting these data. Electronic methods have the advantage of being able to pull information stored in the patient's chart, such as allergies or pertinent lab values.

### Patient Identification

■ At first contact with the patient, the technologist must be careful to accurately identify the patient. Many cases have occurred in which technologists confused patients with similar-sounding names and performed the wrong examination.
  • At least two methods of verifying a patient's identity are required.

### Patient Safety

■ Questions should be asked to ensure that the ordered examination can be safely performed. These questions will look for risk factors related to the administration of iodinated contrast media and, in women, chance of pregnancy.

■ The administration of contrast media is contraindicated in some situations. In other situations, contrast media is administered only after a patient is premedicated to reduce the risks of an adverse event. Patients are questioned regarding renal impairment and previous allergies to assess whether they can be safely given an intravenous iodinated contrast agent. Knowing a patient's previous allergies is also necessary should an unexpected reaction occur that necessitates immediate pharmaceutical treatment. Questions regarding hyperthyroidism and other diseases of the thyroid also relate to whether the patient can safely receive an iodinated contrast agent.

■ A fetus, exposed to ionizing radiation in utero, is particularly sensitive to its harmful effects. Female patients within childbearing age must be questioned as to the possibility that they may be pregnant. If the woman is uncertain, the examination should be delayed while pregnancy status is determined. In the event that the patient is pregnant, a careful analysis of the risks and benefits of the examination must be considered. This discussion should include the patient, the referring doctor, and the radiologist.

### Protocol Selection

■ Ideally, enough patient information is provided by the ordering clinician to guide the selection of examination protocol. In some institutions, additional information can be obtained through electronic health records, or archived paper records. Unfortunately, this is not always the case. In many situations, information obtained from the patient once they arrive at the imaging center will determine what examination protocol is applied. Questions regarding the symptoms that a patient is experiencing, whether the symptoms are new or chronic, and the onset of those symptoms are frequently used to select the appropriate protocol.

### Diagnostic Information

■ Many diseases or conditions have similar findings on CT images. A medical history may aid the radiologist in narrowing down, or pinpointing exactly, the disease or condition from which the patient suffers. Questions that include the patient's past surgeries, significant medical issues, and current symptoms augment other clinical data in helping radiologists to accurately interpret CT images.

### Laboratory Values

■ The laboratory values most frequently reviewed before routine CT examinations are estimated glomerular filtration rate (eGFR), serum creatinine, and blood urea nitrogen (BUN). These values provide information about a patient's kidney function, which is important if the patient will receive an intravenous contrast agent.

■ The normal range of these values can vary slightly from laboratory to laboratory, and also among adult men, adult women, and children. Laboratory reports typically provide guidance as to when a value is outside of the normal limit for a specific patient.

■ As a general guide, the normal range for eGFR is greater than 60 mL/min/1.73 m², BUN is typically between 7 and 25 mg/dL, and the normal range for serum creatinine is 0.6 to 1.7 mg/dL.

■ Many institutions have a policy for when a radiologist is consulted before intravenous contrast medium is administered to patients in whom the BUN is greater than 30 mg/dL, the creatinine value is greater than 2 mg/dL, or the eGFR is less than 30 mL/min/1.73 m².

■ Examinations such as biopsies and fluid drainage carry the risk of excessive bleeding. Before these examinations are performed, it is important to check laboratory values that indicate problems with the blood's ability to form clots (coagulate). Tests most often used are prothrombin time (PT), partial thromboplastin time (PTT), and platelet count.

■ Although the normal range may vary slightly from laboratory to laboratory, a typical range for PT is 11 to 14 seconds, PTT is 25 to 35 seconds, and platelet count is 150,000 to 400,000 mm³.

Table 11-1 lists laboratory values relevant to CT examinations and their approximate normal ranges.

## Patient Education and Informed Consent

■ CT technologists have a professional responsibility to provide patient education. At a minimum, the technologist should describe
  ● How the procedure is carried out
  ● The approximate time the procedure will take

● Whether contrast agents will be administered
  ◆ If contrast media is planned, then an explanation of how it will be administered (e.g., oral, IV) and any potential side effects is required
● What is expected of the patient
● Any follow-up necessary after the examination has been completed

■ Basic (or simple) consent involves letting the patient know what you plan to do and asking them whether they agree.

■ Many facilities have the patient sign a consent form before the examination is performed, particularly when an intravenous contrast material is to be administered, although the practice is not universal.

■ In the case of CT examinations of a more invasive nature, such as biopsies, there is universal agreement that a signed consent form is necessary. When a consent form is required, it must be signed by the patient before the administration of any medication used for pain relief or sedation. In the case of pediatric patients, a parent or legal guardian must sign the consent form.

## Immobilization and Patient Restraint Devices

■ Immobilization and restraint devices are used in CT both for patient safety and to improve the quality of the examinations. For example, straps are used to protect patients from falling from the CT table and to remind them to remain still during the procedure. Beanbags can be placed alongside lower limbs to prevent motion that will degrade the CT images.

■ Technologists should be sensitive to the patient's feelings regarding such devices. Before using any immobilization or restraining device, the technologist must explain to the patient (or the patient's guardians) the need for the device and show them exactly how it will be used in their care. Whenever possible, basic consent for the use of the device should be given.

### Table 11-1 Laboratory Values

| Laboratory Test | Approximate Normal Range* | Indicates |
|---|---|---|
| Blood urea nitrogen (BUN) | 7–25 mg/dL | Renal function |
| Serum creatinine | 0.6–1.7 mg/dL | Renal function |
| Estimated glomerular filtration rate (eGFR) | >60 mL/min/1.73 m² | Renal function |
| Prothrombin time (PT) | 11–14 seconds | Blood coagulation ability |
| Partial thromboplastin time (PTT) | 25–35 seconds | Blood coagulation ability |
| Platelet count | 150,000–400,000 mm³ | Blood coagulation ability |

* The range of normal values varies slightly from laboratory to laboratory and, in many cases, among adult men, adult women, and children. Laboratory reports typically indicate whether a specific value is out of range for that laboratory and that particular patient.

- In some situations, consent cannot be obtained, such as for an unaccompanied patient who is unconscious, delirious, or mentally disabled. Technically, a clinician's order is required to use a restraining device for a patient who cannot provide consent. However, the short-term use of restraints to complete an imaging examination is often done without consulting the patient's physician.
- When restraining devices are used in CT, the following rules should be strictly adhered to:
  - The patient must be allowed as much mobility as is safely possible.
  - The areas of the body to which immobilizers are applied must be padded to prevent injury to the skin beneath the device.
  - Normal anatomic position must be maintained.
  - Knots that will become tighter with movement are prohibited.
  - The immobilizer must be easy to remove quickly if necessary.
  - Neither circulation nor respiration must be impaired by the immobilizer.
  - If leg immobilizers are necessary, wrist immobilizers must also be applied to prevent the patients from either unfastening the device or, in an attempt to leave the table or gurney, unintentionally hanging themselves.

## Assessment and Monitoring Vital Signs

- Technologists should begin to assess the patient when they first introduce themselves. It is important to notice the patient's breathing, skin coloration, and overall health before the patient ever lies on the CT table. This will help the technologist notice signs should adverse effects occur during the scan process.
- Throughout the CT examination, the patient should be monitored visually and spoken to frequently using the scanner's intercom system. This reassures the patient and allows the technologist to intervene quickly should problems arise.
- Patients may become acutely ill while in the radiology department. In addition to the medical symptoms that necessitated the examination, patients may also have adverse reactions to the intravascular contrast agent used for the examination. Adverse reactions are random and unpredictable; therefore, technologists must be alert for physiologic changes in their patients.
- The best early indicators of a problem are changes in body temperature, pulse, respirations, and blood pressure. Collectively, these are called the vital signs (or cardinal signs). The normal range of vital signs may vary somewhat with age, sex, weight, exercise tolerance, and condition. Other important indicators include pain, pulse oximetry values (indicates blood oxygenation), and pupil size, equality, and reactivity.

## Body Temperature

- Body temperature is most often taken by placing the thermometer in the mouth, the ear (using a tympanic infrared thermometer), the axilla, or the rectum. Oral, rectal, and tympanic temperature measurements are higher than are axillary measurements because the measuring device is in contact with the mucous membrane. More recently, devices called temporal artery thermometers provide temperature assessment by sweeping a small scanner first across the patient's forehead, then behind the patient's ear. An advantage of these devices is that they are entirely noninvasive as they do not need to be inserted in a body cavity. Table 11-2 lists the average temperature and the normal range for each temperature site.

## Pulse

- Pulse is defined as the alternate expansion and recoil of an artery. By counting each expansion of the arterial wall in a given time frame, the pulse rate can be determined.
- In general, the pulse can be felt wherever a superficial artery can be held against firm tissue, such as a bone. Some of the specific locations where the pulse is most easily felt are as follows (Fig. 11-1):
  A. Temporal pulse (superficial temporal artery)–just anterior to the ear
  B. Facial pulse (facial artery)–the lower margin of the mandible, about one-third anterior to the angle
  C. Carotid pulse (carotid artery)–along the anterior aspect of the neck, to the right or left of midline
  D. Radial pulse (radial artery)–at the thumb side of the wrist
  E. Brachial pulse (brachial artery)–on the medial side of the elbow cavity, located between the biceps and triceps muscle, frequently used in place of the carotid pulse in infants

| Table 11-2 Average and Normal Range of Body Temperature | | |
|---|---|---|
| **Route** | **Average** | **Normal Range** |
| Oral | 98.7°F (37.0°C) | 96.8°F–100.4°F (36.0°C–38.0°C) |
| Rectal | 99.1°F (37.7°C) | 97.2°F–100.8°F (36.7°C–38.7°C) |
| Axillary | 97.7°F (36.4°C) | 95.8°F–99.4°F (35.4°C–37.4°C) |
| Tympanic* | Calibrated to oral or rectal scales | |
| Temporal artery | 99.1°F (37.7°C) | 97.2°F–100.8°F (36.7°C–38.7°C) |

* Research is inconclusive as to the accuracy of readings and correlations with other body temperature measurements.

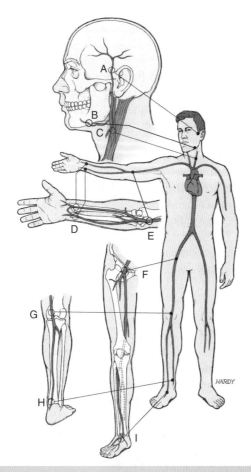

**FIGURE 11-1** Locations where pulse can be taken.

F. Femoral pulse (femoral artery)–in the groin
G. Popliteal pulse (popliteal artery)–behind the knee
H. Pedal pulse (tibialis posterior artery)–posterior ankle, behind medial malleolus
I. Pedal pulse (dorsalis pedis artery)–top of the foot

- The average adult pulse rate ranges from 60 to 100 beats per minute. However, in athletic adults, a normal pulse rate can range between 45 and 60 beats per minute.
- The average pulse rate for a child ranges from 95 to 110 beats per minute; infants, from 100 to 160 beats per minute.
- When a pulse is being counted, the rate, rhythm, and volume should be noted. An irregular pulse is one that has a period of normal rhythm broken by periods of irregularity or skipped beats. The volume (or strength) of the pulse is often described as full and bounding if it seems regular and with good force, or if it is difficult to palpate and irregular, it is often described as weak or thready.

## Respirations

- The respiratory rate is the number of breaths a person takes per minute. It is usually measured when the patient is at rest and simply involves counting the number of breaths for 1 minute by counting how many times the chest rises.
- Normal respiratory rates vary according to age. Commonly accepted normal ranges are as follows: adults, 14 to 20; adolescent youth, 18 to 22; children, 22 to 28; infants, 30 or greater. The ratio of respiration to pulse is fairly constant at approximately one breath to four heart beats.

## Blood Pressure

- Blood pressure may be defined as the pressure exerted by circulating blood on the walls of the vessels. The term blood pressure generally refers to arterial pressure, that is, the pressure measured in the larger arteries. Blood pressure is continually changing depending on activity, temperature, diet, emotional state, posture, physical state, and medications used.
- Blood pressure is most commonly measured by a sphygmomanometer (often condensed to sphygmometer), which uses the height of a column of mercury to reflect the circulating pressure. Although many modern blood pressure devices no longer use mercury, values are still universally reported in millimeters of mercury (mm Hg).
- The systolic pressure is defined as the peak pressure in the arteries. The diastolic pressure is the lowest pressure, and is recorded at the resting phase of the cardiac cycle.
- Although there are large individual variations, typical values for a resting, healthy adult are approximately 120 mm Hg systolic and 80 mm Hg diastolic. This would be written as 120/80 mm Hg, and spoken as "one twenty over eighty."
- Hypertension refers to blood pressure that is abnormally high, whereas hypotension refers to blood pressure that is abnormally low.
- In children, the observed normal ranges are lower; in the elderly, they are often higher. Sex and race also influence blood pressure values.
- In the CT department, blood pressure is used as an indicator of acute problems. Therefore, technologists need only be concerned about measurements that fall outside of a relatively broad range of values considered "normal." For adults, the normal range of systolic pressure is 90 to 140 mm Hg, diastolic, 60 to 90 mm Hg. For children, the normal range of systolic pressure is 65 to 130 mm Hg, diastolic, 45 to 85 mm Hg.
- The technologist should take care to use a blood pressure cuff of the appropriate size (i.e., small cuffs for pediatric patients, larger cuffs for obese patients).

## REVIEW QUESTIONS

1. Regarding an order for a CT examination, all of the following statements are true EXCEPT:
   a. CT examinations can only be ordered by a physician.
   b. Before beginning any examination, the technologist must verify that the correct examination is planned by checking the clinician's order.
   c. In many facilities, clinician orders for CT examinations are transcribed by clerks; this process introduces the potential for transcription errors.
   d. Ideally, some patient screening should occur at the time the examination is scheduled.

2. Which of the following is NOT an acceptable method of verifying a patient's identity?
   a. Call the patient by the full name and then ask the patient to recite his or her birth date and year, so that it can be checked against the CT order.
   b. Use the patient's armband to check the patient's name and medical record number.
   c. Ask family members who accompany the patient to verify the patient's name and address and check that against the CT order.
   d. Use the sign on the door of the patient's room or ask the patient what hospital room they are assigned to.

3. Why is a patient questioned regarding whether he or she has a history of an overactive thyroid?
   a. To select the correct protocol
   b. To determine whether an iodinated contrast agent can be administered intravenously
   c. To help the radiologist diagnose a goiter
   d. To determine whether a female patient could be unknowingly pregnant

4. Blood urea nitrogen (BUN), serum creatinine, and eGFR provide information about a patient's
   a. thyroid function.
   b. kidney function.
   c. risk of allergy to iodinated contrast media.
   d. cardiac function.

5. For which of the following examinations is it common to check laboratory results for prothrombin time (PT), partial thromboplastin time (PTT), and platelet count?
   a. Coronary CT angiography
   b. Postmyelography CT studies
   c. CT-guided biopsy
   d. CT abdomen and pelvis

6. Which of the following is a TRUE statement regarding signed consent forms?
   a. In most states, a signed consent form is required before any CT examination.
   b. Once a patient signs a consent form, he or she can no longer file a malpractice claim.
   c. If written consent is required, it must be signed by the patient before the administration of any medication for pain relief or sedation.
   d. A signed consent form is not necessary for any CT examinations.

7. All of the following are true statements regarding patient restraints EXCEPT:
   a. The immobilizer must be easy to remove quickly if necessary.
   b. Patients are restrained primarily as a convenience for the technologist.
   c. If leg immobilizers are necessary, wrist immobilizers must also be applied.
   d. A doctor's order is necessary when a patient is to be restrained against his or her will.

8. Why is it important for the technologist to note the patient's breathing, skin coloration, and overall health before the examination begins?
   a. The technologist can accurately chart each of these factors on the patient's chart.
   b. It will help determine whether the patient is healthy enough to proceed with the study.
   c. If a patient has even a small problem in any of these areas, he or she will not be given IV contrast material.
   d. It will help the technologist notice signs should adverse effects occur during the scan process.

9. Which of the following is NOT considered one of the vital signs?
   a. Weight
   b. Pulse
   c. Respirations
   d. Blood pressure

10. Where is a pedal pulse felt?
    a. Behind the knee
    b. Along the dorsal aspect of the great toe or arch of the foot
    c. Anterior ankle
    d. Posterior ankle or top of the foot

11. What is the normal range for the respiratory rate of an adult?
    a. 14 to 20
    b. 21 to 26
    c. 26 to 30
    d. 30 to 34

12. The normal range of blood pressure in children is
    a. lower than that in adults.
    b. about the same as that in adults.
    c. about the same as that in the elderly.
    d. is twice that of either adults or the elderly.

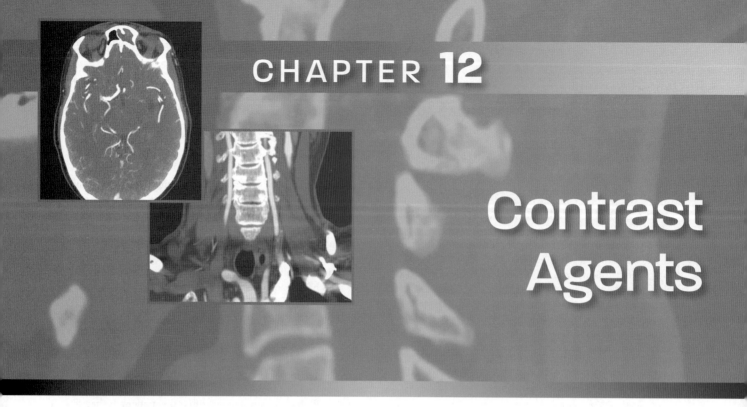

# CHAPTER 12

# Contrast Agents

To distinguish adjacent tissues on a CT image, the tissues must have different densities. These varying densities will result in distinct attenuation coefficients, which produce an image that clearly displays the different tissues.

An oral or intravenous administration of a contrast agent is often used to create a temporary, artificial density difference between objects. The goal is to make differing tissues readily visible on the image.

In CT, enhancement falls into the two main categories of intravascular and gastrointestinal. Less commonly, contrast agents can be administered intrathecally (i.e., in the subarachnoid space of the spinal cord), intraarticularly (directly into a joint space), intraperitoneally (into the abdominal peritoneal space), into a hollow organ via catheter (e.g., into the urinary tract via a percutaneous nephrostomy catheter or into the bladder via a Foley catheter), or into a drain to visualize the space being drained.

In all categories, contrast agents fill a structure with a material that has a different density than that of the structure.

In the case of most agents that contain barium and iodine, the material is of a higher density than the structure. These are typically referred to as positive agents.

Low-density contrast agents, or negative agents, such as air, can also be used.

## INTRAVASCULAR CONTRAST AGENTS

- Iodinated agents are universally used for a variety of radiology examinations because they are water soluble, easy to administer intravascularly, and have a high safety index.

## Properties of Iodinated Agents

- Radiographic contrast material increases the ability of the enhanced structure to attenuate the x-ray beam. The iodine atoms in the contrast material are responsible for this increase in attenuation. Iodine is particularly useful as a contrast agent because it has a relatively high atomic number (i.e., 53).
- The minimal visible detectable difference to identify normal versus pathologic tissue is 10 Hounsfield units (HU). Because different tissues often enhance differently, and because intravascular contrast material is handled differently in normal versus abnormal tissue, contrast agents can serve to widen the difference in attenuation. This difference often allows tissues, tumors, and disease processes to be more easily discernible.
- Contrast agent administration varies significantly from other pharmaceuticals that are administered intravascularly. Unlike other medications, iodinated agents are not used for their therapeutic qualities, but rather for their distribution and elimination from the body. The difference is even more dramatic when dose and delivery are considered. Therapeutic agents are given in very small quantities at regularly spaced intervals, whereas relatively large quantities of contrast media are typically given in a bolus lasting only a minute or two, with the intention of having no untoward physical effects.

### Osmolality

- Most intravascular drugs are nearly isotonic; that is, they have nearly the same number of particles in solution, per unit of liquid, as blood. Contrast agents may have up to seven times the number of particles in solution, per unit of liquid, as blood.

- The structural property of a liquid regarding the number of particles in solution, per unit of liquid, compared with blood is known as osmolality. Osmolality is measured in milliosmoles per kilogram (mOsm/kg) of water. The osmolality of blood plasma is approximately 290 mOsm/kg water.
- Most brands of iodinated contrast medium have a greater osmolality than does blood plasma. Therefore, most contrast agents are said to be hyperosmolar or hypertonic solutions.
- Older iodinated agents, now rarely used for intravascular injections in the United States, are considered high-osmolality contrast media (HOCM). The osmolality of these agents ranges from approximately 1,300 to 2,140 mOsm/kg.
- Contrast agents introduced in the 1980s contain much lower osmolality, from 600 to 850 mOsm/kg. Hence, these agents have been classified as low-osmolality contrast media (LOCM).
- Although the exact mechanisms of adverse reactions are still not completely understood, it is certain that the osmolality of the agent does play a role in contrast media safety.
- In 1996, a contrast agent (Visipaque, GE Healthcare) was introduced with an osmolality equal to that of blood. It is referred to as an isosmolar contrast media (IOCM). Its main benefit is reduced sensation of heat and pain compared to other agents when injected intra-arterially into peripheral arteries.
- Osmolality is universally recognized as playing a major role in nonallergic reactions to contrast medium.
  - A bolus injection of a hypertonic contrast agent causes a rapid increase in the osmolality of the plasma. Effects to the patient occur as the osmolality equalizes in the body, including mild dehydration.

## Viscosity

- Contrast material is much more viscous than most other intravascular agents.
- Viscosity is a physical property that may be described as the thickness or friction of the fluid as it flows.
- It is an important property that will influence the injectability of intravascular agents through small-bore needles and intravenous catheters.
- Molecular structure and concentration affect viscosity; therefore, different brands of iodinated contrast media will possess varying viscosities.
- The viscosity of the contrast material can be significantly decreased by heating the liquid to body temperature for injection.

- The concentration of iodine in the agent also affects its viscosity; the higher the concentration of iodine, the more viscous the solution.

## Ionicity

- Intravascular contrast agents can also be classified as to whether the molecules they contain will separate into charged particles (i.e., ions) when dissolved in an aqueous solution.
- Ionic contrast agents are composed of molecules that will dissociate into ions when in solution.
- The molecules contained in nonionic contrast media do not dissociate; the entire molecule remains intact as it passes through, and is excreted from, the body.
- Although most nonionic contrast agents also have low osmolality, the two terms are not synonymous.

## Clearance

- Once injected, all types of iodinated contrast media undergo very rapid distribution throughout the entire extracellular space. They are not metabolized and are excreted by the body nearly exclusively by the kidney. In patients with normal renal function, half of the dose is eliminated from the body in approximately 2 hours.

## Dose

- To accurately assess the dose of iodinated contrast agent to be delivered, both the iodine concentration and the volume must be considered.
- The beam attenuation abilities of contrast media are directly related to the concentration of iodine. Many concentrations are commercially available.
  - LOCM are measured in milligrams of iodine per milliliter (mgI/mL) of solution, whereas
  - HOCM are measured in percent weight per volume.
- When comparing doses between different contrast concentration and volumes, it is often useful to look at the total grams of iodine delivered.
- Different CT scan protocols require different doses of iodine. In some instances, the injection rate and the delay from injection to scanning will affect the contrast dose selected for the examination. In addition, the iodine concentration of the contrast may influence the selection of injection flow rate.
  - A concentration of 400 mg/mL injected at 3 mL/s will provide the same enhancement as a concentration of 300 mg/mL injected at 4 mL/s.
- Although it rarely occurs, an overdose of iodinated contrast media is possible. Because of the risk of overdose, most facilities set guidelines as to the upper limit on the total volume of contrast media

given for routine adult examinations, regardless of the patient's size. Individual factors, such as a patient's level of hydration, can influence what is a safe dose.

- The upper limit is often quite cautious, typically 200 mL of an agent with a concentration of 320 mgI/mL (a total of 64 g of iodine). It should be noted, however, that specific circumstances may necessitate exceeding this 200-mL guideline.

- Regardless of the type of iodinated contrast agent, the lowest dose necessary to obtain adequate visualization should be used. A lower dose may reduce the possibility of an adverse reaction, particularly those affecting renal function.

- In most clinical practices, the dose used to perform CT examinations on pediatric patients is calculated by weight. The most common formula used is 2 mL/kg.

- On adult patients, the dose is most often standardized to protocol and does not take patient weight into account. However, there may be some advantages in cost and image quality if weight-based dosing protocols are used for adult patients.

## Iodinated Contrast Media During Pregnancy and Lactation

### Pregnancy

- As a result of concerns about exposing the fetus to ionizing radiation, CT examinations using iodinated contrast medium are seldom done during pregnancy. Occasionally, such an examination may be vital for the mother's health. Effects of contrast medium on the human embryo or fetus are unknown. Laboratory and animal tests of HOCM and LOCM, respectively, found no mutagenic effects. Iodinated contrast media do cross the human placenta and enter the fetus.

- The ACR Committee on Drugs and Contrast Media recommends that all imaging facilities should screen patients so as to identify pregnant patients before the performance of any diagnostic examination involving ionizing radiation. If the patient is known to be pregnant, both the potential radiation risk and the potential added risks of contrast media should be considered before proceeding with the study. Although no risks to the fetus have been identified, there is insufficient evidence to be certain that contrast agents pose no risk. Consequently, the Committee recommends that when a patient is known to be pregnant, a radiologist should confer with the referring physician before proceeding with the CT examination.

### Lactation

- Little has been published regarding the excretion of iodinated contrast media into breast milk; however, some important facts are known.
  - Less than 1% of the dose of contrast agent given to the mother is excreted into breast milk. Moreover, less than 1% of the contrast medium in breast milk ingested by an infant is absorbed from the gastrointestinal tract.
  - Therefore, the expected dose of contrast medium absorbed by an infant from ingested breast milk is extremely low, and is just a small fraction (<1%) of the dose that would be given if the infant were to undergo an imaging study.

- Any potential risks to the infant are theoretical only; no adverse effects have been reported. Theoretical risks include allergic sensitization or reaction.

- The ACR recommends that breast-feeding mothers be given the opportunity to make an informed decision as to whether to continue or temporarily abstain from breast-feeding after receiving intravascularly administered iodinated contrast media. Because of the very small percentage of iodinated contrast medium that is excreted into the breast milk and absorbed by the infant's gut, it is believed to be safe for the mother and infant to continue breast-feeding. However, if the mother remains concerned about any potential ill effects to the infant, she may wish to abstain from breast-feeding for 24 hours.

## Adverse Effects of Iodinated Contrast Medium

- Fatal reactions are extremely rare in both HOCM and LOCM, estimated at 0.9 per 100,000 (<0.001%).

- However, adverse reactions sometimes occur and no methods exist that can accurately predict which patients will have an adverse reaction. The drugs and equipment needed to treat acute reactions must be readily available, and staff must be trained to respond quickly.

### Mechanism of Adverse Reactions

- The term "contrast reaction" can be confusing because it is used in a variety of different ways in relation to the effects of iodinated radiologic contrast agents.
  - In some instances, it is used to describe all undesired effects including the many subjective side effects experienced to some degree by most patients to whom contrast is administered. These subjective effects include the feeling of heat, nausea, and mild flushing.

- In other instances, the term contrast reaction is used to describe the less common, more serious side effects that may require treatment or even be life threatening.
- There is variation in the literature among quoted incidences of adverse reactions to contrast media. This is attributable to a number of reasons, but mainly because there is no standard definition of an adverse reaction or standard system to classify their severity.
- To simplify the discussion of adverse reactions to injectable contrast media, it is useful to separate reactions into two categories: chemotoxic reactions and idiosyncratic reactions. However, in clinical practice, it can be difficult to characterize some reactions into one group or the other.
- Chemotoxic reactions result from the physicochemical properties of the contrast media, the dose, and speed of injection. All hemodynamic (i.e., relating to blood circulation) disturbances and injuries to organs or vessels perfused by the contrast medium are included in this category. Contrast-induced nephropathy is an example of a chemotoxic reaction.
- Idiosyncratic reactions include all other reactions. These reactions are largely unpredictable, most often occur within 1 hour of contrast medium administration, and are not related to the dose. The mechanisms by which idiosyncratic reactions occur are not precisely understood.
  - The origin of these reactions is rarely, if ever, "an allergy." True allergic reactions result in the production of antibodies. These are not found after reactions to contrast media.
  - If the reaction were an allergy, it would be expected that patients would consistently suffer a similar or more severe adverse event with subsequent contrast injections. But researchers have not found this to be true; instead, the incidence of recurrent reactions appears to be relatively low, about 7% when LOCM are used.
  - Even though the underlying cause is likely different, symptoms of idiosyncratic reactions resemble allergic (or anaphylactic) reactions and are, therefore, often called "allergic-like" or "anaphylactoid" reactions.
- Children have a lower frequency of contrast reactions than do adults. When they do occur, they tend to be idiosyncratic in nature. Infants and young children are unable to verbalize discomfort or symptoms, posing additional challenges for the CT staff.
- Most adverse reactions occur within minutes of injection, but delayed reactions have also been reported. It is not clear whether delayed reactions are idiosyncratic or chemotoxic in nature. It is likely that both factors play a role; that is, some delayed reactions are idiopathic and others chemotoxic.

### Idiosyncratic Reactions

- Side effects of intravascular contrast media administration that are common, and can be expected to occur in many, if not most, patients are nausea, vomiting, altered taste (often described as metallic), perspiration, warmth, flushing, and anxiety.
  - These side effects are much less common when LOCM are used.
  - In the most common usage of the term, these effects are not considered a contrast reaction; they are generally of no clinical consequence. However, although they do not endanger the patient, some side effects (such as vomiting) may delay the start of scanning and thereby affect the quality of the examination.

### Classifications of Idiosyncratic Reactions

- Acute idiosyncratic reactions are usually characterized as mild, moderate, or severe.
- Although a mild reaction does not require treatment, the patient should be carefully monitored for at least 20 to 30 minutes, as symptoms of a mild reaction may become a more severe reaction.
  - Symptoms of a mild reaction are cough, itching, rash (hives), pallor, nasal stuffiness, minimal swelling in the eyes and face, and facial rash. Mild reactions are usually of short duration and self-limiting.
- Moderately adverse reactions are not immediately life threatening, although they may progress to be so.
  - Symptoms require treatment and include respiratory difficulties (bronchospasm, dyspnea, wheezing, mild laryngeal edema), pulse change, hypertension, and hypotension.
  - Treatment may include diphenhydramine (i.e., Benadryl) for symptomatic hives, leg elevation for hypotension, use of a β-agonist inhaler for bronchospasm, or epinephrine for laryngeal edema.
- Severe reactions are potentially or immediately life threatening.
  - Symptoms include substantial respiratory distress, unresponsiveness, convulsions, clinically manifested arrhythmias, and cardiopulmonary arrest. Although life-threatening reactions are rare, it is imperative that all technologists be aware that they can occur and that they require prompt recognition and treatment.
  - Most severe reactions occur soon after administration and can begin with any number of signs and symptoms, ranging from anxiety to diffuse erythema to cardiac arrest. Complete cardiovascular collapse requires prompt cardiopulmonary resuscitation, advanced specialized life-support equipment, and trained personnel.

- Although idiosyncratic contrast reactions are not truly anaphylactic in origin (because antibodies to contrast agents have not been demonstrated), the clinical presentation is often identical to that of acute anaphylaxis and the treatment is the same, that is to say, the "ABCs" (airway assessment, breathing, and circulation) followed by appropriate advanced cardiac life support (ACLS) treatment.

### Incidence and Risk Factors for Idiosyncratic Reactions

- The majority of idiosyncratic adverse side effects are mild, non–life-threatening events that require only observation, reassurance, and support.
- The reported rate of all types of reactions for HOCM is from 5% to 12%. Of those, 98% to 99% are classified as mild.
- Reported reactions from LOCM are much lower than from HOCM, by a factor of approximately four to five times.
- Because death from either HOCM or LOCM is very rare, it is difficult to accurately assess the mortality rate.
  - Some data suggest that there is no significant difference in mortality between the types of contrast agents, but other data suggest a lower mortality with LOCM.

### Previous Contrast Medium Reaction

- When considering the risk of subsequent contrast-enhanced examinations in patients who have had a previous reaction to contrast media, it is important to recall that contrast media reactions are not true allergic reactions, but are "allergic-like."
  - In a true drug allergy, the first time a medication is administered the immune system launches an incorrect response against a substance that is harmless in most people. The next time the medication is given the body produces antibodies and histamine. Although first-time exposure may only produce a mild reaction, repeated exposures may lead to more serious reactions. Once a person is sensitized (has had a previous reaction), even a very limited exposure to a very small amount of allergen can trigger a severe reaction. The recommendation is that individuals avoid medications that have caused an allergic reaction, even a mild one, in the past.
  - Idiosyncratic contrast reactions are not true allergies, and repeat administration does not carry the same certainty of a reaction as does repeat exposure to a true allergen.
  - Nonetheless, the reaction rate is higher among individuals who have had a previous reaction to contrast medium compared with those who have no history of a reaction.

- With HOCM, the risk of a reaction in a patient who reacted previously has been stated to be 16% to 35% and to be 11 times greater than the risk in a nonreactor. When a patient who previously reacted to a high-osmolality contrast medium is given a low-osmolality contrast medium, the risk of a repeat reaction is reduced to approximately 5%.
- So, although a previous contrast medium reaction is a poor predictor of subsequent reactions, it must still be considered because it is impossible to know which patients will react.
- Of the relative risks of a contrast reaction, a previous contrast reaction is considered to be the most important.

### Asthma

- Asthma is also considered a risk factor. Although there is some variation in the reported incidence, patients with asthma had approximately eight times the risk of reaction to HOCM, and about five times the risk of reaction to LOCM, when compared with the population of patients without asthma.

### Allergies

- A history of allergy to food, drugs, or other substances is associated with an increased risk of adverse reaction to contrast media. Allergic conditions such as hay fever and eczema are also associated with an increased risk of reaction. In most reports, these are less of a risk than is asthma; a twofold risk is commonly sited.
- A patient with a history of allergies to foods that contain iodine (e.g., seafood) is often of particular concern in the CT department. However, this worry is unfounded.
  - Seafood allergy results from hypersensitivity to a protein within the seafood and has no association with iodine.
  - Many years of data substantiate that allergy to seafood is no more significant than is allergy to other foods.
  - In addition, allergy to topical iodine skin preparations (e.g., Betadine) does not increase the risk of contrast medium reactions.

### Drugs

- There is speculation that patients taking β-blockers may be at increased risk for idiosyncratic contrast medium reactions, but this has not been proved. However, it is agreed that the use of β-blockers can impair the response to treatment, should a reaction occur.

### Prevention of Acute Idiosyncratic Reactions

- In patients identified as being at increased risk of adverse reaction to contrast medium, the possibility of performing the CT examination without the benefit of a contrast agent or using an alternative diagnostic method (e.g., ultrasonography, magnetic resonance imaging) should be considered.

- The technologist should bring all relevant information to the attention of a radiologist. If iodinated contrast medium is deemed essential, steps can be taken to reduce the associated risks.

■ Although the majority of severe reactions occur within the first 20 minutes after contrast medium injection, it is prudent to have high-risk patients remain monitored in the radiology department for 1 hour.

■ Idiosyncratic reactions are not dose dependent; reactions have resulted from very small volumes of iodinated contrast media.

- Test injections are of no predictive value and are not recommended.

Use LOCM

■ The most important method of reducing the risk of idiosyncratic contrast medium reaction is to use LOCM.

- The risk associated with these agents are four to five times lower than that of HOCM.
- Patients with a history of contrast reaction to HOCM and subsequently given LOCM had less incidence of adverse reaction than did patients without a history of allergy and given HOCM. Hence, the use of LOCM is now considered the standard of care for IV contrast media administration in CT departments.

Role of Premedication

■ There is good evidence that pretreatment with steroids will reduce the rate of idiosyncratic contrast medium reactions when HOCM are given.

■ When LOCM are used, there is less certainty that premedication with steroids is helpful in reducing moderate or severe adverse reactions.

- Some radiologists believe that steroid pretreatment in conjunction with LOCM is only effective in preventing minor reactions; others conclude that it is likely that moderate and severe reactions are reduced as well.

■ When the decision to premedicate is made by the radiologist, a variety of regimens can be used.

- When steroid premedication is used, it is important that the steroids be started at least 6 hours (but preferably 12 hours) before contrast medium administration.
- Prednisone and methylprednisolone are equally effective.
- If the patient is unable to take oral medication, 200 mg of hydrocortisone intravenously may be substituted for oral prednisone.
- In addition to the steroids, the administration of an $H_1$ antihistamine (e.g., diphenhydramine), given either orally or intravenously, may reduce

the frequency of urticaria, angioedema, and respiratory symptoms.

- When there has been a previous reaction to LOCM, the use of a different brand of LOCM has been recommended to lower the risk of a repeat adverse event.

Documentation

■ An adverse reaction to contrast medium administration must be documented. At a minimum, elements that must be captured are

- Amount and type of the contrast injected
- Signs and symptoms of the reaction
- Interventions or medications given during the reaction and the patient's response to treatment, and
- Final outcome (e.g., was the patient sent home or admitted to the hospital?)

### Chemotoxic Reactions

■ Contrast reactions that stem from the contrast agent's pharmacologic properties are broadly referred to as chemotoxic or physiologic. Like idiosyncratic reactions, the exact mechanism responsible for all types of chemotoxic reactions is not completely understood.

■ The types of chemotoxic reaction are variable, and the underlying etiologies are multifactorial.

### Contrast Media–Induced Nephropathy

■ It is well documented that intravascular iodinated contrast agents may affect kidney function in some patients.

■ Although newer research indicates that iodinated agents are responsible for far less nephropathy than previously thought, iodinated agents can result in significant nephrotoxic effects, particularly in patients who are considered to be at high risk for nephropathy.

■ Contrast media–induced nephropathy (CIN) has been reported to be the third leading cause of acute renal failure (ARF) in hospitalized patients, but this claim of high frequency of CIN has been strongly challenged. Although often treatable, ARF (whether caused by contrast media or something else) is a serious complication associated with high mortality.

■ LOCM are less nephrotoxic than are HOCM. IOCM may be even less nephrotoxic than LOCM, but research is not yet conclusive.

Renal Physiology

■ The kidneys play an essential role in maintaining homeostasis. It is not a static state, but rather the minute-to-minute state of balance of water, electrolytes (such as sodium, potassium, chloride, and bicarbonate), and pH.

- The kidneys represent approximately 0.5% of the total weight of the body, but receive 20% to 25% of the total arterial blood pumped by the heart.
- The basic functioning unit of the kidney is the nephron, a tube that is closed at one end and open at the other. Each kidney contains from one to two million nephrons. The nephron consists of Bowman capsule, glomerulus, proximal convoluted tubule, loop of Henle, distal convoluted tubule, and a collecting tubule. Each component provides a specialized function.
- The nephron produces urine by filtering out from the blood small molecules and ions and then reclaiming the needed amounts of useful materials. Surplus or waste molecules and ions are discarded as urine.
- The overall function of the kidney is often described as clearance, a reference to the ability of the kidney to remove a substance from the blood. Clearance is the volume of plasma that is cleared of a specific substance in a given time.
- It is difficult to use the clearance rate for a direct measure of kidney function as a result of the lack of a perfect compound to measure.
- One method of estimating kidney function is by calculating the glomerular filtration rate (GFR) and the effective renal plasma flow (ERPF). Although accurate, these methods are too cumbersome to use routinely.
- Measuring serum creatinine (SeCr) is a fast and inexpensive way to assess renal function. Creatinine is a by-product of muscle protein metabolism generated by the body at a fairly steady rate and excreted entirely in the urine. However, there are significant limitations in using SeCr as an accurate measure of renal function.
  - The amount of creatinine excreted in the urine is the composite of both the filtered and secreted creatinine. Because of this, creatinine clearance systematically overestimates GFR. In healthy people, this overestimation is relatively predictable, but is greater and less predictable in patients with chronic kidney failure.
  - Another limitation stems from the fact that the generation of creatinine is proportional to total muscle mass. This leads to differences in SeCr according to sex, age, and race, even after adjusting for GFR. Muscle wasting (often from malnourishment) produces a lower SeCr than expected for the level of GFR. Creatinine generation can also be affected by the consumption of cooked meat. Therefore, SeCr is lower than expected for the level of GFR in patients following a low-protein diet.
  - Numerous formulas have been developed that incorporate factors such as patient age, weight,

and height with the reported SeCr level. These have been proved to provide a reasonably accurate estimate of GFR.
  - Despite its drawbacks, SeCr is a good reflection of any major drug-induced fluctuation in GFR and remains a useful clinical tool in assessing kidney function.
- Calculated estimated glomerular filtration rate (eGFR) is more accurate than is serum creatinine at predicting true GFR. As a result, eGFR is gaining attention as a potentially better marker of CIN risk. However, the formula for estimating GFR rely in part on serum creatinine, and therefore are subject to some of the limitations listed above. In addition, because serum creatinine levels lag behind changes in renal function, eGFR is only applicable to stable levels of renal dysfunction.
- The inability of the kidney to maintain homeostasis can result in the accumulation of nitrogenous wastes and is referred to as *renal failure*. The exact biochemical or clinical criteria for a diagnosis of renal failure are not clearly defined.
- The term renal failure is distinguished from *renal insufficiency*, in which renal function is abnormal but capable of sustaining essential bodily function.
- The term *nephropathy* technically denotes any condition or disease affecting the kidney; however, it is sometimes used synonymously with renal impairment.
- Postcontrast acute kidney injury (PC-AKI) is a general term used to describe a sudden deterioration in renal function that occurs within 48 hours following the intravascular administration of iodinated contrast media.
- CIN is a specific term used to describe a sudden deterioration in acute impairment of renal function subsequent to the intravascular administration of contrast material (for which alternative causes have been excluded).
  - Characteristically, the presentation of CIN is an acute, progressive rise in SeCr within 24 hours of contrast administration, although this elevation may take up to 48 hours. The SeCr level generally peaks at 4 to 5 days and then begins to return toward baseline within 7 to 10 days.
  - In most cases, CIN is reversible.
  - To make the diagnosis of CIN, alternative causes must be eliminated. This is an important step because there are many causes (more than 50) that can trigger the pathophysiologic mechanisms that lead to ARF.

CIN Incidence and Risk Factors
- In the random population undergoing contrast-enhanced imaging, the incidence of CIN is low, historically thought to be between 1% and 6% although these percentages have been criticized

as too high. However, a number of factors, such as renal impairment and diabetes, place patients at a higher risk of CIN. Identifying patients at higher risk of developing CIN and intervening with preventive measures may diminish their risk of CIN.

- Most patients who have CIN suffer little morbidity and recover to near-baseline renal function within 7 to 10 days.
- Some patients require temporary dialysis. Even more worrisome, in rare patients, CIN precipitates the need for chronic dialysis.
- The development of CIN appears to increase the risk of death from nonrenal causes such as sepsis, bleeding, respiratory failure, and delirium.
- There is a cumulative effect of multiple risk factors in increasing the risk of CIN.
- Preexisting renal insufficiency is a significant risk factor for CIN.
- Diabetes mellitus is considered a risk factor for CIN. Diabetic patients with normal renal function are probably not at a significantly increased risk of CIN. However, there is a strong association between diabetes mellitus with preexisting renal dysfunction and CIN.
- In summary, although patients with diabetes and normal renal function should be evaluated carefully, most appear to be at fairly low risk for experiencing CIN. However, patients with diabetes mellitus and preexisting renal insufficiency represent a group with an extremely high risk of experiencing CIN.
- There is a direct correlation between the volume of contrast administered and the risk of CIN. Therefore, procedures that require a higher volume of contrast material place a patient at higher risk.
- Patients who are dehydrated before the imaging examination have an increased risk of CIN.
  - Although multiple myeloma has traditionally been regarded as a risk factor for CIN, many researchers now believe that the risk is primarily related to the dehydration of the multiple myeloma patient.

Prevention of CIN in High-Risk Patients
- Use LOCM or IOCM
- Hydration
- Use the smallest amount of contrast agent possible
- Allow at least 48 hours to elapse between procedures in which contrast material is used to allow the kidneys to recover
- Consider temporarily discontinuing other medications that are known to be nephrotoxic

Metformin Therapy
- Metformin is an oral medication given to non–insulin-dependent diabetics to lower blood sugar.

- Metformin is available as a generic drug; it is also sold under a variety of brand names (e.g., Glucophage, Riomet, Fortamet, Glumetza, Diabex, Diaformin).
- Metformin is also available in combination with other drugs (e.g., Avandamet, ActoplusMet, Metaglip, Glucovance).
- The most serious adverse effect of metformin therapy is the potential for the development of lactic acidosis in susceptible patients. Although the incidence of metformin-associated lactic acidosis is very low (<1 case per 10,000 patient-years), when it does occur it is fatal in about 50% of patients. Metformin is excreted primarily by the kidneys; any factors that decrease metformin excretion are risk factors for lactic acidosis. Therefore, renal insufficiency is a risk factor.
- For patients with an eGFR less than 60, it is recommended that metformin be temporarily discontinued after any examination involving iodinated contrast. Metformin therapy can be resumed after 2 days, assuming kidney function is normal.
- Iodinated contrast media does not cause lactic acidosis. Nor does metformin cause renal impairment. Rather, when renal dysfunction occurs in patients taking metformin, the drug can accumulate and result in lactic acidosis.

Dialysis and Contrast Media
- Patients may be started on dialysis after an episode of acute renal failure, with the hope that their kidneys will recover sufficiently so that dialysis can be discontinued. In these situations, the conventional wisdom is that iodinated contrast media should not be given. The aim is to avoid any risk of further renal insult that could diminish residual renal function and result in the renal failure becoming chronic with the need for ongoing hemodialysis.
- In patients with end-stage renal failure, it is not expected that renal function will return. Therefore, contrast-enhanced CT examinations are often performed with the recognition that the kidneys cannot be damaged further. Patients with end-stage renal failure typically receive hemodialysis three times per week; therefore, the contrast media can remain in the blood for prolonged periods. It is not necessary to coordinate the patient's schedule so that dialysis is performed immediately after the administration of contrast media.
- The half-life of iodinated contrast media in patients with normal renal function is approximately 2 hours, but in patients with severe renal dysfunction, it can be extended to more than 30 hours depending on the extent of the renal impairment.
- Contrast media can be efficiently removed from the blood by hemodialysis.

■ Peritoneal dialysis is also effective in removing contrast agents from the body, but takes longer.

### Other Organ- or System-Specific Adverse Effects
Effects on Thyroid Function

■ In the absence of thyroid disease, the administration of iodinated contrast agents will have no significant impact on thyroid function.

● In patients with hypothyroidism, particularly those with autoimmune (Hashimoto) thyroiditis, there may be a small, temporary reduction in thyroid function, which does not require additional treatment.

● In patients with a history of hyperthyroidism, iodinated contrast media can intensify thyrotoxicosis (excessive thyroid hormone). In rare cases, iodinated contrast media can precipitate a thyroid storm (or thyrotoxic crisis), which is a severe, life-threatening condition resulting when thyroid hormone reaches a dangerously high level.

● Hyperthyroidism is not a common condition in the United States; it is seen much less frequently than hypothyroidism. Nonetheless, patients should be questioned as to their thyroid status before the administration of an iodinated contrast agent. When a patient with a history of hyperthyroidism is identified, this fact should be brought to the attention of the radiologist before proceeding with the examination. If the examination is performed, the patient may be instructed to see their endocrinologist for monitoring.

● Iodinated contrast material can interfere with the results of a radioactive thyroid uptake study performed in the nuclear medicine department. Therefore, CT studies that use iodinated contrast material should not be scheduled sooner than 2 weeks before the nuclear medicine thyroid study.

Pulmonary Effects

■ Several potential pulmonary adverse effects have been documented after the IV administration of iodinated contrast agents. These include bronchospasm, pulmonary arterial hypertension, and pulmonary edema. Patients with a history of pulmonary hypertension, bronchial asthma, or heart failure are at increased risk.

Central Nervous System

■ The blood-brain barrier (BBB) is a semipermeable structure that protects the brain from most substances in the blood, although still allowing essential metabolic function. Iodinated contrast agents will not cross an intact BBB.

■ The use of iodinated contrast media has been shown to provoke seizures in patients who have diseases that disrupt the BBB. For unknown reasons, the risk of seizures after contrast administration is greater for patients with metastasis to the brain than those with primary brain tumors, although both tumors disrupt the BBB.

■ The risk of seizure can be substantially reduced by a one-time oral dose of 5 to 10 mg of diazepam (i.e., Valium), 30 minutes before contrast administration.

■ Seizures can also be controlled with diazepam.

Contrast Extravasation

■ Because of the routine use of IV contrast material in the CT department, extravasation of contrast medium into the subcutaneous tissue sometimes occurs. The prevention and management of extravasated iodinated contrast media is discussed in Chapter 13.

### Delayed Reactions

■ Delayed reactions to intravascular iodinated contrast media are defined as reactions occurring between 1 hour and 1 week after contrast medium injection.

■ Accurate statistics regarding late reactions are inherently difficult to collect, because as the time interval increases between the contrast medium injection and the onset of symptoms, so does the difficulty of being certain that the symptoms are directly related to the contrast medium.

■ Although the exact rate is not known, it is certain that delayed reactions do sometimes occur.

● Skin reactions appear to account for the majority of true late reactions. Most are minor and last only a short time, but severe reactions can occur. Types of late skin reactions include maculopapular rash (red spots or bumps), angioedema (weltlike swelling), and urticaria (hives). In general, there is no relationship between the volume of contrast administered and the frequency or severity of delayed cutaneous events.

● Less frequently reported, iodide "mumps" (salivary gland swelling) and a syndrome of acute polyarthropathy (pain in multiple joints) are other possible delayed reactions. These can occur after either HOCM or LOCM and may be more frequent in patients with renal dysfunction.

● Patients who are receiving or have received interleukin-2 can have delayed reactions after the administration of contrast media. Interleukin-2 (brand name Proleukin, Chiron Corporation) is an immunotherapy used to treat some cancers. After the administration of iodinated contrast media, patients may experience symptoms that recall the side effects of the interleukin-2 therapy, such as fever, nausea, vomiting, diarrhea, itching, and rash.

■ Like other types of reactions, delayed reactions occur less frequently with LOCM. The exact nature of delayed reactions is unclear; it is likely that some can be attributed to chemotoxicity, whereas others are idiosyncratic in nature. Unlike other contrast-related adverse events, there is some evidence that suggests that delayed cutaneous reaction may be immune mediated (stemming from a true allergy or an autoimmune response).

## GASTROINTESTINAL CONTRAST MEDIUM

■ In the gastrointestinal tract, contrast medium is essential to distinguish loops of bowel from a cyst, abscess, or neoplasm. For this reason, oral contrast material is used in most CT scans of the abdomen and pelvis. For some indications, the rectal administration of contrast material is useful.

■ In general, contrast media is classified as positive if it appears bright on the image, and negative if it appears dark on the image.

■ The most common definition classifies gastrointestinal agents as positive or negative depending on the density of the material relative to the walls of the gastrointestinal tract.

● Using this definition, water is a negative agent, because with an HU of 0, it is less dense than the wall of the gastrointestinal tract.

■ Less commonly, contrast media is classified in accordance to its HU.

● Agents with positive HU values are considered positive agents; those with negative HU values are called negative agents. Using this definition, water is considered a neutral agent.

■ Options for the gastrointestinal tract available in oral preparations include barium sulfate solutions or iodinated water-soluble agents. Options available for rectal preparations include air, carbon dioxide, barium sulfate, or iodinated water-soluble solutions.

■ The ideal agent should provide adequate differentiation of bowel from surrounding structures without creating artifacts.

### Barium Sulfate Solutions

■ Conventional radiography barium suspensions cannot be used in CT because they would produce unacceptable streak artifacts. Products are available specifically for use in CT.

● The most commonly used are positive agents that contain a 1% to 3% barium sulfate suspension and are specially formulated to resist settling.

■ A higher dose of oral contrast material provides greater bowel opacification. Timing and dose are largely dependent on the area to be opacified.

■ In patients who cannot take fluids by mouth, a nasogastric tube may be inserted. The contrast medium can be introduced through the tube.

■ The typical low-concentration, low-viscosity barium sulfate solutions may not be adequate for an esophageal study. In such cases, the high-viscosity, low-concentration pastes designed for this purpose are recommended.

■ One disadvantage of positive contrast media is that they make mucosal surfaces more difficult to evaluate after IV administration of contrast material. Another problem is that the density of positive contrast material may create streak artifacts or impede three-dimensional modeling.

● A low-HU oral barium sulfate suspension (VoLumen, E Z EM) was developed to overcome these difficulties. With just 0.1% barium sulfate, the agent resembles water on CT but provides improved distention (as compared with water), faster transit than positive barium sulfate solutions, and more effective visualization of both the bowel wall and the mucosa. On CT images, VoLumen measures from 15 to 30 HU, a density lower than the wall of the GI tract. Hence, it is most often considered a negative agent as defined by attenuation compared with the bowel wall, but by some definitions it is called a neutral agent.

■ Barium sulfate should not be given if perforation of the gastrointestinal tract is suspected. Barium leaking into the peritoneal cavity can result in inflammation of the peritoneum that is referred to as barium peritonitis. The mortality rate from this complication is significant. It can be prevented by substituting a water-soluble iodinated oral contrast agent whenever perforation is suspected.

■ Barium sulfate is an inert substance that passes through the gastrointestinal tract basically unchanged. Allergic reactions to oral barium sulfate solutions are rare (approximately 1 in 500,000) and are usually attributed to the additives, such as flavorings.

■ Although procedural complications are rare, they include aspiration pneumonitis, barium impaction, and intravasation.

■ Fewer complications from aspiration appear to occur with barium sulfate than with high-osmolality iodinated agents.

### Iodinated Agents

■ Both HOCM and LOCM are positive agents that can be diluted and administered orally. Because of the unpleasant taste of HOCM, flavoring is normally added to the solution.

- A 2% to 5% solution of a water-soluble agent is normally used.
- Given orally, iodinated contrast agents usually stimulate intestinal peristalsis. Therefore, patients may experience diarrhea.
- Dosages are similar to those used with barium sulfate. However, water-soluble oral contrast material tends to pass through the gastrointestinal tract slightly faster.

■ In most situations, HOCM is used for oral administration because they are less expensive than LOCM and provide equivalent gastrointestinal opacification.

- In selective cases, LOCM have advantages over HOCM that justify their increased expense. If aspirated, LOCM cause less pulmonary edema than do HOCM.
- LOCM should be used in infants and young children under the following conditions: 1) when the possibility of entry of contrast agent into the lung exists; or 2) when the possibility of leaking of contrast agent from the gastrointestinal tract exists.
- Another advantage is that LOCM has a neutral taste when diluted, so patient cooperation is often greater.

■ When rectosigmoid abnormality is suspected, rectal administration of contrast material may be necessary. In these cases, 150 to 200 mL of dilute water-soluble agent (1%–3%) can be given by enema.

### Comparison of Positive Oral Contrast Agents

■ Barium sulfate and water-soluble contrast material cause comparable bowel opacification.

■ Because of the low concentrations used, neither coats the mucosa significantly. Instead, most visible contrast is attributed to the agents filling the bowel. Barium sulfate, in small amounts, tends to cling to the intestinal wall, providing a minimum of visible contrast. In comparison, a small quantity of water-soluble oral contrast is usually absorbed by the bowel.

## Water

■ Water is sometimes used in place of positive contrast agents. As a negative (or neutral) agent, water will not obscure mucosal surfaces or superimpose abdominal vessels on 3D images. However, water transits quite rapidly and distends the bowel poorly. It will not provide sufficient detail if the bowel is not fully distended.

## Air and Carbon Dioxide

■ Room air or carbon dioxide can be used to produce a very high negative contrast on images of the gastrointestinal tract.

■ Negative contrast agents are particularly useful in CT colonography in which adequate colonic distention is critical for effective polyp detection. Poorly distended segments of bowel may also be mistaken for carcinoma.

■ Room air or carbon dioxide is administered via a small flexible rectal catheter.

- Room air is delivered using a standard handheld air bulb insufflator. This air bulb can be controlled by either the patient or the CT technologist.
- Carbon dioxide is delivered using an automated insufflation system.

■ Both room air and automated carbon dioxide provide reliable colonic distention and produce only slight postprocedure discomfort.

■ However, carbon dioxide has some advantages over room air in that it is readily absorbed by the body and is eliminated by respiration. It induces less spastic response of the bowel wall and is therefore better tolerated by most patients.

■ The antispasmodic medication, glucagon hydrochloride, is sometimes given by intravenous injection to further improve bowel distention.

## INTRATHECAL CONTRAST ADMINISTRATION

■ Although rarely performed in the CT department, contrast media can be injected into the intrathecal space surrounding the spinal cord.

■ Only certain iodinated contrast media can be safely used intrathecally. Serious adverse reactions have been reported as a result of the inadvertent intrathecal administration of iodinated contrast media that are not indicated for intrathecal use.

■ Patients are frequently sent to the CT department for a postmyelogram CT while the contrast agent is still in the intrathecal space. Therefore, the contrast agent is injected before the patient arrives for the CT study.

■ To reduce the incidence of headache, keep the patient's head elevated (approximately 30°). The CT examination is typically done from 1 to 3 hours after the intrathecal injection. If the examination is done too soon, the contrast material may be too dense and generate streak artifacts.

■ Rolling the patient once or twice before scanning is recommended to mix the contrast material that may have settled since the myelogram.

## Intraarticular Contrast

- Contrast media can be injected directly into a joint space to better visualize the soft tissue structures of the joint.
- Arthrography can be performed with fluoroscopy in the general radiography department, or more commonly, in magnetic resonance. However, CT arthrography has the advantage of allowing the simultaneous evaluation of bone and soft tissue.
- Intraarticular contrast injections are performed by the radiologist, most often under fluoroscopic guidance. Once the contrast has been injected into the joint space, the patient is transported to the CT department.

## Intravesical Contrast

Contrast media can be used to opacify the bladder for a CT cystogram. Contrast media is diluted to avoid streak artifact. 350 mL of the dilute solution is instilled via urinary catheter or until the bag stops dripping.

### REVIEW QUESTIONS

1. To distinguish adjacent tissues on a CT image, the tissues must
   a. have different densities.
   b. have different functions.
   c. have sharply defined edges.
   d. be abnormal.
2. A contrast material that is of a substantially higher density than that of the surrounding structures can be referred to as a _____ agent.
   a. low-attenuation
   b. positive
   c. negative
   d. gastrointestinal
3. The structural property of a contrast agent regarding the number of particles in solution compared with blood is known as
   a. ionicity.
   b. osmolality.
   c. valence.
   d. viscosity.
4. The intravenous infusion of HOCM may result in
   a. a sharp drop in blood sugar.
   b. severe fetal abnormalities if given to a pregnant woman.
   c. dehydration.
   d. a sensitivity to seafood.
5. Which factors affect the viscosity of an intravenous iodinated contrast agent?
   1. Iodine concentration
   2. Lipid solubility
   3. Total volume delivered
   4. Temperature of the agent
   a. 1 and 2
   b. 2 and 3
   c. 1 and 4
   d. 1, 3, and 4

6. An imaging center's protocol for a routine body CT on an adult patient calls for the administration of 100 mL of a low-osmolality contrast medium with a concentration of 320 mgI/mL. A particular patient has very poor veins, necessitating venipuncture with a smaller-than-recommended caliber of indwelling catheter. Concerns about the precarious venous access have resulted in the decision to use a lower concentration (less viscous) contrast agent. What volume of a low-osmolality contrast medium with a concentration of 240 mgI/mL will deliver an equivalent amount of iodine to that of the dose called for in the protocol?
   a. 84 mL
   b. 100 mL
   c. 125 mL
   d. 133 mL
7. Why is there such a wide variation in the literature among quoted incidences of adverse reactions to contrast media?
   a. There is no standard definition of adverse reactions or standard system to classify their severity.
   b. Adverse reactions are not reported because of fears about possible litigation.
   c. Adverse reactions are so rare that statistics are difficult to collect.
   d. The pharmaceutical companies that produce contrast agents do not allow statistics regarding the incidence of adverse reactions to be published.
8. Which is an example of a chemotoxic reaction to intravascular contrast media?
   a. Hives
   b. Contrast-induced nephropathy
   c. Coughing
   d. Nasal stuffiness
9. Contrast reactions that are accompanied by a temporary drop in blood pressure, bronchospasms, facial edema, urticaria, and laryngeal edema are generally classified as
   a. side effects.
   b. minor reactions.
   c. moderate reactions.
   d. severe reactions.
10. Comparing the reported rate of adverse reaction,
    a. LOCM are somewhat lower than HOCM, by a factor of approximately two times.
    b. LOCM are much lower than HOCM, by a factor of approximately four to five times.
    c. LOCM and HOCM have similar reaction rates, but LOCM reactions are less severe.
    d. some data suggest a lower mortality rate with HOCM.
11. When a patient who previously reacted to HOCM is given LOCM for a subsequent study, the risk of a repeat reaction is approximately
    a. 5%.
    b. 40%.
    c. 80%.
    d. 95%.
12. What is the single best method of reducing the risk of idiosyncratic contrast medium reaction?
    a. Premedicate the patient with steroids.
    b. Use LOCM.
    c. Reduce the dose.
    d. Perform a test injection.

13. The basic functioning unit of the kidney is the
    a. cortex.
    b. nephron.
    c. medulla.
    d. collecting tubule.
14. Which statement is true concerning the use of serum creatinine (SeCr) to assess renal function?
    a. SeCr is a highly accurate measure of renal function.
    b. SeCr uniformly overestimates the glomerular filtration rate; therefore, the values can be easily adjusted for an accurate measure of renal function.
    c. Measuring SeCr is a fast and inexpensive way to estimate renal function.
    d. SeCr values are not affected by patient demographics.
15. Which of the following are considered at high risk for developing CIN?
    a. Patients older than 65 years of age
    b. Male patients with a history of atherosclerotic disease
    c. Patients with diabetes mellitus and preexisting renal insufficiency
    d. Patients with a history of renal calculi
16. Which is a TRUE statement regarding the risks posed by intravascular contrast media in combination with the drug metformin?
    a. Iodinated contrast media can cause lactic acidosis, which is only dangerous if the patient is also taking metformin.
    b. Metformin causes renal impairment, exacerbating the risk of CIN.
    c. Iodinated contrast media in combination with metformin will result in acute (and, in some instances, chronic) renal failure requiring dialysis.
    d. When renal dysfunction occurs in patients taking metformin, the drug can accumulate and result in lactic acidosis.
17. After the injection of an iodinated contrast medium, patients with brain metastasis have an increased risk of
    a. seizures.
    b. dehydration.
    c. anaphylactoid reaction.
    d. renal failure.
18. What is the most common type of delayed reaction to intravascular contrast medium?
    a. Fever
    b. Headache
    c. Skin reactions
    d. Salivary gland swelling
19. Barium leaking into the peritoneal cavity is referred to as
    a. barium peritonitis.
    b. barium impaction.
    c. aspiration pneumonitis.
    d. barium obstruction.
20. Given **orally**, compare LOCM with HOCM.
    a. LOCM offer no advantage and are much more expensive.
    b. LOCM offer a clear advantage in all patients.
    c. LOCM have not been approved for oral administration.
    d. In some instances, particularly with infants, LOCM may provide significant advantages over the HOCM agents.

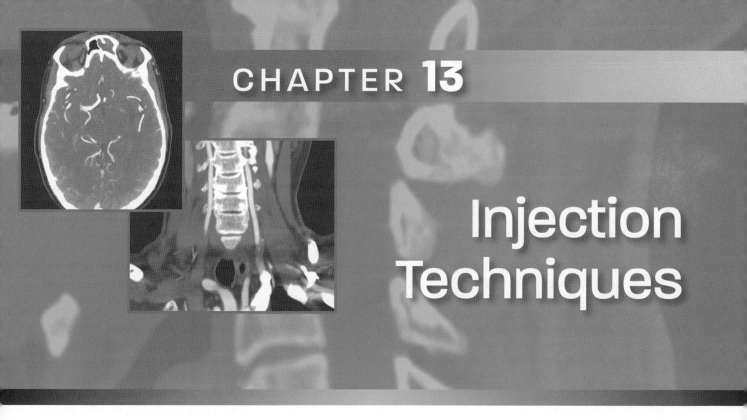

# CHAPTER 13

# Injection Techniques

Many factors must be taken into account when selecting the injection parameters to be used for a specific intravenous contrast-enhanced CT examination. Injection techniques will vary depending on the vascular access available, the type of examination, and the specific clinical indications for the examination. These factors will determine whether the injection will be performed by hand or with the use of a mechanical injector. They will also influence the contrast volume and concentration used, the flow rate at which the contrast will be injected, the delay between injection and scanning, and whether a saline flush is advantageous. This chapter examines issues surrounding the intravascular injection of iodinated contrast medium for CT examinations.

- Subject to the requirements of state law, a radiologist, radiologic technologist, or nurse may administer contrast media.
- The American College of Radiology (ACR) approves of the injection of contrast material by certified or licensed radiologic technologists and radiologic nurses under the direction of a radiologist or his or her physician designee who is personally and immediately available, if the practice is in compliance with institutional and state regulations.

## VASCULAR ACCESS

- Stable intravenous (IV) access is necessary for contrast media administration. In many instances, the IV line must be placed while the patient is in the CT department. In other instances, patients arrive in the CT department with IV access.

- In addition to standard indwelling peripheral catheters (e.g., BD Angiocath, BD Medical, Franklin Lakes, NJ), patients may arrive with central venous access devices (CVADs).
- Although CVADs are not optimal for contrast administration, in some cases, they are the only option available. Therefore, CT technologists must have a working knowledge of the different types of CVADs, including when and how they can be used to administer iodinated contrast media.

## Starting a Peripheral Intravenous Line

- Starting an IV line requires a venipuncture technique, in which a needle is inserted into a vein.
- Before beginning the process, the basic consent of the patient is obtained by explaining the procedure and asking whether the patient consents.
- Sterile technique must be observed for all intravenous procedures.
- For the protection of the patient and the healthcare worker, universal precautions must be strictly adhered to.
- An indwelling catheter set with a flexible plastic cannula should be used whenever a mechanical injector will be used for contrast media injection. The use of metal needles (i.e., butterfly infusion sets or straight needles) should be avoided.
- Steps to venipuncture include the following:
  - Assemble needed supplies.
  - Choose the gauge of the IV indwelling catheter. The anticipated flow rate of the contrast injection should be appropriate for the gauge of the

catheter used. Although 22-guage catheters may be able to tolerate flow rates up to 5 mL/s, a 20-gauge or larger catheter is preferable for flow rates of 3 mL/s or higher.

- Verify the patient's identity, explain the procedure, and answer any questions the patient may have.
- Choose the site. An antecubital or large forearm vein is the preferred venous access site when a mechanical injector is used. However, if the patient will be required to lift the arms for scanning, it is important that the patient is able to keep the arm somewhat straight while above the head. Bending at the IV site may kink the IV line and cause it to fail during the injection of contrast media. If a more peripheral site, such as the hand or wrist, is used, it may be necessary to limit the flow rate to 2.0 mL/s or less.
- Place the needle.
  - Apply a tourniquet 1 to 2 inches proximal to the chosen site.
  - Wearing gloves, prepare the area selected for puncture with antiseptic solution.
  - Puncture the skin. As soon as the needle enters the vein, blood will enter the flashback visualization chamber. Advance the catheter hub slightly away from the needle hub and release the tourniquet set. Continue to advance just the catheter hub three-quarters of the way over the needle, but not completely off of the needle.
  - Place a piece of gauze under the end of the catheter to absorb any small volume of blood that might be lost. Hold direct pressure just proximal to the insertion site, release the needle from the catheter (setting the needle in plain sight), and attach the saline-filled syringe or connector to the catheter hub. After flushing the IV with the saline to demonstrate the patency of the IV line, cover the site (except the end of the connector) with sterile covering. If there was difficulty in threading the catheter through the vein, try to continue threading the catheter while flushing with saline. This procedure often allows the catheter to pass along the inside lumen without further difficulty.
- Secure the connector to the arm with tape. Secure any extension tubing to the arm with tape.
- Properly dispose of the needle.

## MANAGING PATIENTS WITH EXISTING VASCULAR ACCESS

- If the patient arrives in the CT department with an existing indwelling peripheral venous catheter, it must be carefully evaluated before it can be used to administer a contrast agent.

- An ideal IV access site for administering contrast media is well located; was established in the past 1 or 2 days; contains a connecting hub or port that is not yet accessed, or if it is accessed has a saline (0.9% sodium chloride) or a solution of 5% dextrose in water (D5W) running; and does not show evidence of redness, blanching, or swelling in the skin surrounding the puncture site.
- Before injecting contrast media, ensure the patency of the line by flushing with a small amount of saline solution.
- Contrast media should not be mixed with, or injected in, IV administration lines containing other drugs or total nutritional admixtures.
  - If medications are being given through the port at the time of the examination, an additional bag of saline can be hung (i.e., "piggybacked") and connected to an open port on the existing IV tubing.
  - Existing medications should be turned off only long enough to complete the contrast injection. The line should be flushed with saline before the contrast injection. Once completed, the line should once again be flushed with saline solution before medications are restarted. It is important to restart the patient's medication at the identical preexamination rate.

## Using a Central Venous Access Device

- A CVAD is a venous catheter designed to deliver medications and fluids directly into the superior vena cava (SVC), inferior vena cava (IVC), or right atrium (RA).
- Compared with a standard indwelling catheter, a CVAD is more durable and does not become as easily blocked or infected.
- There are several kinds of CVADs. They may contain one, two, or three lumens. Each lumen is an independent catheter port so there is no mixing of injected medications.
- Catheters may have an open end or closed end. Open-ended peripherally inserted central catheters (PICCs) must be clamped when not in use. Many manufacturers recommend that between uses they be flushed with a heparinized saline flush to maintain the catheter's patency. Closed-end catheters contain a valve that controls fluid flow and prevents reflux of blood into the catheter. Closed-end catheters require only a saline flush to maintain patency.

### Peripherally Inserted Central Catheters

- A PICC is a long catheter that is inserted through the large veins of the upper arm (i.e., cephalic and basilic veins) and advanced so that its tip is located in the lower third of the SVC.

- PICCs are intended to provide central venous access for several weeks, but can remain in place as long as several months. They can be either single or double lumen.
- A midline catheter is a similar, but considerably shorter, version that is placed so that it terminates in the upper arm near the axilla. Because midline catheters do not extend into the large central vein, they are considered peripheral, not central catheters.
- The external appearance of a midline catheter is often difficult to distinguish from a PICC. The type of catheter should be noted in the patient's chart.
- Many PICC lines cannot tolerate the pressure required to inject contrast media (which are more viscous than most intravenously administered medications) at the high injection rates typical of CT examinations that use mechanical injectors. In these cases, it is recommended that a separate IV be inserted for the administration of contrast media.
- When no other options exist and the PICC must be used for contrast injection, the injection rate must be slowed and the injection should be performed by hand bolus rather than by mechanical injector.
- In recent years, specific PICC lines have been designed to withstand up to 300 psi–more than enough for power injectors. Many manufacturers produce these special PICC lines in colors that make them readily distinguishable from the traditional PICC lines.
- The practice for flushing PICCs after contrast administration is variable among facilities. To maintain patency of the PICC and decrease the potential for occlusion, PICCs are typically flushed with normal saline, heparinized saline, or a combination of both.
- A popular method for PICCs and other CVADs is the SASH method: saline flush, administer medication or draw blood, saline flush, heparinized saline flush. Technologists should assure that they are administering a premixed heparin flush solution and not concentrated heparin sodium injection; the latter could result in serious hemorrhagic complications for the patient.
  - However, practice will be different if the PICC contains a Luer-activated device. The Luer-activated device is a saline-only device and does not require flushing with heparinized saline after infusion.
  - Technologists should become familiar with their facility's written policy regarding PICC lines.

### Nontunneled and Tunneled Central Venous Catheters

- Central venous catheters (CVCs) are catheters with tips in the central venous system; they differ from PICCs in having a larger caliber because they are designed to be inserted into a relatively large, more central vein such as the subclavian or jugular. The peripheral end of a CVC may be an external bug in a nontunneled or tunneled CVC, or may be a subcutaneously implanted port. Nontunneled catheters usually have three ports, are open ended, and typically remain in place for a few days to 2 weeks.
- Tunneled CVCs are inserted into the target vein (often the subclavian) by "tunneling" under the skin. This reduces the risk of infection, because bacteria from the skin surface are not able to travel directly into the vein. Examples of tunneled catheters include Hickman, Broviac, and Groshong catheters. The tunneled catheter is the best choice when access to the vein is needed for long periods and when the line will be used many times each day. It is secure and easy to access.
- Implantable ports consist of a single- or double-lumen reservoir attached to a catheter. The reservoir hub is implanted in the arm or chest subcutaneous tissue, and the catheter is tunneled to the accessed vein. The port is accessed by use of a special noncoring hooked needle. Accessing and deaccessing an implanted port requires special training and is beyond the scope of a CT technologist. However, once a port is properly accessed, it can be used for infusion by technologists.
- No established guidelines exist for using CVCs for the mechanical infusion of contrast media. Therefore, whenever possible, a standard peripheral IV access is preferred for contrast media injection. However, using central lines for injecting contrast medium may be the only option in some cases.
  - In general, most CVCs may be infused at rates of 1.5 to 2 mL/s.
  - More rapid injection could potentially result in catheter perforation. When a CVC is used, the technologist should carefully examine the insertion site and report any drainage, oozing, redness, or swelling to the radiologist before injecting into the line.
- Just as with any form of IV access, cleansing solution should be used to clean all junctions and connections. All cleansing solutions should be allowed to completely dry to provide maximum disinfection. The injection cap cannot be touched once it has been cleaned. Only sterile devices or needles are used to access CVADs.

- Before administering any substance, the patency of a central line must be verified. This can be done by demonstrating blood aspiration. The inability to aspirate blood can indicate catheter malposition or occlusion.
  - To aspirate a central line, clean the injection cap and attach an empty 10-mL syringe. Gently pull back on the plunger just enough to see blood, and then flush with normal saline solution. If there is any doubt concerning the patency of a CVC, do not inject into the catheter. If there is resistance to flushing a CVC, no further attempt should be made as doing so may cause the catheter to rupture.
- After injection, the catheter should be flushed with 10 mL of normal saline.
- Institutions vary in their policies regarding the use of CVCs for contrast medium infusion. For example, some facilities prohibit the use of ports for contrast infusion, whereas it is common practice in others.
- There are several types of large-bore tunneled catheters used for dialysis. These should never be used for contrast media injection.
- Manufacturers label the external portion of catheters by printing the size and type on the catheter hub or external tubing. If the catheter type is in doubt, do not use it to inject contrast media.

## BASIC PRINCIPLES OF INTRAVENOUS CONTRAST ADMINISTRATION

- Injection parameters include the volume and concentration of contrast, the flow rate(s) at which the contrast will be delivered, and the timing between the start of the injection and the start of scanning.
- Documentation of intravenous contrast administration is a legal necessity and should include the name of the agent, the dose (volume and concentration), the flow rate(s), and the injection site.
- Controversy exists about the optimal method of administering contrast material. The overarching goal is to select parameters that will consistently improve images and will facilitate reproducible studies.
  - It is important that studies be reproducible because CT is often used for follow-up care and in cancer staging. It is difficult to determine whether a lesion has actually changed in size (even if it appears so on the image) if the technical factors used during scanning vary widely from study to study.

### General Phases of Tissue Enhancement

- Three general phases of tissue enhancement are commonly discussed in CT: the bolus phase, the nonequilibrium phase, and the equilibrium phase.

- The difference between these phases is predominantly determined by the rate at which the contrast material is delivered and the time that elapses from the start of the injection and when scanning is initiated.
- The phases are frequently compared by the arteriovenous iodine difference (AVID). In practice, this is done by comparing a Hounsfield unit (HU) measurement taken within the aorta to that of a measurement taken in the inferior vena cava on the same slice.
- The bolus phase is the earliest phase–that which occurs just seconds following an IV bolus injection. It is characterized by an attenuation difference of 30 or more HUs between the aorta and the inferior vena cava.
  - In the bolus phase of contrast enhancement, the arterial structures are filled with contrast medium and brightly displayed on the image.
  - It is also commonly called the arterial phase.
  - Initially, contrast medium has not yet filled the venous structures.
  - CT angiography images are taken while contrast is in the bolus phase.
- The second phase is the nonequilibrium phase. It follows the bolus phase and is characterized by a difference of 10 to 30 HU AVID.
  - The contrast agent is still much brighter in the arteries than in the parenchyma of organs, but now the venous structures are also opacified.
  - It is also called the venous phase.
  - This phase begins approximately 1 minute after the start of the bolus injection and lasts only a short time, approximately 1 minute. This window can be manipulated to some degree by varying conditions such as the volume and flow rate of the injected contrast medium.
  - Most routine (nonangiographic) body images are acquired while contrast is in the nonequilibrium phase.
- The last phase of tissue enhancement after the IV injection of contrast medium is known as the equilibrium (or delayed) phase. It can begin as early as 2 minutes after the bolus phase or after a drip infusion. It is characterized by an attenuation difference between the aorta and the inferior vena cava of less than 10 HU.
  - In this phase, no new contrast medium is being introduced, and the contrast medium already in the body has soaked the organ parenchyma; structures with no vascularity (such as cysts or fluid in the CT tract) remain unenhanced. As blood circulates continuously through the body, the contrast material becomes evenly diluted in the blood, resulting in similar enhancement (and thus attenuation) within arteries and veins.

In this phase, blood and interstitial concentrations of contrast material equilibrate and decline at an equal rate. The exception is the kidneys (which concentrate the contrast material) and the lumen of the urinary tract (where the concentrated contrast is excreted in the urine).

- The equilibrium phase is the worst phase for acquiring scans of the abdomen, particularly the liver.
- Compared with noncontrast examinations, visualization of tumors in the liver is improved in both the bolus and nonequilibrium phases, but not in the equilibrium phase.
- In some instances, scanning in the equilibrium phase is worse than is simply scanning without IV contrast enhancement. Because in this phase contrast material disperses more equally in the hepatic parenchyma and the tumor's interstitial space, the tumor can become isodense (i.e., the same density as the surrounding tissue) and be indistinguishable.
- Scanning in the equilibrium phase does not improve visualization of hepatic tumor compared with a precontrast examination and carries a considerable risk of masking the tumor enhancement.

- On older, slower, CT scanners, it was impossible to obtain all scans through the liver before contrast media reached equilibrium. In these situations, liver lesions were often difficult, or impossible, to detect with only the contrast-enhanced study. For this reason, patients were often first scanned without contrast enhancement through the liver, and then the entire abdomen was scanned after the injection of contrast media. Modern scanners are much faster, and all scans can easily be obtained before the equilibrium phase. As a result, precontrast scans are now seldom needed for routine abdomen studies.
- The exact timing of the start and end of each of the three phases are affected by many factors, including injection parameters and the condition of the patient.
- With the fast scanners now available, the bolus and the nonequilibrium phases can be subdivided into shorter (but more numerous) phases.
  - The terms early arterial phase, late arterial phase, hepatic arterial phase, portal venous phase, hepatic venous phase, and nephrographic phase have all been used. Frequently, the various terms are used inconsistently.
- Contrast material remains concentrated in organs and vessels for a very short time. Injection protocols are designed by first determining the time window from when contrast material is likely to first arrive in the organ or vessel of interest to when most of the contrast has vacated. Once this is estimated, equipment can be programmed so that scans are acquired within the window.

- Because patient factors can significantly influence the estimated window, tools such as bolus triggering and timing a test bolus are often incorporated into specific examination protocols.
- It is important to note that arrival time indicates when contrast material is likely to first be present in the organ or vessel. Therefore, arrival time represents the earliest possible time to acquire scans; images acquired before the contrast arrival times will appear unenhanced.
- Contrast enhancement typically reaches a near peak in the aorta from 24 to 45 seconds after the start of the injection. The time it takes to reach peak attenuation is affected by the cardiac output of the patient. As more contrast medium reaches the aorta, the aortic enhancement rises only slightly more, creating a type of plateau. The peak aortic enhancement is reached at the end of this phase when all of the contrast has been delivered, then drops off dramatically.
  - The plateau can be extended by adding a saline flush, which will push forward the contrast material left in the tubing and in the veins leading to the aorta.
  - Scanning within this enhancement plateau is ideal for imaging the arteries.
  - Because the true peak enhancement point is short-lived (often < 2 seconds), variable, and difficult to predict, scanning protocols are most often designed so that images are acquired within the plateau (which typically lasts 10–15 seconds) and not the peak.
- Most organs have an exclusively arterial blood supply. The peak organ enhancement for such organs (e.g., pancreas, bowel, bladder) occurs about 5 to 15 seconds after peak aortic enhancement.
- The kidneys are an exception because their excretion of contrast medium must also be considered. Kidney scans are often acquired in the nephrographic phase, which is 80 to 120 seconds after injection.
  - This can be accomplished by incorporating a slight scan delay between scans of the liver and that of the kidney.
- The liver has a dual blood supply. It is supplied primarily by the portal vein, contributing approximately 75%; the remainder is supplied by the hepatic artery. Although liver scanning is sometimes repeated to capture more than one phase of contrast enhancement, at a minimum, it should be scanned in the portal venous phase. This phase occurs approximately 60 seconds after a bolus injection and, by definition, includes both arterial and venous enhancement.

- Routine brain scanning (for metastases or primary central nervous system tumors) provides a notable exception to the general rules of contrast media injection.
  - The enhancement of most brain lesions is caused by blood-brain barrier disruption, not the intrinsic vascularity of the tissue.
  - Therefore, the injection rate is not important, and scan delay is primarily important in that scans are not performed too soon after injection.
  - A scan delay of 4 minutes or greater is typical to allow sufficient time for contrast to leak across a disrupted blood-brain barrier into the abnormal tissue.
  - However, specialized brain scanning such as CT angiography or CT brain perfusion studies require careful adherence to contrast injection protocols.

## Methods of Contrast Media Delivery

- The two methods of administering contrast material are the drip infusion and bolus techniques.

### Drip Infusion

- In the drip infusion technique, an IV line is initiated and contrast medium is allowed to drip in during a period of several minutes. Scanning begins after most, or all, of the contrast agent is administered (roughly 2–3 minutes).
  - Because this method relies on gravity, the actual flow rate delivered is quite variable and affected by many factors (e.g., bottle height, contrast volume, tubing length, IV catheter size, contrast media viscosity).
  - This variability prevents the injection from being uniformly reproduced in subsequent follow-up studies.
- This method is not recommended for scans of the neck, chest, abdomen, or pelvis because all of the scans acquired with this technique are taken in the equilibrium phase.
- The drip infusion method is the least effective injection method for abdominal imaging, and in some respects, it is even inferior to scanning without contrast enhancement.
- The drip infusion method cannot produce peak enhancement of sufficient magnitude for CT angiography.
- However, it can be used for routine brain scanning.

### Bolus Techniques

- The bolus technique of contrast enhancement uses scanning after a rapid injection of contrast material. A volume of contrast of 50 to 200 mL is injected at a rate (or combination of rates) between 1 and 6 mL/s; scanning begins after a short delay.

- The interval between the initiation of the injection and the start of scanning (the scan delay) is critical. The contrast bolus can be delivered by hand (using syringes) or by a mechanical injection system.

### Hand Bolus Technique

- When contrast medium is injected by hand, the flow rate is subject to many factors, including syringe size, contrast viscosity, IV catheter size, and operator strength.
  - Smaller size syringes require less operator strength to inject but must be serially disconnected when empty and reattached with replacement syringes. This delay will cause a drop in the peak enhancement.
  - Higher viscosity agents and smaller indwelling catheters will require more operator strength for injection.
- The advantages of the hand bolus method:
  - Relatively inexpensive
  - Does not require any special equipment to implement
  - Allows the injection site to be closely observed so that the injection can be immediately stopped should there be signs of extravasation of contrast into the soft tissue
  - Often the recommended method for injecting into standard PICC lines
- There are many disadvantages to the hand bolus method:
  - The operator will be exposed to scatter radiation from standing in the room during the scanning process.
  - Because someone must stay in the scan room, this method requires two operators.
  - The primary disadvantages are that the flow rate is variable and the scan delay cannot be precisely controlled. These two factors result in inconsistent images that are not readily reproducible in subsequent studies.
- Although the hand bolus method is an improvement over the drip infusion method, significant disadvantages limit its use to special circumstances.

### Mechanical Injection Systems

- Mechanical injection systems are standard in CT suites for the following reasons:
  - They deliver the precise flow rates and volumes specified by the operator, regardless of the viscosity of the solution and the gauge of the indwelling catheter.
  - Injections are consistent and can be reproduced in subsequent examinations (providing the parameters from studies are properly recorded and repeated).
  - They are programmable, providing broad clinical utility for a wide range of indications.

- Mechanical injectors, or power injectors as they are frequently called, are made by a variety of manufacturers, come in different models, and offer various features.
  - CT injectors may have a single head for affixing the syringe, or they may accommodate two syringes.
  - Dual-head injectors are designed so that saline can be given immediately before or after the contrast media injection.
  - Most models of mechanical injector include a programmable pressure limit. This allows the operator to set an upper pressure limit, along with an injection rate. Contrast medium is then administered at the selected rate, unless the pressure reaches the maximum set. If the pressure reaches the selected limit, the injector reduces the flow rate to prevent exceeding the pressure limit and an alarm sounds to notify the operator. A common reason for reaching the pressure limit is when the IV tubing becomes kinked, restricting the flow of contrast medium.
  - Another feature available on some models is a device designed to aid in the detection of contrast medium extravasation.
  - Extravasation is the leakage of fluid from a vein into the surrounding tissue during IV administration.
  - There is particular concern that mechanical injectors may increase the severity of extravasation when they occur. Because mechanical injectors typically deliver contrast at fast flow rates and the operator does not remain in the room throughout the injection to quickly intercede should signs of extravasation appear, there is worry that a large volume of contrast extravasation could more readily occur when a mechanical injector is used.
  - However, when appropriate precautions are taken, the risk of serious extravasation can be substantially reduced.
  - The extravasation detection feature available on some injector models is designed to augment, rather than supplant, such precautions.
  - Most extravasations involve small volumes and are not clinically significant. Slight swelling and erythema may develop and usually subside without complication. However, severe tissue necrosis and ulceration may occur.
    - Infants, young children, and unconscious and debilitated patients are at higher risk of contrast media extravasation.
    - LOCM are less injurious to cutaneous and subcutaneous tissue than are HOCM.
    - There is no universally accepted treatment for contrast extravasation. The best method of reducing injury is prevention.
  - Guidelines for preventing contrast medium extravasation
    - An indwelling catheter set with a flexible plastic cannula should be used; 18 to 20 gauge is preferred.
    - The use of metal needles (i.e., butterfly infusion sets or straight needles) should be avoided.
    - Monitor the injection site, preferably a medially directed antecubital vein, during the initial moments of injection. Swelling at the site of injection indicates extravasation, and the injection should be stopped immediately.
    - Warm the contrast medium to body temperature to reduce contrast viscosity.
    - Use LOCM.
- Although it rarely occurs, when a mechanical injector is used, large air embolism can result from the incorrect preparation and inadequate connection of the injector syringe and tubing. Large air emboli can cause seizures, permanent neurologic damage, or occasionally death.
  - These large air emboli occur only as a result of human error. Safeguards have been built into injection systems, which are successful in preventing most errors of this type.
- The exact process of preparing the injector varies depending on the type of injection system, whether the facility uses prefilled syringes, and the specific injection protocol. Therefore, each facility should develop a protocol for preparing the mechanical injector(s) used in that department. The protocol should clearly specify the steps taken to prepare the injector for use.
- In summary, the use of mechanical injectors produces the best results. However, precautions must be taken to prevent contrast media extravasation, and care must be taken in the preparation and connection of the injector and cannula to avoid the risk of large air emboli.

## Factors Affecting Contrast Enhancement

- Many factors affect the degree of contrast enhancement in human tissue. These factors can be broadly categorized as pharmacokinetic factors, which are largely controllable, and patient or equipment factors over which technologists have little, or no, control.

### Pharmacokinetic Factors

- Pharmacokinetic factors include contrast medium characteristics (e.g., iodine concentration, osmolality, viscosity), contrast media volume, flow rate, flow duration, scan delay time, and total scan time.

- Although many concentrations are commercially available, most facilities use one concentration for the majority of their CT examinations. Higher concentration agents may be reserved for specialized studies, such as CT angiography.
- Contrast enhancement depends on the iodine concentration in the vasculature or tissues. In the vessels, this concentration depends on the injection rate of iodine in mg/s. Therefore, a concentration of 400 mg/mL injected at 3 mL/s will provide the same total iodine as a concentration of 300 mg/mL injected at 4 mL/s. In spite of the relatively equal enhancement they produce, there are advantages and disadvantages associated with different concentration agents.
  - To maintain the same vascular and organ enhancement, lower concentrations of contrast medium require an increase in the injection rate and an increase in the volume (to maintain the same iodine dose).
  - When IV access is not ideal (e.g., small-gauge catheter in the back of the hand), extravasation of contrast material is more likely when a higher injection rate is used.
  - Lower concentrations of contrast medium have the advantage of possessing slightly lower osmolality, which is associated with fewer adverse effects.
  - Theoretically, lower concentration solutions will produce fewer high-contrast (streak) artifacts in the injected vein.
  - In comparison, injecting a higher concentration agent (≥350 mg iodine/mL) will deliver the same amount of iodine at a lower flow rate. Higher concentration contrast agents are well suited for examinations with a short scan duration, particularly when multislice scanners are used.
  - The viscosity of contrast agent increases with its iodine concentration. Prewarming of the contrast material to body temperature can help to reduce the viscosity so that it can flow more easily through indwelling IV catheters.

## Contrast Media Volume, Flow Duration, Flow Rate

- As scan acquisition speed has increased with new technology, scan duration has dramatically decreased. This increased speed has had an impact on the volume of contrast media used for typical CT studies.
  - When scanners were slower, a larger volume of injected contrast served to extend the flow duration and expand the window of opportunity for acquiring scans while tissues were optimally enhanced.
  - Shorter acquisition times often allow the contrast volume to be reduced. The degree to which contrast volume can be decreased depends on the study, however. Whether, and how much, contrast volume can be cut during liver imaging is controversial. A certain amount of iodine is needed to achieve adequate parenchymal enhancement; dropping below that volume will reduce lesion conspicuity.
- The rate at which contrast medium is injected largely determines the time needed for it to reach peak enhancement and will influence how dramatically enhancement falls off once this peak is reached.
- The effects of variation in injection rates are more pronounced for aortic enhancement than for hepatic enhancement.
- The consequences of varying injection parameters can be graphically depicted using a time-density curve.
  - The $x$ axis of the graph depicts the time elapsed (in seconds) after the start of injection, whereas the $y$ axis charts the relative enhancement levels achieved, in Hounsfield units.
- For a constant injection rate, as the contrast dose is increased (by increasing contrast volume), the magnitude of the peak enhancement increases and the time required to reach that peak also increases.
- For a constant volume and concentration of contrast medium, as the flow rate is increased, there is a decrease in the time to peak aortic enhancement.
  - In practice, this means that the scan delay must be adjusted according to flow rate.
  - For a constant volume of contrast medium, increasing the flow rate shortens the duration of the contrast injection.
  - It should be clear that to capture optimal vascular enhancement for CT angiography studies, the scan timing must be precise. Image acquisition that is too soon will miss the contrast bolus, whereas scanning too late may not provide adequate opacification, particularly of small vessels.
  - Manipulating the flow rate during an injection can improve the likelihood of scanning during optimal vascular enhancement; it is sometimes referred to as "bolus shaping."
  - The typical time-density curve for aortic enhancement using a single injection flow rate (uniphasic) may not be ideal for CT angiography. A uniphasic injection results in a single peak of aortic enhancement that is generally much greater than necessary, but of a very short duration. Ideally, injection techniques would achieve an adequate level of aortic

enhancement and then maintain that level for a longer period of time, thereby increasing the window of opportunity for scanning and allowing the scan timing to be less precise. This is particularly useful when using a slower scanner, when using very narrow collimation, or when scanning a longer area. In addition, more uniform vascular enhancement is beneficial for postprocessing.

- In practice, bolus shaping is accomplished by beginning the injection with a relatively high flow rate and then decreasing the flow rate throughout the injection period.

- When two flow rates are used, the technique is often referred to as biphasic; when more than two flow rates are used, the technique is referred to as multiphasic. Often, the final flow rate is to deliver a saline flush.

■ However, for most clinical applications, a uniphasic contrast injection with a constant flow rate is sufficient.

■ Although considerably less pronounced, many of the same principles apply to hepatic enhancement:

- Increasing the flow rate will shorten the time to peak enhancement.

- Increasing the dose will increase the magnitude of the hepatic enhancement.

■ However, compared with aortic enhancement, the slope of the contrast-timing curves for hepatic enhancement is less steep with a longer horizontal portion during which contrast enhancement remains relatively constant.

- In practice, this allows a wider window of opportunity for scanning; therefore, the timing of scans for routine abdominal imaging does not need to be as precise as those designed to capture peak aortic enhancement.

### Patient Factors Affecting Contrast Enhancement

■ Many patient factors have important effects on contrast enhancement. These include the patient's age, sex, weight, height, cardiovascular status, renal function, and the presence of other disease.

■ Although patient factors are largely uncontrollable, it is important to recognize their potential effects on contrast enhancement. In some cases, injection parameters can be adjusted to help mitigate patient factors.

■ The patient's weight has a pronounced effect on the degree of aortic and parenchymal enhancement. Although peak enhancement is reached at nearly identical times, as patient weight increases, the magnitude of contrast enhancement diminishes.

- In large patients, arterial enhancement can be increased by increasing the injection rate (by either increasing the flow rate or increasing the iodine concentration). Because hepatic parenchymal enhancement is determined primarily by the total iodine dose, increasing the dose can also improve hepatic enhancement in large patients.

- Some institutions use a weight-based system for determining the contrast medium dose for routine body scans. Typically, a maximum dose limit is present, however.

■ A patient's cardiac output status can have a significant effect on the time it takes injected contrast medium to reach peak aortic enhancement.

- As cardiac output is reduced, there is a progressively longer delay in the time required for the contrast bolus to reach the aorta, thus delaying peak aortic enhancement. This requires the scan delay to be extended in proportion to the degree of cardiac impairment; practically, this can only be done by using a method (i.e., test bolus, or bolus tracking) that individualizes the scan delay to the patient.

### Equipment Factors Affecting Contrast Enhancement

■ Contrast administration and scan timing must also be modified according to the type and capabilities of the CT scanner used.

- As a general rule, the scan delay is increased as scan duration decreases. Adding 5 to 20 seconds to the scan delay when using a 64-detector row scanner (as compared with a single-detector row scanner) helps to ensure that imaging occurs during peak arterial enhancement. In this way, it is possible to keep all other contrast injection parameters constant, thereby achieving the same aortic enhancement curves, by simply adjusting the scan delay according to scanner speed.

- For some applications, a faster scanner may allow the use of a smaller volume of contrast material.

### Automated Injection Triggering

■ Two methods exist for individualizing the scan delay; the injection of a test bolus and bolus triggering. Both techniques require the CT scanner to have specialized software. These methods are particularly useful for vascular imaging, in which it is critical that the timing of scan acquisition coincides with peak contrast enhancement. These methods effectively accommodate individual differences in circulation time attributable to heart rate, age, and illnesses.

### Test Bolus

- This method consists of administering 10 to 20 mL of contrast medium by IV bolus injection and performing several trial scans to determine the length of time from injection to peak contrast enhancement in a target region, such as the aorta.
  - Using a mechanical injector, the test injection is delivered at the same rate as the diagnostic scans. Trial scans are taken using the lowest possible mAs settings, typically at 2-second intervals, at the same slice location, for 20 to 30 seconds (i.e., 10–15 scans). Trial scans begin from 8 to 15 seconds after the start of the injection. The test bolus is evaluated by identifying the image that shows the maximum enhancement in the target region.
  - The optimal scan delay time for the actual study is presumed to be equal to the time that elapsed from the start of the test injection to that of the image showing maximum enhancement. Experience shows that the best results are achieved by adding 3 seconds to this calculated delay.
  - Scan delay time can be calculated from the test injection using the following formula:

trial scan delay + (2 × the image number showing maximum enhancement) + 3 seconds

### Bolus Triggering

- This method of determining the scan delay is called bolus triggering, bolus tracking, or automated triggering. It is a more efficient method than the test bolus because it uses the contrast bolus itself to initiate the scan. This technique uses a series of low-radiation scans to monitor the progress of the contrast bolus.
  - A single cross-sectional slice is taken, and an area of interest is determined. The injection is initiated, and low-radiation scans begin from 8 to 10 seconds later. Once an adequate level of enhancement is achieved (determined visually or by a curser placed on the area of interest), the table moves to the starting level and scanning begins. Scanning can be triggered automatically by setting a predetermined threshold CT number, or it can be initiated manually by the technologist.
  - Because the table must move to the correct position and the mAs must be set to the appropriate level for diagnostic scanning, there is a 3- to 9-second delay between the last monitor scan and the start of scanning. This lag time is seen by many as a significant drawback to the technique. Recognizing the delay, many facilities use a relatively low trigger threshold (approximately 50 HU) or manually start the scan as soon as the contrast material is seen in the target region.
  - An important drawback to bolus triggering is that technologists cannot stay with the patient for even a short time after the contrast injection begins, or they will be exposed to radiation from the monitor scans. For this reason, bolus tracking is typically reserved for vascular imaging but not for routine examinations of the chest or abdomen, in which timing is not as critical.
  - For routine studies, most facilities rely on preset scan delays.

## REVIEW QUESTIONS

1. Which is NOT a true statement regarding the placement of a peripheral IV line for the administration of an iodinated contrast agent for a scan of the abdomen?
   a. Standard precautions must be adhered to.
   b. Sterile technique must be followed.
   c. An indwelling catheter, butterfly infusion set, or straight needle can be used, depending on the preference of the technologist.
   d. Basic consent must be obtained from the patient.
2. What type of catheter do most manufacturers recommend be flushed with a heparinized saline solution after their use?
   a. Open-ended CVAD catheters
   b. Closed-end CVAD catheters
   c. Standard peripheral indwelling catheters
   d. PICCs that contain a Luer-activated device
3. Which is a TRUE statement regarding implantable ports?
   a. Implanted ports are typically used for short-term injections that require high flow rates, such as blood transfusion or contrast media administration.
   b. Among CVADs, ports have the lowest incidence of infection because they are completely buried under the skin and there is no site for microorganisms to enter.
   c. The port can be easily accessed using standard straight needles; no special training is required.
   d. The port is placed so that only the face of the device shows through an opening in the skin.
4. The difference between the bolus phase, the nonequilibrium phase, and the equilibrium phase of contrast enhancement is primarily determined by the
   a. brand of iodinated contrast agent used.
   b. injection rate and scan delay.
   c. type of pathology present.
   d. film processing time.
5. The arteriovenous iodine difference is calculated by
   a. taking an HU measurement of the liver before and after the contrast injection.
   b. comparing an HU measurement of the pancreas to that of the liver.
   c. comparing an HU measurement of the aorta to that of the inferior vena cava.
   d. dividing the concentration of iodine by the volume used.

6. Another name for the bolus phase of contrast enhancement is the
   a. arterial phase.
   b. venous phase.
   c. portal venous phase.
   d. delayed phase.

7. Iodinated contrast is administered at a rate of 3 mL/s for a routine abdominal scan in which the protocol calls for a delay of 60 seconds between the start of injection and the start of scanning. Soon after the start of the contrast injection, the patient begins to experience an intense warm feeling and, being surprised by this, calls for the technologist. How long, beyond the 60 seconds, can the technologist delay the scan acquisition (so that he might comfort the patient) without risk of degrading the diagnostic utility of the study?
   a. 5 to 10 seconds
   b. 30 to 40 seconds
   c. 5 to 8 minutes
   d. 12 to 15 minutes

8. The general rules of contrast media injection regarding injection rate and scan delay do not apply to
   a. routine brain scanning.
   b. coronary angiography.
   c. routine abdominal scanning.
   d. thoracic scanning.

9. When can a drip infusion technique for contrast media administration be used?
   a. For a study of the chest when the clinical indication is suspicion of pulmonary emboli
   b. For an angiographic study of the brain performed to demonstrate a suspected middle cerebral artery occlusion
   c. For a study of the brain when the clinical indication is suspicion of tumor
   d. A drip infusion technique can never be used for contrast-enhanced CT studies

10. All of the following are disadvantages of the hand bolus technique of contrast administration EXCEPT:
    a. Flow rate is variable.
    b. Scan delay cannot be precisely controlled.
    c. It requires two operators.
    d. It cannot be used for injecting into standard PICC lines.

11. The volume of contrast administered is increased from 100 to 150 mL. The flow rate is unchanged at 3 mL/s. What can be expected?
    a. The time to reach peak aortic enhancement is decreased.
    b. The magnitude of the peak enhancement is decreased.
    c. The duration of the contrast injection is increased.
    d. The duration of the scan acquisition is increased.

12. Because of the patient's IV access, the flow rate of a contrast injection is reduced from the protocol of 4 to 2 mL/s. What other adjustment is likely to be made?
    a. The scan delay is increased.
    b. The scan delay is decreased.
    c. The volume of contrast is decreased.
    d. The volume of contrast is increased.

13. What injection technique is used for most clinical applications?
    a. A drip infusion technique
    b. A uniphasic injection with a constant flow rate
    c. A biphasic injection in which the initial 50-mL bolus is delivered at a higher flow rate
    d. A multiphasic injection with two or more contrast flow rates, followed by a saline flush

14. What effect does a patient's cardiac output status have on contrast enhancement?
    a. As cardiac output is reduced, the magnitude of the peak aortic enhancement is diminished.
    b. As cardiac output is reduced, the magnitude of the peak aortic enhancement is increased.
    c. As cardiac output is reduced, there is a progressively longer delay in the time required for the contrast bolus to reach peak aortic enhancement.
    d. As cardiac output is reduced, there is a progressively shorter delay in the time required for the contrast bolus to reach peak aortic enhancement.

15. The test bolus method is used to determine the scan delay for a CT angiography study. Ten trial images are taken at 2-second intervals beginning 12 seconds after the start of the test injection. Maximum enhancement in the selected region of interest is seen on the fourth image. What scan delay range is optimal?
    a. 5 to 8 seconds
    b. 20 to 23 seconds
    c. 32 to 35 seconds
    d. 100 to 120 seconds

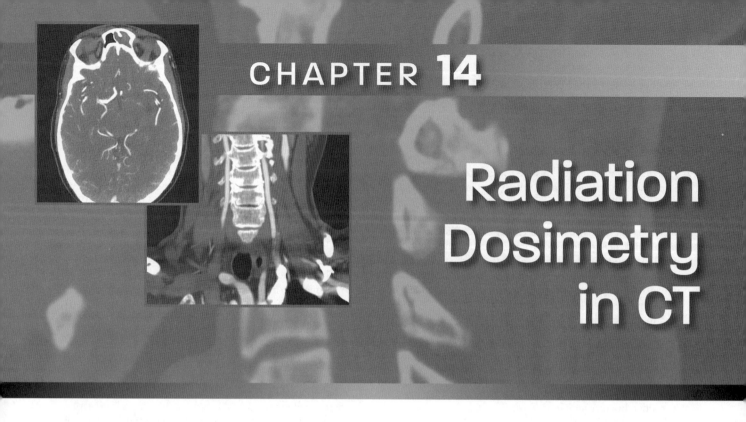

# CHAPTER 14

# Radiation Dosimetry in CT

## BASIC DOSE CONCEPTS

- The rational use of CT relative to patient care involves two components: appropriate patient selection and minimization of the radiation dose without compromising diagnostic image quality.
- There is no consensus regarding a single expression of dose. Effective dose, organ dose, absorbed dose, multiple scan average dose, and CT dose index, among other measurements, are all used.

## Measurement Terminology

- The ionizing radiation used in CT is an x-ray with a range of energy from 80 to 140 kVp and an average energy near 70 keV.
- The unit of x-ray exposure in air is the roentgen (R).
- The International System of Units (abbreviated SI from the French Le Système International d'Unités) is used in the field of radiation dosimetry. The SI unit of absorbed dose is the gray (Gy). This unit describes the amount of energy absorbed per unit mass at a specific point.
- The older unit of absorbed dose is the radiation absorbed dose, or rad. This unit is now obsolete.
- A centigray (cGy) equals 1 rad. There are 100 rad in 1 Gy.
- In recognition of the health effects of x-ray, another conversion factor, called the quality factor (Q), is applied to the absorbed dose. This factor accounts for the different health effects produced from different types of ionizing radiation. The quality

factor is 1 for the diagnostic x-rays that are used in CT. The radiation weighting factor ($w_R$) is a newer term that is very similar to the quality factor.
- When the quality factor has been applied to the radiation absorbed dose, the new quantity is the dose equivalent, expressed in units known as the sievert (Sv). The old unit was the rem, or roentgen equivalent man. There are 100 rem in 1 Sv.
- Another measurement, referred to as effective dose, or effective dose equivalent, attempts to account for the effects particular to the patient's tissue that has absorbed the radiation dose. This unit is a weighted average of organ doses. The weighting factors are set for each radiosensitive organ. Effective dose is reported in Sv or rem. Determining the radiation dose to radiosensitive organs is problematic and is a barrier to accurate calculation of the effective dose.
  - Effective dose is a measure of energy deposited per unit mass and provides a mean to gauge the potential for biologic effects.

## Dose Geometry

- In projection radiography, either film-screen or digital, the skin of the entrance plane receives 100% of the radiation, and the percentage falls rapidly as the x-ray beam is attenuated by the patient's tissue. By the time the beam exits the patient, most of the radiation has been absorbed or scattered. In conventional radiography, it is common for the exit dose to be only 1% (or 1/100) that of the entrance dose.

- In CT, the difference between the dose at the center and the dose at the periphery is not nearly as great as that of conventional radiography. In CT studies of the head, the dose to the skin is close to that in the center of the slice.
- The dose is more uniform in CT than in projection radiography for two reasons. First, in CT, the beam is heavily filtered as it exits the x-ray tube. Because the filtered beam consists of only higher energy photons, a lower percentage of the beam will be absorbed or scattered as it passes through patient tissue. In addition, the CT exposure comes from all directions, creating a more uniform exposure.
- The uniformity of the dose decreases as the scan field of view and patient thickness increase. Therefore, body scans are less uniform than are head scans. The central dose for a body scan is approximately one-third to one-half that of the peripheral dose.
- To a great degree, the more uniform beam accounts for the fact that, for a given set of machine parameters (mAs, slice thickness, pitch), organ doses are clearly higher for children compared with (larger) adults. This is attributable to the partial shielding that inherently occurs in larger subjects.

## Z Axis Variations

- In addition to the variations within the scan plane, variations along the length, or $z$ axis, of the patient, are described by the $z$ axis dose distribution (or radiation profile).
- To understand this concept, let us first look at a traditional axial scan sequence (a full gantry rotation at one table position) with contiguous slices (slice thickness is equal to the table increment; therefore, no overlapping slices, no gapped slices). If there were no scatter radiation, the radiation dose would be equal throughout the study.
- For the sake of illustration, let's assume that there is no scatter inherent in CT. In this case, if a single CT slice delivered a dose of 1 cGy, then the total radiation dose from a 30-slice CT examination that was performed with contiguous slices would also deliver 1 cGy. This would be true because no area of the patient is exposed more than once.
- In reality, there is some scatter inherent in CT. However, it is important to recognize that although there is some radiation that is scattered, the overall amount is low, and the distance it travels is quite short, particularly when compared with projection radiography. In this discussion of scatter radiation, we are considering scatter that affects adjacent

slices. Therefore, we are referring to a distance of only 1 to 10 mm.
- In CT, the amount of scatter radiation that travels greater distances, such as to the door of the scan room, is small. However, to accurately assess the $z$ axis dose distribution, the dose to a single slice must be added to the radiation that scatters into adjacent slices.
- The areas of scatter into adjacent tissue are sometimes called tails.
- The total dose will be higher when multiple scans are performed. How much the scatter radiation will contribute to the dose depends on factors such as patient size and physical makeup and the image acquisition parameters such as kVp, slice thickness, rotation time, and mA used.
- In general, the tails will contribute approximately 25% to 40% additional dose to the entire study. Therefore, if a single slice of the chest delivered a dose of 4 cGy, the entire dose from 30 contiguous slices is approximately 5 cGy (i.e., 4 cGy + 1 cGy) to 5.6 (i.e., 4 cGy + 1.6 cGy). As compared with the dose from a single slice, the overall radiation dose will be higher when multiple scans are performed.
- Because most CT applications involve multiple scans with adjacent slices, dose is usually calculated from multiple scans. Measurements are made at the center of the slice and several points around the periphery with plastic phantoms. This procedure accounts for the effect of scatter from the tails of each slice into the neighboring slices.
- The multiple scan average dose (MSAD) is the central slice radiation dose, plus the scatter overlap (or tails). The MSAD will increase if slices overlap and decrease if there are gaps between slices.
- Another type of radiation dose measurement in CT is the computed tomography dose index (CTDI). The CTDI is what manufacturers report to the U.S. Food and Drug Administration (FDA) and prospective customers regarding the doses typically delivered for their machines.
- The CTDI can only be calculated if slices are contiguous, that is, there are no overlapping or gapped slices. If there is slice overlap or gaps, the CTDI is multiplied by the ratio of slice thickness to slice increment. This would technically be the MSAD, because the CTDI conditions would no longer exist. Equipment manufacturers report CTDI doses for typical head and body imaging techniques. These are equivalent to the dose a patient receives if multiple scans are taken.
- In an effort to expand the use of CTDI to scans with variable parameters, such as slice thickness and pitch, other indices were created.

- The $CTDI_{100}$ is calculated using a dosimeter called a pencil ionization chamber. It is a 100-mm-long cylindrical device. Measuring dose in this way accounts for the variable pitches commonly used in helical scan sequences.
- $CTDI_{vol}$ is the preferred expression of radiation dose in CT dosimetry.
- Dose-length product (DLP) is an expression of radiation dose that accounts for the length of scan. DLP values are affected by variances in patient anatomy, and therefore DLP is not as useful as is $CTDI_{vol}$ when making comparison among different protocols.

## Comparison of Dose From CT With Doses From Conventional Radiographic Studies

- The modalities are significantly different; therefore, a simple comparison between doses delivered from CT and projection radiography cannot be conducted.
- However, it is important for technologists to have a general idea of the dose being delivered to the patient and how it relates to other modalities.
- The radiation dose for CT examinations is substantially higher when compared with projection radiography.
- For example, comparing a supine view of the abdomen done in projection radiography with an abdominal study done in CT, the skin (surface) dose is approximately 10 times higher in CT, and the average absorbed dose is approximately 100 times higher.
- Special procedures such as angiography and interventional radiography may produce radiation doses near or exceeding those from CT. Actual doses are highly variable and are affected by many factors, including type and manufacturer of scanner.

## Factors Affecting Dose

### Radiation Beam Geometry

- Theoretically, a rotation arc of only 180° is all that is required to satisfy most reconstruction algorithms. Most scanners use a 360° tube arc to compensate for radiation beam divergence and patient motion. The extra scanning information improves image quality but increases radiation dose.
- Additionally, overscanning, which is the process of using more than a 360° tube arc, is sometimes used–particularly in fourth-generation CT systems. Overscans will increase the radiation dose. It is important to differentiate overscanning from the term *overranging*, which is an extension of exposure in the *z* axis and is discussed later.

### Filtration

- Filtration affects the radiation dose by removing some of the soft (i.e., low-energy) x-rays. These low-energy x-rays are quickly absorbed by the patient. Adding metal filters to the beam permits selective removal of x-rays with low energy and reduces the radiation dose while maintaining contrast at an acceptable level.

### Detector Efficiency

- Detector absorption efficiency affects radiation dose to the patient. Less-efficient detectors will require a higher radiation exposure to produce an adequate image. Solid-state detectors are from 90% to 100% efficient, whereas the xenon gas detectors used in older model scanners are significantly less efficient.

### Slice Width and Spacing

- In considering a single cross-sectional slice, as slice thickness increases, the volume of tissue irradiated increases, and the dose may increase slightly in the slice. However, for multiple slice examinations, decreasing slice thickness and using contiguous slices will increase the MSAD because of the increased amount of scatter radiation to adjacent slices. Also, to maintain image quality at the same level, additional radiation is needed for thinner slices.
- Multiple slice examinations using overlapping slices will produce a higher overall dose, whereas gapped slices will produce a lower overall dose.
- Although the effects of beam collimation are small for single-detector row scanners, that is not the case with MDCT. The radiation doses delivered with these systems are much more dependent on x-ray beam collimation. These effects result from differences in x-ray beam collimation–even when the same reconstructed section thickness is used.

### Pitch

- The spacing of CT slices obtained with a helical (or spiral) scan process is called pitch. Helical scans performed with a pitch of 1 deliver approximately the same dose as that of conventional axial CT studies–provided the kVp and mAs values are the same for each mode. Selecting a pitch greater than 1 will spread the radiation more thinly over the slices. That is, although there are no areas along the *z* axis that are skipped completely, the gantry will not make a full rotation in a given slice location. The pitch has a direct influence on patient radiation dose because as pitch increases, the time that any one point in space spends in the x-ray beam is decreased.

- The pitch values must be interpreted differently for MDCT scanners. For example, the table may be incremented 30.0 mm per rotation to image several simultaneous 10.0-mm slices; however, if the CT system collimates the x-ray beam for four 10.0-mm slices simultaneously (effective pitch, 0.75), there is an overlap of irradiated tissue.
- MDCT scanners typically have several modes that allow the technologist to select whether to overlap slices or extend the pitch.
- Generally, the radiation doses to patients are approximately 30% to 50% greater with earlier models of MDCT, primarily as a result of scan overbeaming, positioning of the x-ray tube closer to the patient, and possible increased scattered radiation with wider x-ray beams.

### Overranging

- Overranging is a phenomenon that occurs only with helical scan sequences and cannot be avoided by the technologist. To reconstruct a CT image, data are required from at least half a rotation around the patient. This means that data from before and after each imaging section are needed to create the first and last section of the imaged volume. This requires the scanner to make at least an extra half rotation at the beginning and end of the desired image volume. The added dose from these partial rotations is defined as the overrange dose. The greater the number of detector rows, the greater the overrange length.
  - The parameters that have the greatest effect on the degree of overranging dose are detector collimation and pitch.
  - The extent to which overranging contributes to the radiation dose in helical CT is highly protocol and manufacturer dependent.

### Scan Field Diameter

- Scan field diameter affects the dose. Phantoms are frequently used to measure radiation dose. Phantoms of two diameters—16 and 32 cm—are used to simulate head and body scans, respectively. Holding all technical factors constant, a scan of the head phantom will result in a higher radiation dose than that of the body phantom. Smaller objects always absorb a higher dose; the difference is at least a factor of two. Thus, smaller patients would be expected to absorb much higher amounts of radiation than would larger patients. This effect is primarily attributed to the fact that total exposure is made up of both entrance radiation and exit radiation. For smaller patients, the patient has less tissue to attenuate the beam, which results in a much more uniform dose distribution. Conversely, for a larger patient, the exit radiation is much less intense as a result of its attenuation through more tissue.

### Radiographic Technique

- As in projection radiography, the technique used to create the CT image affects radiation exposure to the patient. The higher the mAs and kVp settings used to create the image, the higher the dose to the patient.
- The relationship between mAs and dose is linear. That is, if the mAs settings were doubled, the doses and risks would be doubled. Likewise, if the mAs settings were halved, the doses–and therefore the risks–would be halved.
- However, a reduction in dose is associated with a subsequent increase in image noise. For example, first assume that the minimum dose to obtain acceptable image quality has been determined. If this dose is halved by halving the mAs, a noise increase of 41% can be expected.
- X-ray tube potential (or kVp) also affects the radiation dose, although the effect is not linear. With the mAs kept constant, changing from 120 to 140 kVp increases the radiation dose approximately 30% to 45%.

### Patient Size and Body Part Thickness

- Large patients or thick body parts require radiographic techniques that increase the radiation dose to avoid an unacceptable level of image noise. In addition, the patient size and body composition may affect the degree of scatter radiation.

### Repeat Scans

- Areas of the patient that are rescanned to visualize various stages of intravenous contrast enhancement or for other technical or clinical reasons receive additional radiation. The effect is cumulative.

### Collimation

- Lead collimators are used near the x-ray tube to control the size of the beam striking the patient. If the beam were not controlled to match the detector size, there would be additional scatter radiation to degrade the image; this scenario would result in a higher radiation dose to the patient. Collimators may also be used near the detectors for scatter rejection and aperture use.

### Localization Scans

- The localization scan performed before scanning, which is often referred to as the scout image, delivers a very low dose. The radiation dose for the scout image is much lower than that used to produce cross-sectional slices.

## WHY THE GROWING CONCERN?

### Commonly Used and Relatively High Radiation Doses

- CT scanning is a relatively high-dose procedure that contributes disproportionately to the overall radiation dose from all radiologic sources.
- CT examinations represented approximately 11% of all diagnostic radiologic procedures but accounted for 67% of the effective dose from diagnostic radiologic procedures.
- This unbalanced distribution of dose is simply because the dose associated with CT is higher than that from other radiologic examinations.
- To offer the reader a point of comparison, the radiation dose from one abdominal CT scan has been commonly reported to be equivalent to that of 100 to 250 chest radiographs.
- Recent high-speed MDCT technology creates more-defined images in shorter times and has allowed for new clinical indications such as CT angiography. In addition, the faster scan speed has reduced the need for sedation in pediatric patients, thus spurring this modality's use in that population.
- Comparing MDCT with older, single-detector row helical scanners, effective radiation dose is estimated to be 27% to 35% higher with MDCT, whereas organ dose (i.e., kidneys, uterus, ovaries, and pelvic bone marrow) is estimated to be 92% to 180% higher.
- Therefore, new CT technology results in two concerns: 1) expanded technology resulting in more CT studies being performed, and 2) higher radiation doses associated with the newer scanners.

## INFORMATION CONCERNING THE EFFECTS OF LOW-DOSE RADIATION

- Information concerning the effects of low-dose radiation on atomic bomb survivors who were irradiated as children became available in the year 2000. It prompted a change of thinking among both physicists and healthcare professionals.
- These research findings have shown that the effective doses with diagnostic CT are associated with a small but statistically significant increased risk of developing cancer as a result of the radiation.
- On the basis of predictions from these data, radiation doses from typical pediatric CT studies may cause the eventual cancer-related death of 1 in 1,000 children examined.
- It is important to note that the validity, applicability, and utility of extrapolating data from the data collected from high-dose atomic bomb survivors to apply to low-dose diagnostic radiologic studies is hotly debated.

## A NEED FOR EDUCATION

- Parents, pediatricians, technologists, and even radiologists often lack basic information regarding the dose delivered during CT examinations.
- Research done in the early 2000s revealed that most children were routinely being imaged with parameters suited for adults and that adjustments were not being made to compensate for the smaller size of children. No adjustments were made on the basis of patient age or size; mA settings were no less for the youngest infants and children than those used for teenaged patients. It was found that many infants were being imaged at a tube current greater than that used for adolescent patients.
- The results suggested that pediatric patients were being exposed to unnecessarily high radiation doses from CT.
- A more recent study showed that progress is being made. In this study, it was found that most pediatric radiologists practicing in children's or university hospitals do practice age-adjusted helical CT.

### Extra Images

- "Extra" images are defined as those images obtained beyond the desired area of interest.
- Assuming that other scanning parameters are held constant, the radiation dose is directly proportional to the scan volume. Therefore, restriction of the scan volume to the area of interest can help avoid unnecessary radiation.
- Research has shown that a substantial number of extra images are acquired beyond the borders of the area of interest with abdominal or pelvic CT examinations.
- These extra images added approximately 10% to the patient's radiation dose from the examination, but contributed no additional information.
- Researchers confirm that extra images are routinely obtained, both above the diaphragm and below the pubic symphysis, regardless of the clinical indications, patient age, or patient sex.
- In some cases, the inclusion of images beyond the strict area of interest may be justified. At the supradiaphragmatic level, the acquisition of extra images may be justified to ensure that even if the patient's breathing is irregular, the entire liver and spleen are included in one phase of contrast enhancement. Infrapubic extension of routine abdominal or pelvic CT examinations without appropriate clinical request or reason, especially given the risks of radiation to the gonads, cannot be as easily justified.

- Although the acquisition of extra images might be acceptable in uncooperative or breathless patients, it adds no diagnostic information to that provided by images in the area of interest for routine abdominal or pelvic CT and should be restricted when not indicated or requested for specific clinical reasons.

## Need for Awareness

- Historically, awareness regarding the radiation dose and possible risks associated with CT is low among patients, emergency department physicians, and radiologists.
- Most patients are not informed of the risks and benefits before their CT examinations.
- The growing concern about the risks associated with diagnostic CT examinations can be linked to five main factors: 1) higher use; 2) new scanners that deliver higher radiation doses; 3) information correlating the effects of low-dose radiation to a higher lifetime cancer risk; 4) lack of knowledge concerning the radiation dose among radiologists, technologists, attending physicians, and patients; and 5) studies showing that some facilities are not adjusting scanning parameters for pediatric patients, therefore exposing infants and children to a higher-than-necessary radiation doses.

## Perception of Risk

- It is important to put the increased risk that pediatric radiation exposure poses into perspective so that we are better able to effectively communicate with patients and their families.
- Inherent in the discussion of risk is an understanding that the public may have a different perception of risk than that of scientists or researchers.
- In general, people are more concerned about unfamiliar or poorly understood risks. They are more concerned about risks that are not under their personal control. People are more concerned about risks that are perceived to disproportionally affect children.
- Some generalizations can still be made regarding people's willingness to accept risk. A yearly risk of death of one in a million is generally ignored (e.g., being struck by lightning), whereas a risk of death of one in a hundred is totally unacceptable (e.g., accident and disease in coal miners at the turn of the century).
- The risk level associated with pediatric CT falls into the more ambiguous intermediate level. This level of risk can be considered acceptable if 1) the individual is aware of the risk; 2) the individual receives some commensurate benefit; and 3) everything reasonable has been done to reduce the risk.

- These general principles of risk are applied to the specific case of pediatric CT through the following recommendations:
  - The patient—or the parent in the case of a patient who is a child—should be told of the small risk involved.
  - The procedure should be restricted to cases in which it is specifically indicated and conveys a commensurate diagnostic benefit that is difficult to obtain by any other means. Pediatric CT involves too large a dose to be used indiscriminately as a screening procedure.
  - Every effort should be made to decrease the radiation dose by adjusting the kVp and mAs to a suitable level according to the size of the child being scanned. "One size fits all" is no longer appropriate now that the risks have been identified.

## Special Consideration for the Pediatric Population

- There are three primary factors of special relevance to the use of CT in pediatric radiology: increased sensitivity, higher effective dose, and increasing use.
- Children are much more radiosensitive than are adults. For example, a 1-year-old infant is approximately six times more likely than is a 50-year-old adult to develop a malignancy from the same dose of radiation.
- There are two reasons for this increased sensitivity. One is that because of their younger age, children have more time to develop cancer than do adults. Remembering that the latency time for cancer induction in the dose ranges used in CT is estimated to be between 10 and 30 years, it is clear why radiation exposure to a child is of greater concern than that to an adult. In addition, exposure is cumulative, and many patients have multiple CT examinations over their life spans.
- Radiation for older adults and the elderly does not carry the same cancer risk because many radiation-induced cancers, particularly solid malignancies, will not be evident for decades and thus would develop beyond the life span of many of these older persons.
- Also, children are inherently more sensitive to radiation simply because they have more dividing cells and thus suffer more adverse radiation effects on dividing cells.
- Research shows that children are four to six times more sensitive to the effects of radiation than are middle-aged adults.
- Because of the absence of partial shielding, organ doses are larger in a child compared with an adult (assuming the adult is larger).
- The use of helical CT is increasing even faster in children than in adults.

- A fetus is particularly sensitive to the harmful effects of ionizing radiation.
  - The radiosensitivity of a developing fetus is greatest from conception to 3 months' gestation because this is the time of organ and neural crest development.
  - The ACR recommends that when imaging is required in the evaluation of the pregnant woman, nonionizing techniques, such as sonography and MRI, be used as the first choice.
  - However, CT is often used for such indications as suspected pulmonary embolus (PE), appendicitis, renal colic, or trauma.
  - The major concerns regarding risks to the fetus with the low levels of exposure associated with body CT are neurologic and carcinogenic in nature.
  - Standard body protocols using MDCT scanners should not result in significant neurologic impairment.
  - However, the correlation between prenatal radiation exposure and carcinogenesis is less clear. The doses delivered in some body protocols could theoretically double the chance of developing childhood cancer.

## STRATEGIES FOR REDUCING DOSE

### General Strategies

- Because a combination of factors is responsible for the total radiation dose delivered to the patient during a CT examination, a variety of methods for reducing dose are available. The following options can be used in any combination according to the specific clinical situation.
  - Adjusting mAs–small bodies require a lesser dose, and large bodies require a greater dose. Adjustments can be made based on the patient's weight or on the diameter of the patient. Either approach has proved successful.
  - Equipment options–manufacturers have recently provided users with another method to reduce patient dose. Newer systems may have an option that will make changes in tube current (mA) based on the estimated attenuation of the patient at a specific location. The estimations are derived from scout views done in both the anteroposterior and lateral projections.
  - Avoid increasing kVp–increasing the x-ray tube potential increases both the radiation dose and penetration of the x-rays through the body. In general, increases beyond 120 kVp should be avoided, except when imaging obese patients. However, an increase in kVp could be accompanied by a reduction in tube current to offset the increased dose.
  - Increased pitch–increasing pitch will reduce the radiation dose without loss of diagnostic information.
  - Limit the use of thin slices–using a large number of thin adjacent CT slices results in 30% to 50% more radiation dose to the patient than using fewer thicker slices to scan the same anatomy. Although it is not always possible to avoid using thin slices, technologists and radiologists should be aware of the consequences.
  - Limit repeat scans–because the effects of repeat scans of the same area are cumulative, redundant or multiphase studies should be performed only when clinically indicated. Although multiphasic studies are clearly indicated in some situations, they should not be done in all circumstances. Triple-phase studies for the evaluation of kidney lesions should be reserved for patients in whom a question arises on a routine study or other examination rather than as a standard protocol.

### Additional Strategies for Dose Reduction in Pediatric Patients

- Use CT only when clinically indicated.
- Consider alternative modalities.
- Customize the CT examination. One way of tailoring the examination to the specific diagnostic need is for the radiologist to limit the examination to the region in question. For example, routine scanning of the pelvis as part of an abdominal CT is not always necessary. In addition, specific clinical indications may allow the region of the examination to be limited. For example, in follow-up examinations, the region scanned could be limited to just the area of interest (e.g., pseudocyst, lung, or abdominal abscess).
- Limit the use of multiphase examinations. In the rare instance when multiple phases are necessary, scan parameters–including length of scan, slice thickness, and tube current–should be adjusted to minimize the additional radiation received.
- Adjust mAs according to region scanned. Appropriate selection of mAs is important for all patients, but it is imperative in children. Patient size is the primary criterion in the selection of mAs, but the region scanned and the clinical indication that prompted the scan are also considerations. Lower tube currents are adequate in evaluating lung parenchyma. Because bone intrinsically has high contrast, the tube current should be lowered when a bone is of primary interest.
- Adjust mAs according to clinical indications. The cost of reducing mAs below a threshold point is that the signal-to-noise ratio decreases because the number of image-forming photons decreases.

The resulting noisier images have decreased spatial resolution. In many cases, this decrease in image quality will affect diagnosis, but in some cases, the reduction may be acceptable. For example, in a child for whom a large abnormality is being evaluated, such as a retroperitoneal hematoma or an abscess, the noisier image will probably be sufficient. Therefore, tube current should be adjusted for patient size, region scanned, and scan indication.

■ When feasible, use patient shielding. Although lead shielding is standard in general radiography, it is less beneficial in CT. Because of narrow collimation, radiation to areas outside that of the selected scan area is minimal and usually attributable to the internal scattering of photons that are unaffected by surface shielding. However, shielding of the breast tissue and thyroid gland can be a valuable dose-reduction strategy. Perhaps what is more important is that patient shielding may play a role in the perception of risk; that is, it would assure the child's family that every effort was being taken to reduce the radiation dose.

## Initiatives to Raise Awareness

■ In response to concerns about exposure to radiation from a lifetime of diagnostic radiologic test, several national organizations have initiated campaigns to raise awareness.

● The goals of the *Image Gently* program are to educate radiology providers about "child-size" radiation delivered to pediatric patients and to increase awareness among referring pediatricians and other physicians about ordering alternatives to CT scans when appropriate.

● The *Image Wisely* campaign has similar goals although the focus is primarily on raising awareness among radiology professionals.

### REVIEW QUESTIONS

1. The rational use of CT involves which two key components?
   a. Halving the mAs and doubling the kVp
   b. Eliminating most pediatric examinations and requiring a second physician's opinion to order adult examinations
   c. Reducing the use of helical scanning and increasing the frequency of visits by physicists to assess radiation dose delivered
   d. Appropriate selection of patients and the minimization of the radiation dose without compromising diagnostic quality
2. Which unit universally expresses dose?
   a. Effective dose
   b. Organ dose
   c. Absorbed dose
   d. There is no consensus regarding an expression of dose, and many units have been used

3. The unit of ionizing radiation exposure in air is the
   a. roentgen (R).
   b. radiation absorbed dose (rad).
   c. gray (Gy).
   d. sievert (Sv).
4. The unit of absorbed dose is the
   a. roentgen (R).
   b. radiation absorbed dose (rad) or gray (Gy).
   c. computed tomography dose index (CTDI).
   d. multiple scan average dose (MSAD).
5. The Système International d'Unités (SI) for ionizing radiation
   1. is used internationally.
   2. replaces the unit known as the rad.
   3. replaces the unit known as the rem.
      a. 1 only
      b. 1 and 2
      c. 1 and 3
      d. 1, 2, and 3
6. The quality factor (Q) is used to
   a. account for the different health effects produced from different types of ionizing radiation.
   b. account for the pitch in helical CT.
   c. describe exposure from scatter radiation.
   d. convert older units to SI units.
7. Which of the following statements is TRUE concerning the measurement referred to as effective dose?
   a. It is measured in rad or Gy.
   b. It is a weighted average of organ doses.
   c. There is no agreement on the weighting factors to be applied to each radiosensitive organ.
   d. It is relatively easy to calculate accurately and is therefore used universally.
8. The areas of scatter radiation into adjacent tissue are sometimes called
   a. tails.
   b. overflow.
   c. excess.
   d. collimation.
9. The dose to the central slice plus the dose from the scatter into nearby slices equals the
   a. MSAD.
   b. Sv.
   c. mAs setting.
   d. R.
10. Which is now the preferred expression of radiation dose in CT dosimetry?
    a. R
    b. $CTDI_{vol}$
    c. DLP
    d. MSAD
11. The relationship between mAs and dose is
    a. inversely proportional: the higher the mAs, the lower the dose.
    b. linear: the higher the mAs, the higher the dose.
    c. represented by the equation: dose $= 1/\sqrt{}$ (mAs).
    d. highly variable and impossible to quantify.
12. When looking at the overall radiation dose from radiologic sources, CT contributes
    a. a very low percentage of the total.

b. a proportional amount–that is, CT examinations represent approximately 11% of all diagnostic procedures and account for approximately 11% of the total dose.

c. a disproportionately high percentage of the total.

d. nearly 90% of the total.

13. Keeping in mind how a parent will perceive risk to his or her child, guidelines have been outlined for CT examinations of pediatric patients. Which of the following is NOT one of the recommendations?

a. The parent should be told that the CT examination of a child is associated with a small risk.

b. The parent should sign a consent form acknowledging that out of every 100 children who undergo CT examination, 1 will develop a fatal cancer later in life.

c. The examination should be restricted to cases in which it is specifically indicated and cannot reasonably be substituted for with a diagnostic examination that does not use ionizing radiation.

d. Scan parameters must be customized according to the size of the child being scanned.

14. The latency time for cancer induction in the dose ranges used in CT is estimated to be between

a. 10 and 30 days.

b. 1 and 5 years.

c. 10 and 30 years.

d. 40 and 60 years.

15. Children are more sensitive to radiation than are adults for all of the following reasons EXCEPT:

a. Children have more time to express a cancer than do adults.

b. In children, the latency time for cancer induction is only a few months.

c. Radiation exposure is cumulative, and children may undergo more than one CT examination in their lifetimes.

d. Children have more dividing cells, and adverse effects of radiation act on dividing cells.

16. Which of the following are strategies that may reduce the radiation dose to the patient?

1. Adjusting mAs to suit individual patient size

2. Avoid increasing kVp beyond 120

3. Increasing pitch

4. Performing multiphase studies only when clinical indications exist

a. 1 and 2

b. 1 and 3

c. 2 and 4

d. 1, 2, 3, and 4

# SECTION **III**

# Cross-Sectional Anatomy

# CHAPTER 15

# Neuroanatomy

## HEAD

### Brain

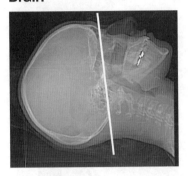

1. Eye, globe
2. Ethmoid sinus
3. Medulla oblongata
4. Eye, lens
5. Foramen lacerum
6. Vomer
7. Clivus
8. Mastoid air cells
9. Occipital bone
10. Mandibular condyle

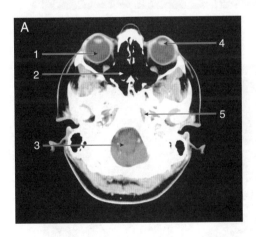

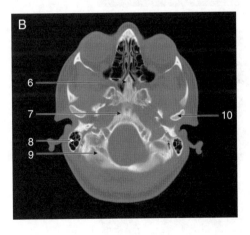

1. Cerebellum
2. Pons
3. Basilar a.
4. Sphenoid sinus
5. Frontal lobe
6. Frontal sinus
7. Crista galli
8. Temporal lobe
9. Fourth ventricle
10. Cerebellum, tentorium
11. Middle cerebral a.
12. Falx cerebri
13. Anterior cerebral a.
14. Infundibulum (pituitary stalk)
15. Cerebellum, vermis
16. Lateral ventricle, inferior horn
17. Pineal body with calcifications
18. Thalamus
19. Putamen
20. Lateral ventricle
21. Caudate nucleus
22. Internal capsule
23. Torcula (confluence of sinuses)
24. White matter
25. Pericallosal aa.
26. Central sulcus
27. Superior sagittal sinus

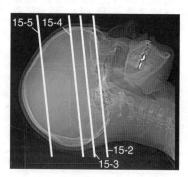

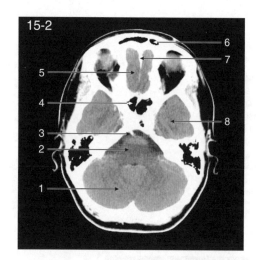

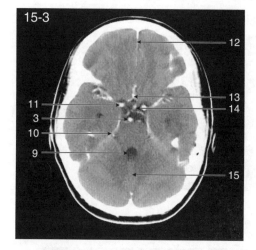

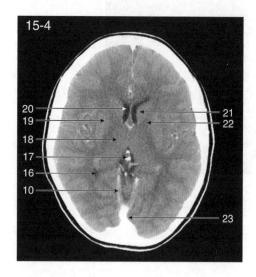

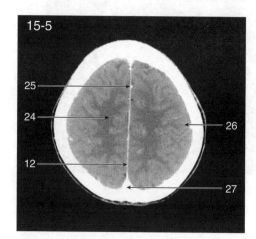

## Sinuses

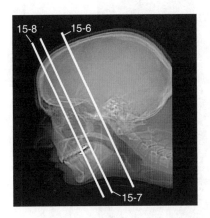

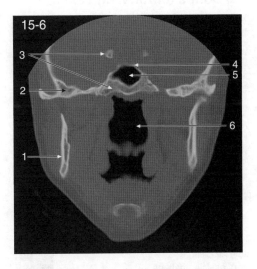

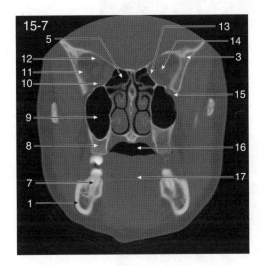

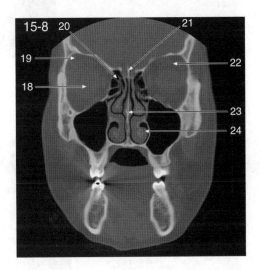

1. Mandible, right side
2. Right zygomatic arch
3. Sphenoid bones
4. Sella turcica, floor
5. Sphenoid sinus
6. Pharynx
7. Tooth
8. Right maxillary bone
9. Right maxillary sinus
10. Right inferior rectus m.
11. Right lateral rectus m.
12. Right levator palpebrae/orbicularis oculi m.

13. Left medial rectus m.
14. Left optic canal / nerve
15. Infraorbital fissure
16. Oral vestibule
17. Tongue
18. Right eye, globe
19. Lacrimal gland
20. Ethmoid sinus
21. Crista galli
22. Left superior rectus m.
23. Nasal septum/nasal bone
24. Inferior nasal turbinate

## Temporal Bones (coronal and axial)

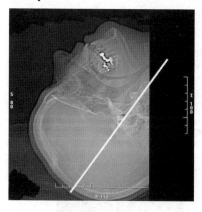

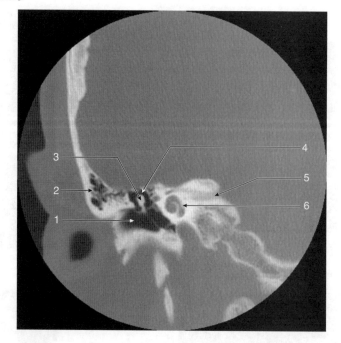

1. Tympanic cavity
2. Mastoid air cells
3. Auditory ossicle, malleus
4. Epitympanum
5. Internal auditory canal
6. Cochlea

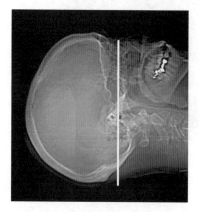

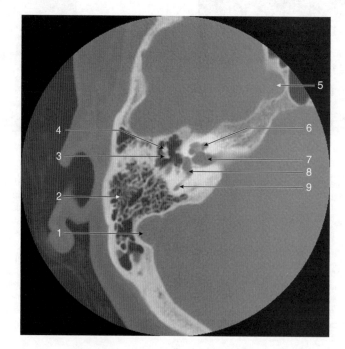

1. Sigmoid sinus
2. Mastoid air cells
3. Auditory ossicle, incus
4. Auditory ossicle, malleus
5. Carotid canal
6. Cochlea
7. Internal auditory canal
8. Vestibule
9. Semicircular canal

# NECK

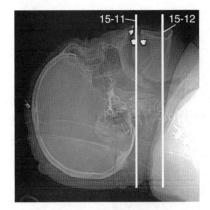

1. Dens
2. Mastoid tip
3. Right parotid gland
4. Right retromandibular v.
5. Pharynx
6. Ramus of mandible, left side
7. Atlas, anterior arch
8. Spinal cord
9. Vertebral a.
10. Sternocleidomastoid m.
11. Submandibular gland
12. Tongue
13. Genioglossus m.
14. Left internal jugular v.
15. Left external carotid a.
16. Left internal carotid a.

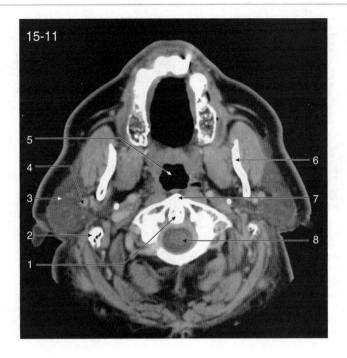

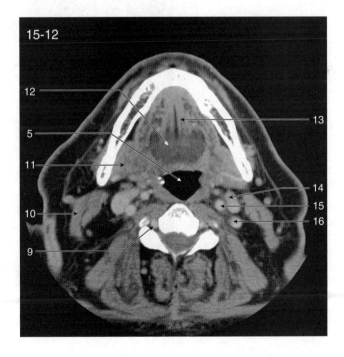

# SPINE

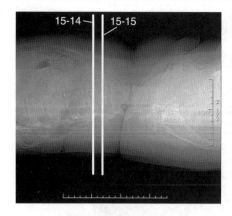

1. L1, spinous process
2. L2, transverse process
3. Lumbar vertebra 2
4. Dural sac
5. Pedicle
6. Articular facet
7. Cauda equine
8. L2, vertebral body
9. Left psoas m.
10. Nerve root
11. L2, lamina
12. Erector spinae m.
13. L2, spinous process

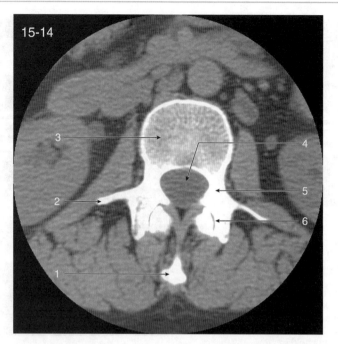

15-14

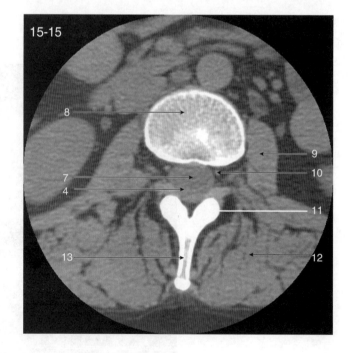

15-15

# CHAPTER 16

# Thoracic Anatomy

## CHEST

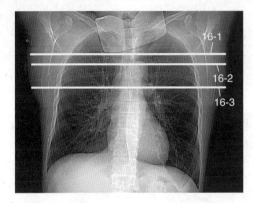

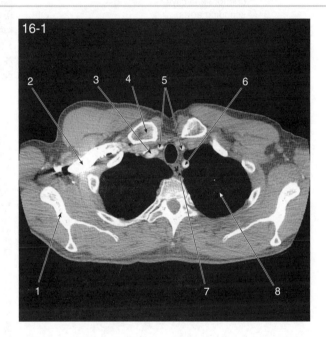

1. Right scapula
2. Right subclavian v.
3. Right subclavian a.
4. Right clavicle
5. Common carotid aa.
6. Left subclavian a.
7. Esophagus
8. Left lung
9. Trachea
10. Right brachiocephalic v.
11. Left brachiocephalic v.
12. Aortic arch
13. Ribs, left side
14. Trachea (carina)
15. Ascending aorta
16. Sternum
17. Left pulmonary a.
18. Pulmonary vessels
19. Descending aorta
20. Intercostal m.
21. Superior vena cava

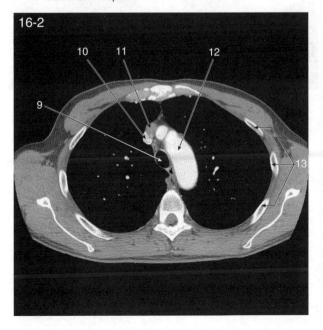

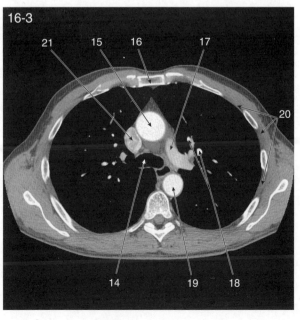

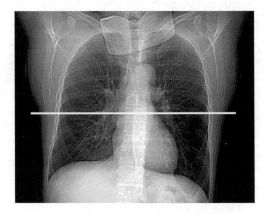

1. Right lower lobe segmental a.
2. Superior vena cava
3. Ascending aorta
4. Main pulmonary a.
5. Left lung
6. Left atrium
7. Left superior pulmonary v.
8. Descending aorta
9. Right bronchus intermedius
10. Right interlobar pulmonary a.
11. Lingula bronchus
12. Left lower lobe pulmonary a.
13. Left lower lobe bronchus

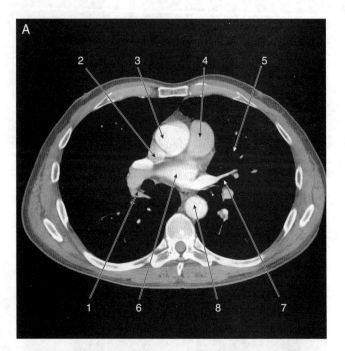

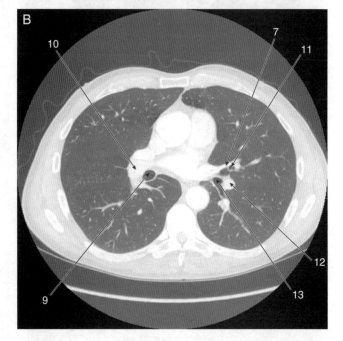

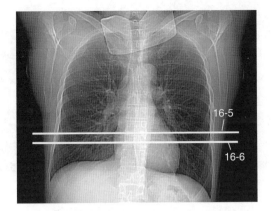

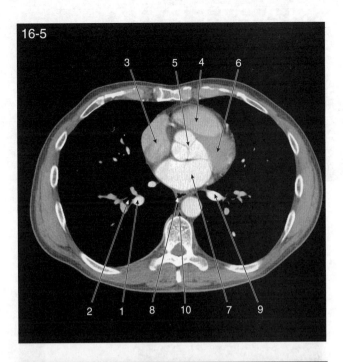

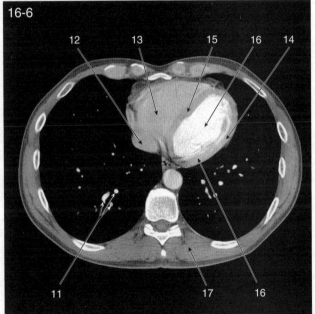

1. Inferior pulmonary v.
2. Right lower lobe segmental bronchus
3. Right atrium
4. Right ventricle
5. Aortic valve
6. Left ventricle
7. Left atrium
8. Esophagus
9. Left inferior pulmonary v.
10. Azygos v.
11. Pulmonary vessels
12. Inferior vena cava
13. Right ventricle
14. Pericardium
15. Interventricular septum
16. Left ventricle
17. Erector spinae m.

# CHAPTER 17

# Abdominopelvic Anatomy

## ABDOMEN/PELVIS

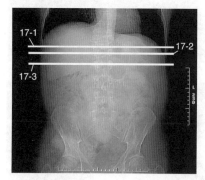

1. Diaphragm
2. Inferior vena cava
3. Hepatic v.
4. Portal v.
5. Liver, right lobe
6. Falciform lig.
7. Left gastric a. and left gastric v.
8. Stomach (barium-filled)
9. Splenic a.
10. Spleen
11. Left lung
12. Left kidney
13. Right adrenal gland
14. Liver, caudate lobe
15. Pancreas
16. Air in stomach
17. Colon, transverse
18. Splenic v.
19. Left adrenal gland
20. Left kidney, cortex
21. Left kidney, medulla
22. Gallbladder
23. Duodenum
24. Pancreas, head
25. Portal v., confluence
26. Jejunum/ileum
27. Left renal v.
28. Aorta, descending

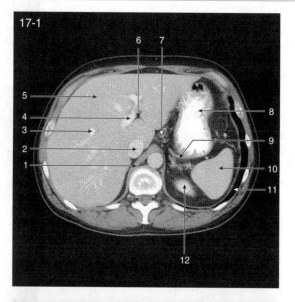

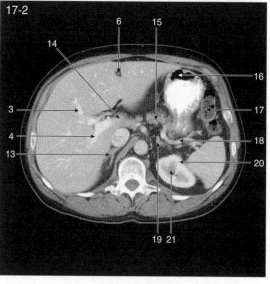

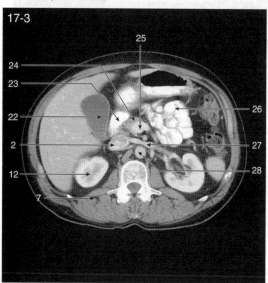

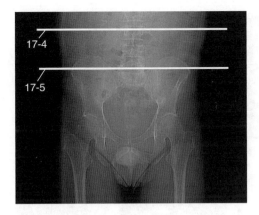

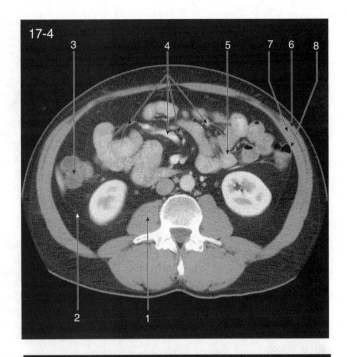

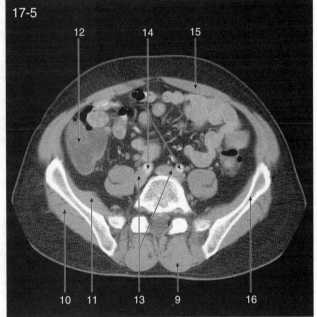

1. Psoas m.
2. Fascia, renal
3. Ascending colon
4. Mesenteric vessels
5. Jejunum/ileum
6. Abdominal wall, external oblique m.
7. Abdominal wall, internal oblique m.
8. Abdominal wall, transverse m.
9. Erector spinae m.
10. Gluteus medius m.
11. Iliacus m.
12. Cecum
13. Common iliac vv.
14. Common iliac aa.
15. Rectus abdominus m.
16. Left ilium

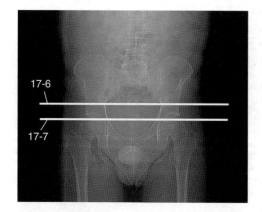

1. Sacrum
2. Gluteus maximus m.
3. Ilium
4. Right external iliac v.
5. Right external iliac a.
6. Bladder
7. Sigmoid colon
8. Left piriformis m.
9. Coccyx
10. Right ischium (ramus)
11. Right femoral head
12. Pubis (body)
13. Seminal vessicles
14. Obturator internus m.
15. Rectum

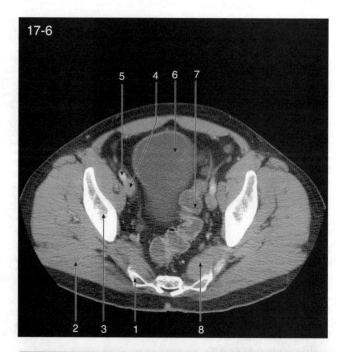

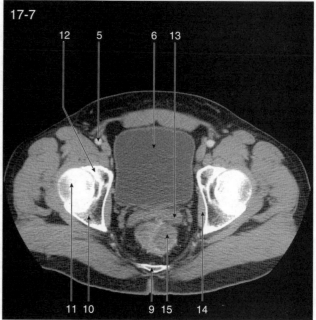

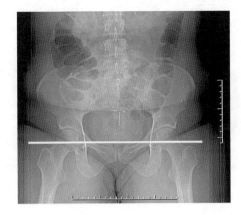

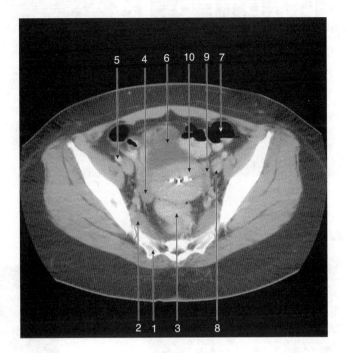

1. Sacrum
2. Piriformis m.
3. Rectum
4. Right ovary
5. Right external iliac a.
6. Bladder
7. Colon, sigmoid
8. Left external iliac v.
9. Left ovary
10. Uterus (with IUD present)

# CHAPTER 18

# Musculoskeletal Anatomy

## WRIST

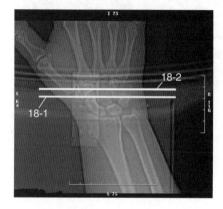

1. Trapezium
2. Scaphoid
3. Capitate
4. Hamate
5. Triquetrum
6. Pisiform
7. First metacarpal
8. Hamate, hook
9. Trapezoid

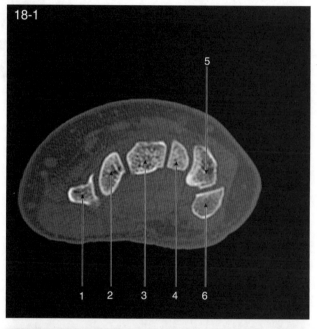

18-1

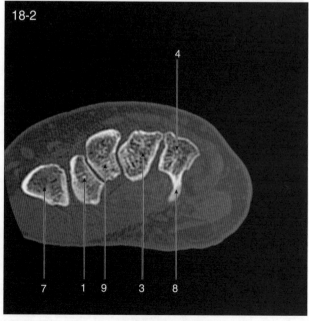

18-2

# HIP

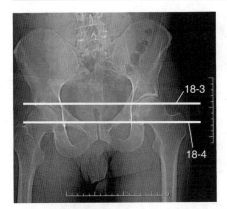

1. Hip joint
2. Fovea capitus femoris
3. Acetabulum (anterior column)
4. Acetabulum
5. Femoral head
6. Acetabulum (posterior column)
7. Ischium
8. Pubis
9. Femoral neck
10. Greater trochanter

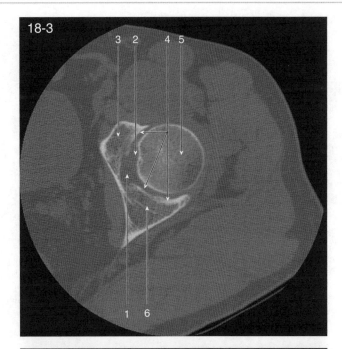

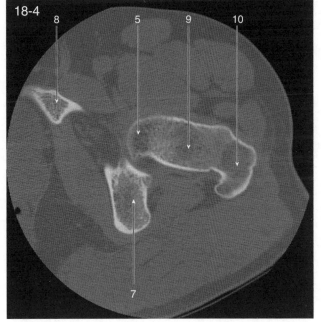

## KNEE (LEFT)

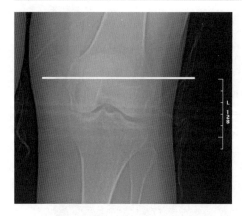

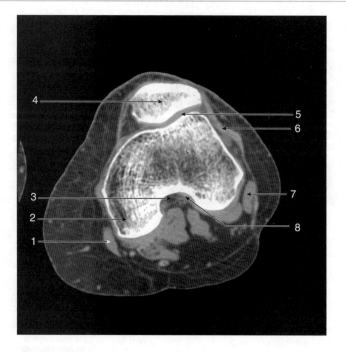

1. Sartorius m.
2. Medial femoral condyle
3. Intercondylar fossa
4. Patella
5. Patellofemoral joint
6. Patellar lig.
7. Biceps femoris m.
8. Anterior cruciate lig.

# FOOT (RIGHT)

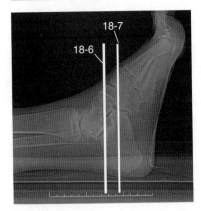

1. Achilles tendon
2. Calcaneus
3. Talus
4. Navicular
5. Calcaneus, sustentaculum
6. Cuboid
7. Cuneiform, lateral (3rd)
8. Cuneiform, intermedial (2nd)
9. Cuneiform, medial (1st)

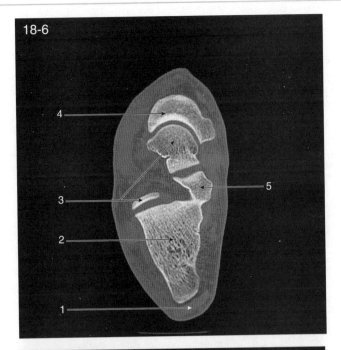

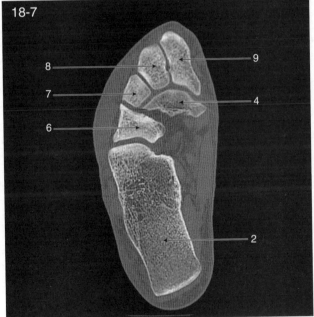

# SECTION **IV**

# Imaging Procedures and Protocols

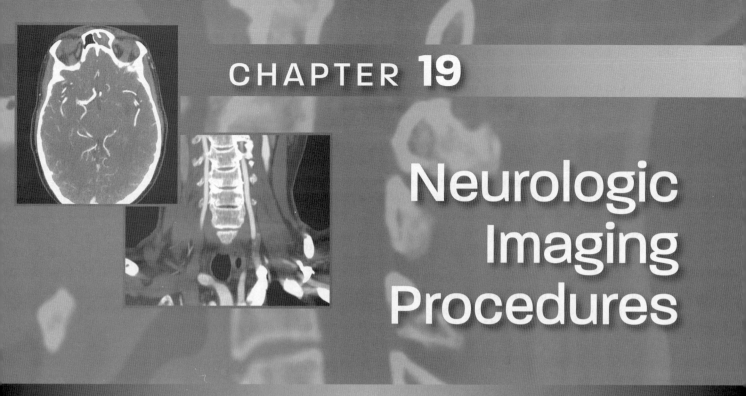

# Neurologic Imaging Procedures

## HEAD PROTOCOLS

### Routine Brain Imaging

■ Before the examination begins, the patient should be made as comfortable as possible and immobilized as effectively as possible to prevent motion artifact on the images. This is often accomplished by placing small wedge sponges on either side of the patient's head.

■ It is not necessary to ask the patient to suspend breathing for CT studies of the head or neck.

■ Anatomy displayed in cross-sectional slices will look slightly different depending on the angulation used.

■ The slice angle is determined by the position of the patient's head (i.e., moving the chin up or down) and the angle of the gantry.

● It was once common to plan the cross-sectional slices of the brain to be parallel to the orbitomeatal line; however, more recent practice favors using the supraorbital meatal line (also called the glabellomeatal line) to avoid radiation exposure to the lens of the eye.

■ A disadvantage of many multidetector CT systems is that they do not allow the gantry to be tilted when in helical mode. Therefore, axial (step-and-shoot) techniques are often used for routine brain imaging.

■ Imaging the posterior fossa of the brain is a challenge in CT scanning. Because of the great difference in beam attenuation ability between the dense bone of the skull and the much less dense tissue of the brain, streak artifacts are common.

● This inherent limitation may be managed by decreasing slice thickness when scanning the posterior fossa and increasing the kVp setting.

■ Modern multislice CT scanners allow studies of the head to be routinely acquired with thinner slices than in the past–1.25 mm thickness is typical. These thin slices help to reduce beam-hardening artifacts. Images are often merged into thicker slices for viewing.

■ In examinations of the head, helical CT is used mainly for the purpose of generating three-dimensional reformations or to minimize motion-related artifacts. In general, routine head studies are done using an axial mode, and CT angiography (CTA) studies of the head and neck are done using a helical mode.

■ Cross-sectional slices of the brain are viewed in multiple window settings. Standard window settings include

● Soft tissue (brain) 160/40 for slices in the posterior fossa, 100/30 for slices above

● Bone (particularly on trauma or postoperative patients) 2,500/400

● Blood 200/60

■ Depending on the clinical indication, CT studies of the brain may be done without contrast or may include a noncontrasted series followed by a series with contrast enhancement.

● Clinical indications for noncontrast brain CT include intracranial hemorrhage (ICH), early infarction, dementia, hydrocephalus, and cerebral trauma.

- Clinical indications for an examination that is performed first without contrast and then with contrast enhancement include mass, lesion, arteriovenous malformation (AVM), metastasis, and aneurysm; also for symptoms of headache and seizure.
- CT is the most frequently used initial examination for imaging of ICH. The appearance of an ICH will change with the passage of time. These changes are complex and depend on many factors. As a general rule, ICH will appear hyperdense to normal brain tissue for approximately 3 days, after which it will gradually decrease in density, eventually becoming hypodense to normal brain tissue.
- When iodinated contrast is indicated, the dose is typically between 90 and 125 mL (300 concentration agent); compared with other CT studies, it is typically delivered somewhat slowly, approximately 1.0 mL/s, and a delay of 5 minutes (from the start of the injection to the initiation of image acquisition) is common.
  - The scan delay allows time for contrast media to leak across a disrupted blood-brain barrier.

### Other Head Protocols

- High spatial resolution is vital for studies of the temporal bones so that the small bones of the inner ear can be adequately displayed. Therefore, temporal bone protocols typically include very thin slices (≤1.0 mm). To further improve spatial resolution, images are often reconstructed using a small display field of view (DFOV) in which each side is displayed separately.
- Depending on the clinical indication, temporal bone studies may be done without contrast enhancement or with contrast enhancement. In some facilities, they are done both without and with contrast enhancement.
  - Clinical indications for noncontrasted temporal bone studies include cholesteatoma, inflammatory disease, fractures, and to evaluate implants.
  - Clinical indications for contrasted temporal bone studies include internal auditory canal tumor, hearing loss, acoustic neuroma, and schwannoma.
  - Temporal bones are most often scanned in both transverse and coronal planes.
  - Data are reconstructed in both a soft tissue and bone algorithm.
- Sinus screening is intended as an inexpensive, accurate, and low radiation dose method for confirming the presence of inflammatory sinonasal disease. If confirmed and the patient will then have endoscopic sinus surgery, the coronal images provide a useful guide to the surgeon.

- Sinus screening is done without IV contrast enhancement.
- Studies of the facial bones and orbits are frequently done after trauma, where they are done without IV contrast enhancement, most often in the transverse plane only (as the trauma patient is unlikely to be able to tolerate the coronal position). When the clinical indication for the study is inflammation, infection, or mass, the study is done with IV contrast enhancement, most often in both the transverse and coronal planes.
- Studies of the dorsum sella are most often done with IV contrast enhancement in both the transverse and coronal planes. Clinical indications for this examination include pituitary mass, microadenoma, and parasellar masses.

## NECK PROTOCOLS

- Routine scanning of the neck is typically performed with the patient supine and the neck slightly extended.
- Neck studies are most often performed in the helical mode.
- Unless contraindicated, IV contrast media is used when scanning the neck. The goals in CT scanning of the neck are to allow sufficient time after contrast administration for mucosa, lymph nodes, and pathologic tissues to enhance, yet acquire images while the vasculature remains opacified. Scanning too early after the contrast media injection could result in certain types of neoplastic and inflammatory diseases going undetected. However, by delaying scan acquisition, the injected contrast agent will no longer fully opacify the vasculature. One strategy for addressing these contradictory goals is a contrast injection technique referred to as a split bolus.
  - The total contrast dose is split, often in half. The first dose is given, and a delay of about 2 minutes is observed. This allows time for structures that are slower to enhance to be opacified. The delay is followed by a second bolus containing the remainder of the contrast; scanning is initiated soon after the second injection is complete. The split bolus injection technique is also frequently used for maxillofacial studies when contrast media is indicated.

## CTA OF THE HEAD AND NECK

- Advances in multidetector CT systems and image postprocessing techniques have expanded the role that CT plays in the evaluation of cervicocranial vascular disease.

- Cerebral catheter angiography or digital subtraction angiography (both performed in the interventional radiology department) is still generally regarded as the gold standard for the imaging of cerebrovascular disorders. However, those techniques are time consuming and are associated with a small, but significant, rate of permanent neurologic complications.
- CT angiography has the advantages of being noninvasive and widely available. The time-saving nature of CTA over traditional angiography is particularly important in the case of patients suspected of suffering an acute stroke in which treatment decisions must be made quickly.
- In addition, cerebral CTA can be combined with brain perfusion imaging to also assess brain parenchyma and its vascular supply.
- Cerebral and carotid CTA techniques provide important information about vessel walls; three-dimensional postprocessing of the image data depicts the spatial relationship of complex vascular lesions to the surrounding structures, providing valuable information for the surgeon.
- Rapid, high-resolution scans are taken while contrast is in the arterial enhancement phase.
- The goals of CTA for cervicocranial vascular evaluation can be summarized:
  - To accurately measure carotid stenosis
  - To evaluate the circle of Willis for completeness using three-dimensional reformations of cerebral vasculature in relation to other structures
  - To detect other vascular lesions, such as dissections
- A modification of CTA, called CT venography (CTV), is used for the depiction of venous anatomy. Scan parameters are quite similar to CTA, except images are acquired while contrast is in the venous enhancement phase.

## SPINE PROTOCOLS

- Compared with conventional radiography, CT examinations of the spine produce images with inherently high soft tissue contrast. This contrast permits the visualization of structures such as the intervertebral disks, ligaments, and muscle, as well as bone detail.
- Visualization of intradural structure is improved by the intrathecal administration of water-soluble contrast material. CT examinations are performed after myelography to enhance or clarify myelographic findings of intradural and extradural abnormalities.
- Most reports suggest a delay of 1 to 3 hours between the intrathecal injection and scanning. This delay allows the contrast material to dilute. If the scans are performed while the contrast material is too dense, intradural structures may be masked. Rolling the patient once or twice before scanning is recommended to mix the contrast material that may have settled since the myelogram.
- In some situations, magnetic resonance imaging (MRI) provides even higher soft tissue sensitivity than does CT, and is the modality of choice when imaging the spine for certain indications such as multiple sclerosis and hydromyelia.
- For some conditions, such as spinal stenosis, MRI is equivalent to CT.
- In some situations, CT is considered superior to MRI, such as in the evaluation of bony abnormalities of the spine.
- Proper localization is essential in scanning the spine.
  - All studies should include scout images in both anteroposterior (AP) and lateral projections. The scouts will permit vertebral levels to be readily counted and classified to ensure that scans are taken at the appropriate levels.
  - When scanning the lumbar spine, it is important to note whether the patient has a sixth lumbar vertebra that requires additional scans.
- CTA of the spine is a newer protocol that can demonstrate the spinal vessels. Clinical indications for spinal CTA include localization of the shunt of spinal dural arteriovenous fistulas, spinal AVM, and blunt trauma suspected of causing spinal vascular injury.

## THE EVALUATION OF STROKE

- A reduction of blood flow for even a short period can be disastrous and is the primary cause of a stroke.
- Therapeutic options, such a thrombolytic therapy (i.e., tissue plasminogen activator or t-PA), can limit the extent of brain injury and improve outcome after stroke when administered to patients who fall within narrow clinical guidelines.
- However, these therapies may result in potentially life-threatening complications, drawbacks that make it crucial that each case be assessed by its individual risk-benefit ratio.
  - Most important, the location and extent of the ischemic lesion, combined with the severity of the blood flow reduction, are the main factors that predict outcome in the treatment of stroke. These factors demand an assessment of cerebral blood circulation to determine whether a conservative or a more aggressive therapy is needed in the early stage of stroke.
  - CT imaging plays an important role in identifying patients who may be candidates for t-PA therapy.

- Stroke may be divided into two main categories: ischemic, caused by a blockage in an artery, and hemorrhagic, caused by a tear in the artery's wall that produces bleeding in the brain.
  - Ischemic strokes are by far the more common, accounting for 80% of all strokes. Ischemia is defined as a deficiency of oxygen in vital tissues. The two main types of ischemic stroke are thrombotic, which are caused from a blood clot or a fatty deposit within one of the brain's arteries, and embolic, which result from a traveling particle that forms elsewhere and is too large to pass through small vessels and eventually lodges in a smaller artery.
- Hemorrhagic stroke occurs from the rupture of a blood vessel in the brain that causes leakage of blood into the brain parenchyma, cerebrospinal fluid (CSF) spaces around the brain, or both. Approximately 20% of strokes occur from hemorrhage. Hemorrhagic strokes are classified by how and where they occur.
  - Intracerebral hemorrhagic strokes occur within the brain parenchyma itself and an actual hematoma often results. These strokes account for more than half of hemorrhagic strokes. Most often, they result from hypertension, which exerts excessive pressure on arterial walls already damaged by atherosclerosis.
  - Subarachnoid hemorrhagic strokes occur when there is bleeding into the subarachnoid spaces and the CSF spaces. These strokes are usually caused by the rupture of an aneurysm.
  - Arteriovenous malformations (AVMs) are composed of tangles of arteries and arterialized veins. When an AVM exists, blood is shunted directly from the arterial system to the venous system. This results in elevated pressure in the vessels and can cause the vessels to rupture, resulting in a hemorrhagic stroke.
- The treatment known as t-PA can only be used for acute ischemic stroke.
- To be effective, t-PA must be administered within 3 hours of the first signs of stroke. This means that the stroke victim must be transported to the hospital, diagnosed, and administered the t-PA treatment before the 3-hour window has expired.
- The target of t-PA therapy is the tissue known as penumbra. After an acute ischemic stroke, areas of tissue death (infarction) occur because of a local lack of oxygen. The penumbra is ischemic tissue that is destined for infarction but is not yet irreversibly injured. It is the penumbra that may be salvageable with the administration of t-PA. The infarcted tissue will not benefit from reperfusion after t-PA and may be at increased risk of hemorrhage. However, if reperfusion of the penumbra occurs expeditiously, the tissue will recover and the patient improves. This is why the timing of t-PA therapy is so critical.
- Stroke experts commonly refer to the sense of urgency in stroke treatment with the expression "time is brain."
- Published guidelines recommend that the time between arriving in the emergency room and actual treatment should be 60 minutes or less. During this hour, various tests must be performed, including a neurologic examination, blood tests, and a CT scan of the head to determine whether hemorrhage has occurred and contraindicates t-PA.
- Fast diagnosis of both the presence and type of stroke is critical in saving lives and reducing the likelihood of severe disability. Patients must be carefully selected because the treatment itself can cause bleeding that can be lethal if the stroke is hemorrhagic in origin.
- Although MRI can also be used to evaluate stroke patients for possible thrombolytic therapy, CT is used more frequently. This is because the imaging tool must be used quickly, and CT is much more available than is MRI. In addition, CT is regarded as more practical because the imaging time is shorter, it is better tolerated by many patients, and all relevant information is provided with only one imaging sequence.
- A noncontrast CT of the brain is routinely performed to assess the state of cerebral circulation and tissue and, secondarily, to assess the underlying disease.
- Although less common, studies such as CT perfusion and CTA are sometimes done in addition to the noncontrast CT scan.

## CT BRAIN PERFUSION SCANS

- CT perfusion techniques measure cerebral blood flow, whereas CTA of the carotid arteries and vessels of the circle of Willis can demonstrate stenosis or occlusion of extracranial and intracranial arteries.
- CT perfusion provides valuable information by calculating blood flow (rCBF) and blood volume (rCBV) and mean transit time (MTT). A workstation equipped with commercially available perfusion software is necessary to perform these calculations.
- Perfusion studies are obtained by monitoring the passage of iodinated contrast through the cerebral vasculature.
- Attractive characteristics of this approach are the widespread availability of CT scanners, their high image quality, and relatively low costs. In addition,

simply extending the routine CT examination eliminates time-consuming transport of patients between scanners that serves to further delay treatment.

■ The goal in performing perfusion studies for patients with acute stroke is to distinguish infarcted tissue from the penumbra.

■ The most common technique associated with CT perfusion scanning is based on the first pass of a contrast bolus through the brain tissue. With this technique, a 50-mL bolus of a low-osmolality IV contrast is injected at 4 to 5 mL/s. A helical scanner is used to produce a dynamic set of images at a single location. A 5-second scan delay is used; slices are typically 5 mm thick. Typical scan durations are in the range of 40 to 45 seconds.

  ● The slices are produced by repeatedly scanning the same region at the same table position, a technique some manufacturers refer to as the cine mode. Scans are typically acquired at 1.25-mm sections to lessen beam-hardening artifacts, then reformatted into 5-mm-thick sections for viewing to improve the signal-to-noise ratio.

  ● The brain perfusion protocol begins with an unenhanced scan of the whole brain.

  ● The most common level for scanning the enhanced portion of the study is that of the basal ganglia. This level contains territories supplied by the anterior, middle, and posterior cerebral arteries, thus offering the opportunity to interrogate each of the major vascular regions.

  ● Brain perfusion studies are frequently ordered with a CTA of the circle of Willis or the carotid arteries. In these situations, the CTA should be performed first; the brain perfusion study can immediately follow.

■ CT perfusion is most frequently ordered in the evaluation of acute stroke. Other clinical indications include vasospasm, tumor grading, and determining cerebrovascular reserve. It can also be used in conjunction with temporary balloon occlusion protocols.

## REVIEW QUESTIONS

1. A patient is being positioned for a routine scan of the brain. Why is he asked to tuck his chin down toward his chest?
   a. So that the scan time can be reduced
   b. To allow immobilization sponges to be used
   c. To reduce the radiation exposure to the lens of the eyes
   d. To eliminate the need to tilt the gantry so that the axial scan mode can be used

2. What is the expected HU value of a measurement taken in a lateral ventricle?
   a. −70 to −60
   b. 4 to 8
   c. 20 to 30
   d. 40 to 50

3. Which is a typical injection protocol for a routine examination of the brain?
   a. 100 mL delivered at 1 mL/s, scan delay of 5 minutes
   b. 150 mL delivered at 2 mL/s, scans begin when injection is complete
   c. Split bolus: 50 mL delivered at 1.5 mL/s, wait 2 minutes, 50 mL delivered at 1.5 mL/s, scans begin when second injection is complete
   d. 60 mL (concentration 370), delivered at 4 mL/s, scan delay from timing bolus using the carotid artery as the reference vessel

4. Compared with a cerebral CTA, what parameter must be changed for a cerebral CTV?
   a. Slice thickness is reduced.
   b. Delay from the start of injection to the start of scanning is increased.
   c. Scans are performed in the axial mode, rather than the helical mode.
   d. kVp is increased.

5. Which is a TRUE statement regarding an emergency department patient who is suspected of suffering from acute stroke?
   a. A CT scan of the head is only done if the patient has a previous history of stroke.
   b. An MRI of the head is the first choice of imaging procedures; a CT of the head is only done if an MRI cannot be done within 24 hours.
   c. A CT scan of the head must be done as soon as possible because it is a necessary examination in determining whether a patient can receive t-PA treatment.
   d. An unenhanced CT scan will provide no useful information in the diagnosis and treatment of acute stroke. Only CTA and CT perfusion studies are indicated.

6. What is the goal in performing perfusion studies for patients with acute stroke?
   a. To determine whether the stroke is hemorrhagic or ischemic
   b. To determine the onset time of the stroke
   c. To depict the spatial relationship of complex vascular lesions to the surrounding structures
   d. To distinguish infarcted tissue from the penumbra

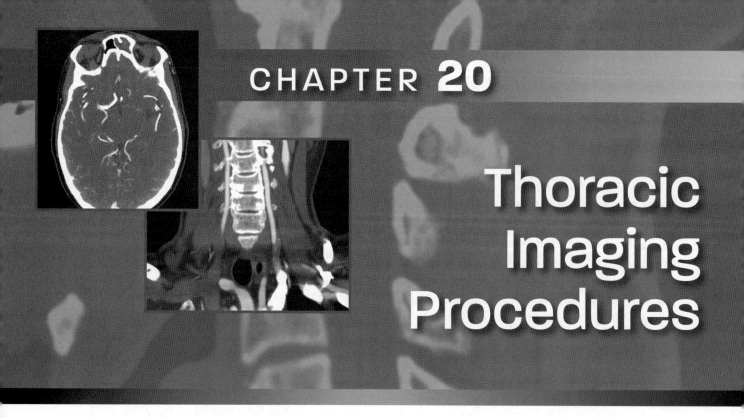

# CHAPTER 20

# Thoracic Imaging Procedures

## GENERAL THORACIC SCANNING METHODS

- CT imaging of the organs of the chest presents unique challenges because of their continuous motion. Improvements in speed and spatial resolution that have been realized as a result of multidetector-row CT (MDCT) and dual source scanners have been particularly valuable in thoracic imaging.
- Postprocessing techniques such as three-dimensional and multiplanar reformation can accurately display the pulmonary and coronary vasculature. These new, noninvasive CT imaging techniques can augment, and sometimes replace, more invasive methods such as coronary angiography.
- Most thoracic protocols are performed while the patient lies in a supine position on the scan table with the arms elevated above the head. In a few instances, primarily high-resolution protocols of the chest, additional scans are obtained with the patient in the prone position.
- Using the shortest scan time possible will help to reduce artifacts created by cardiac motion. Whenever possible, scans of the chest should be acquired within a single breath-hold as this will prevent misregistration caused by uneven patient breathing between scans.
- The thorax has the highest intrinsic natural contrast of any body part. The pulmonary vessels and ribs have significantly different densities from the adjacent aerated lung. In most adults, the mediastinal vessels and lymph nodes are surrounded by enough fat to be easily identified.
  - Because of this intrinsic natural contrast, intravenous (IV) iodinated contrast administration is not necessary for all thoracic indications. For example, scans done for the screening, detection, or exclusion of pulmonary nodes or infiltrates are typically done without IV contrast administration.
- The demarcation of the esophagus can be improved by giving the patient an oral agent, most often a barium suspension, shortly before beginning the scan.

## CT of the Airways

- Technical parameters used for CT imaging of the airways include the use of thin sections (1.25 mm or less), a fast acquisition that allows the entire lungs to be scanned during a single breath-hold, optimal spatial resolution, and the use of postprocessing techniques.
- Overlapping $z$ axis image reconstruction of 50% is typical.
- Neither IV nor oral contrast media are required.
- Airway imaging is routinely performed at expiration.
- Applying postprocessing techniques such as volume rendering is referred to as CT bronchography. Virtual bronchoscopy is accomplished with similar postprocessing techniques but is different in that it offers an internal rendering of the tracheobronchial walls and lumen.

## High-Resolution CT

- High-resolution CT (HRCT) is used for the assessment of the lung parenchyma in patients with diffuse lung disease such as fibrosis and emphysema.
- HRCT protocols use thin sections (1.25 mm or less), a fast acquisition, and optimal spatial resolution.
  - Spatial resolution is further optimized by the selection of an algorithm (such as a bone algorithm) and a display field of view (DFOV) that is just large enough to include the lungs (Chapter 6).
- In many facilities, HRCT protocols are designed so that only 10% of the lung parenchyma is scanned. This is accomplished by obtaining a thin slice, in the axial mode, with an interval of 10 mm or more between slices. This technique is intended to provide representative areas of lung disease. However, because evidence of some types of diffuse lung disease may not be uniform in distribution throughout the lung, this method of sampling may result in characteristic foci of the disease not being imaged.
- More recently, as MDCT scanners have become commonplace, the technique known as volumetric HRCT is replacing the HRCT axial protocols.
  - Volumetric HRCT protocols use a helical mode to acquire images of the entire lung, rather than representative slices.
  - These helical protocols cover the entire lung so they result in a more complete assessment of the lung. In addition, they allow postprocessing techniques such as maximum (MIP) and minimum (MinIP) intensity projection reformation.
  - Although there are clear advantages to the use of volumetric HRCT over an interspaced technique, the increased radiation exposure is a consideration. Many volumetric HRCT protocols decrease the tube current (mA) to reduce the radiation dose.
- HRCT protocols (both volumetric and axial) often include more than one series of scans. When the patient is supine, the effect of gravity results in a gradual increase in attenuation and vessel size from posterior to anterior lung regions.
  - An additional series of prone images can help to differentiate actual disease from densities caused by the effects of gravity that mimic disease in some patients.
  - In addition, anatomic detail is displayed somewhat differently in inspiratory scans compared with expiratory scans. When the lungs are fully expanded, the contrast between low-attenuation aerated air space and high-attenuation lung structure is maximized. However, expiratory images are useful in many instances. For example, expiratory images better depict bronchiolitis and air trapping.
  - Hence, HRCT protocols may include three series of scans: inspiratory supine, expiratory supine, and inspiratory prone. In volumetric protocols, only the inspiratory supine series is done in a helical mode. The additional images are done in the representative axial fashion to reduce the radiation dose.

## CT Lung Volume/Density

- Measurements of lung volume are useful for diagnosing and stratifying lung disease.
- Traditionally, functional lung volume is measured with a pulmonary function test (PFT). With advances in quantitative CT analysis techniques, the use of CT to assess lung volume and analyze lung density has been increasing and playing a role in respiratory medicine.
- Using specialized software images from both the supine inspiration and the supine expiration series are postprocessed using a threshold-based, three-dimensional autosegmentation technique.

# THORACIC CTA

- The MDCT advantages of high temporal and spatial resolution are particularly well suited to accurately image the heart and thoracic vessels and have resulted in many new scanning protocols.
- The discussion of the use of MDCT in the diagnosis of pulmonary embolism (PE) illustrates many of the issues that must be addressed in CT angiography (CTA) examinations of the thorax. However, the detection of PE is just one of many indications for chest CTA.

## CTA of Pulmonary Embolism

- MDCT angiography has become an imaging mainstay in the diagnosis of pulmonary embolism (PE).

### Anatomy and Terminology Review

- The formation, development, or existence of a clot within the vascular system is referred to as thrombosis. If the thrombus occludes a vessel, it can stop the blood supply to an organ.
  - If the thrombus detaches from its original site, it is referred to as an embolus. In addition to clotted blood, an embolus can be formed from fat, air, tumor, or tumor tissue.
  - The embolus is carried through the bloodstream and can ultimately occlude a vessel at

a distance from its origin. For example, thrombus that originated in a patient's leg veins after a hip fracture may travel up the inferior vena cava, through the right atrium, right ventricle, and pulmonary trunk to the right pulmonary artery. There, the thrombus may lodge against the openings of branches too narrow to contain them. This patient is suffering from pulmonary embolism, a life-threatening condition.

- Pulmonary emboli can be caused by clots from the venous circulation, the right side of the heart, tumors that have invaded the circulatory system, or other sources such as amniotic fluid, air, fat, bone marrow, and foreign substances. Pulmonary emboli may arise within the body, or they may gain entrance from external forces, as sometimes occurs after a compound fracture. Most pulmonary emboli are caused from thrombi originating in the lower extremities, known as deep vein thrombosis (DVT).

## Circulation

- The circular pattern of blood flow from the left ventricle of the heart through blood vessels to all parts of the body and back to the right atrium is referred to as the systemic circulation.
- Pulmonary circulation describes venous blood that moves from the right atrium to the right ventricle to the pulmonary artery to the lung and capillaries. Here, exchange of gases between blood and air occurs, which involves conversion of venous blood to arterial blood. This oxygenated blood then flows on through lung venules into four pulmonary veins and returns to the left atrium of the heart. From the left atrium, it enters the left ventricle to be pumped again through the systemic circulation.

## Pulmonary Artery

- The pulmonary artery follows closely the subdivision of the bronchial tree.
- The main pulmonary artery divides into right and left pulmonary arteries. Each of these divides into two branches, one going to the upper lobe, and one supplying the middle and lower lobes. After entering the hilum, the left pulmonary artery divides into many branches.
- According to the angle at which vessels and bronchi leave the hilum or return to it, a CT scan will show them as round, oval, or elongated shapes. Vertical tubular structures will be cut as a round section; those with a gentle slant as oval; and those that lie almost horizontal will be cut as long shadows.

### Other Diagnostic Options

- PE is a relatively common condition. Untreated, PE is associated with a 30% death rate.
  - Compared with PE, DVT is less difficult to diagnose, and alone, it very rarely causes death.
- The timely and accurate diagnosis of acute PE is crucial to providing appropriate patient care and reducing mortality.
- Before the routine use of CTA, the nuclear medicine study ventilation-perfusion scans (or VQ scans) was the imaging study of choice in the diagnosis of PE. VQ studies do not directly visualize the emboli, but instead look for inequalities of perfusion and ventilation. The use of VQ scanning in the diagnosis of PE is declining owing to the high percentage (up to 73%) of studies performed in which the results are indeterminate.
- Pulmonary angiography has long been considered the gold standard in the diagnosis of acute PE. However, it has several shortcomings. It is invasive and expensive and has been associated with a small but significant risk of major complications. In addition, it is not universally available.
- A laboratory test known as D-dimer enzyme-linked immunosorbent assays (ELISA) can play a valuable role in the workup for possible PE. This inexpensive blood test can be used as a screening tool for suspected PE.
  - If D-dimer values are within the normal range, there is a very low likelihood of PE.
  - Unfortunately, an abnormal D-dimer value does not confirm the presence of PE as many other etiologies may result in elevated D-dimer assays, including cancer, myocardial infarction, pneumonia, sepsis, and pregnancy.
  - Therefore, this test is usually done with the understanding that an elevated value indicates the necessity for further diagnostic tests.

### CT Angiography

- Helical CT offers direct visualization of the pulmonary vasculature and, as a substitute for VQ or angiography, plays a major role in the detection of both acute and chronic thromboembolic disease.
- In addition to imaging the pulmonary arterial system, CT venography (CTV) may be performed to assess for venous thrombosis within the pelvis and lower extremities.
- This is accomplished by obtaining a second scan series in a delayed venous phase (180 seconds after IV contrast injection) from the iliac crest through the knees.
- MDCT technology allows scans to be obtained while iodinated contrast in the pulmonary arteries is at its peak. Narrow slices improve spatial resolu-

tion and visualization of small vessels. Slices can be reconstructed at overlapping intervals to further improve resolution.

- Another advantage of CT is that it is often helpful in establishing an alternative diagnosis in the absence of demonstrable PE. It can detect other abnormalities that may be contributing to the patient's symptoms such as congestive heart failure, pneumonia, interstitial lung disease, aortic dissection, malignancy, and pleural disease.
- MDCT in the diagnosis of PE has some limitations. Although larger emboli can still be diagnosed even in technically limited studies, the visualization of smaller arteries can be affected by problems with technique or suboptimal vessel opacification.
  - Breathing motion affects the peripheral (subsegmental) arteries more, although the central and segmental arteries can still usually be evaluated even in studies limited by patient breathing.
  - In some institutions, PE scanning is performed in the caudal-to-cranial direction. Respiratory motion, which is greatest at the lung bases, can make interpretation difficult. Scanning in a caudal-to-cranial direction minimizes respiratory artifact.
  - Overt patient motion will create artifacts that can greatly degrade image quality. A patient must be able to lie still for the length of time required to complete the test.
  - The need for contrast material can limit the use of helical CT. The most common contraindications for evaluating PE with helical CT are contrast material allergy and renal impairment.
- The radiation dose delivered requires careful consideration in developing protocols. For most patients, the benefits of using CT for diagnosing PE outweigh the risks. The decision to use CT for young or pregnant woman, particularly those at low-to-moderate clinical suspicion, requires even greater scrutiny. However, the doses from CT protocols compare favorably with conventional angiography.
  - As in all CT examinations, the decision to perform a study on a pregnant patient belongs to the patient's physician in collaboration with the radiologist. The technologist's role is to identify patients who require additional scrutiny and to bring them to the attention of the radiologist.
- The most reliable sign of an acute embolus is a low-density filling defect projecting into the vessel lumen, outlined by contrast material. This observation makes the dose, rate, and timing of contrast administration critical to the creation of diagnostic examinations.

- Because the time to maximal vascular opacification can vary with age, cardiac output, lung disease, and the position of the IV catheter, the quality of the examination is dependent on the experience of the technologist.
- The use of a saline flush after the injection of the iodinated contrast is recommended for CTA pulmonary studies. This will eliminate beam-hardening artifacts from dense contrast media within the superior vena cava that may obscure small emboli in adjacent vessels, particularly in the right main and right upper lobe pulmonary arteries.
- In patients who are physically larger than average, a slightly wider slice thickness (2.0 to 2.5 versus 1.25 for small or average size patients) can be used to decrease quantum mottle.
- In some institutions, ECG gating is used to reduce cardiac pulsation artifacts. This technique remains controversial because it requires a longer breath-hold and increased radiation exposure.

## CARDIAC CT

- Cardiac CT has emerged as a less-invasive imaging modality for the diagnosis of coronary artery disease. Continuous improvements in CT detector technology and in temporal (speed) and spatial (thin slices) resolution have resulted in clinical results with cardiac CT that are similar to those obtainable with conventional catheter coronary angiography.
- Cardiovascular disease (CVD) is the leading cause of death in the United States. Coronary artery disease is responsible for the majority of these deaths, but also included are noncoronary cardiac diseases such as congenital heart disease and other forms of acquired heart disease (e.g., valvular disease, cardiomyopathies, tumors, and pericardial processes).
- Cardiac CT can provide not only anatomic information but also functional information to aid in the diagnosis and treatment of CVD.
- The technologist's understanding of the structural anatomy and the path and timing of the circulation is essential to the creation of high-quality cardiac CT images.

### Cardiac Anatomy

- The human heart is a four-chambered muscular organ with a size and shape roughly equivalent to a person's closed fist. Lying in the mediastinum, approximately two-thirds of its mass is left of midline. The lower border of the heart lies on the diaphragm, pointing toward the left to form a blunt point known as the apex. The upper border of the heart, or base, lies just below the second rib.

- The heart is enclosed in a loose-fitting, double-layered sac called the pericardium.
  - The outer layer is made of a tough white fibrous tissue known as the parietal layer.
  - The inner, or visceral, layer of the pericardium is composed of a smooth, moist, serous membrane. This visceral layer closely envelops the heart and is also called the epicardium.
  - Between the two layers is the pericardial space, which contains a small amount of fluid that serves to lubricate the constantly rubbing surfaces.
- The heart also consists of distinct layers of tissue.
  - The majority of the wall is composed of cardiac muscle, or myocardium.
  - The outer covering of the myocardium is the epicardium (which is the inner section of the pericardium).
  - The inner lining of the myocardium is the endocardium.
- The interior of the heart is divided into four chambers; the two upper are the atria, and the two lower are the ventricles.
- Systole occurs when the heart contracts and pumps blood out of the heart.
- Diastole occurs when the heart relaxes and fills with blood.
- Heart valves limit the flow of blood to only one direction. They lie at the exit of each of the four heart chambers. When open, the four heart valves ensure that blood always flows freely in a forward direction. When closed, the valves prevent blood from flowing backward to its previous location.

### Coronary Circulation

- Like all other cells in the body, the myocardial cells that make up the heart tissues must also be supplied with nutrients and oxygen and be freed of waste products. Coronary circulation refers to the movement of blood through the tissues of the heart.
- Blood is carried to the heart by the two coronary arteries and their branches.
- Cardiac veins remove deoxygenated blood and waste products.
- The major vessels of the coronary circulation are the left main coronary artery (LM), which divides into the left anterior descending (LAD) and circumflex (LCX) branches, and the right coronary artery (RCA). In about 10% of the general population, an artery arises from the LM between the LAD and LCX. This artery is called the ramus intermedius and is considered a normal variant.
- The left and right coronary arteries originate at the base (or ascending) portion of the aorta. These major coronary vessels lie on the epicardial surface of the heart and function as distribution vessels. Additional arteries branch off from the major coronary vessels and penetrate the myocardium to supply it with blood.
- Most of the blood supplied by the coronary arteries is returned to the right atrium via the coronary sinus. Branches of the coronary sinus include the great cardiac vein (also called the left coronary vein), middle cardiac vein, and small cardiac vein.

### Coronary Artery Grafts and Stents

- The buildup of fat and cholesterol plaque is called atherosclerosis. When one or more of the coronary arteries is atherosclerotic, a partial or total blockage results, and thus the heart does not get an adequate blood supply. This can be called either ischemic heart disease or coronary artery disease (CAD). CAD is one of the leading causes of death in Western societies.
- Coronary artery bypass graft surgery (CABG, commonly pronounced "cabbage") is typically recommended when there is disease of the left main coronary artery or disease of three or more vessels, or if nonsurgical management has failed. Technologists should be familiar with the basics of this procedure because it is a common indication for CT imaging, both in evaluating patients for possible CABG surgery and for assessing graft patency after the surgery is performed.
- Arteries or veins taken from elsewhere in the patient's body are grafted from the aorta to the coronary arteries to bypass atherosclerotic narrowings and improve the blood supply to the coronary circulation supplying the myocardium.
- The terms "single," "double," "triple," or "quadruple bypass" refer to the number of coronary arteries bypassed in the procedure. The arteries or veins used for the graft can be taken from different areas of the body. The choice is highly surgeon dependent.
- Grafts may occlude in the months to years after bypass surgery is performed. A graft is considered patent (open) if there is flow through the graft without any significant stenosis (>70% diameter) in the graft.
- Balloon angiography and coronary stenting are less invasive than is CABG and are options for some patients.
  - Angioplasty is a technique that is used to dilate an area of arterial blockage using a catheter with a small, inflatable, sausage-shaped balloon at its tip. However, angioplasty has some shortcomings. The balloon may not expand areas evenly. In addition, some of the areas compressed by the balloon will bounce back

shortly after expansion, and gradual restenosis of the vessel can occur.

- Coronary artery stents were designed to overcome some of the shortcomings of angioplasty. A common type of stent is made of self-expanding, stainless steel mesh. In many cases, the stent is coated with a pharmacologic agent that is known to interfere with the process of restenosis. These stents are called drug-eluting stents, although patients more often refer to them as "coated" or "medicated" stents.
- Compared with angioplasty alone, stents open the disease segment into a rounder, bigger, and smoother opening. Stents reduce the chance of restenosis.
- However, stents cannot be used in all situations; for instance, stents are difficult to place in vessels that have extreme bends and cannot be used in very small vessels.
- Like coronary grafts, technologists should recognize coronary stents because they are a common finding on CT images.

## CTA Technique

- Studies of the heart and coronary arteries require dedicated cardiac CT acquisition techniques to produce images free of motion artifact.
- In addition, care must be taken with the delivery of contrast medium to ensure optimal enhancement of the targeted structure and the surrounding tissues.
  - Visualization of the coronary arteries, a major application of cardiac CT, is difficult because the coronary arteries are of relatively small caliber, are often tortuous in shape, and are subject to constant, often rapid, heart motion.
- MDCT technology has largely overcome these limitations. Additionally, two other strategies are used to decrease cardiac motion artifacts.
  - First, the patient's heart rate can be temporarily lowered by the administration of β-blockers (pronounced beta-blockers).
  - Second, a technique called cardiac gating attempts to use only those images acquired during periods of lowest cardiac motion.

### Pharmacologic Heart Rate Control

- Many institutions use β-blockers as part of their cardiac CT protocols. β-Blockers are used to lower the heart rate to less than 65 to 70 beats per minute (bpm) and to make the rhythm more regular.
- To avoid complications, guidelines should be followed when β-blockers are considered. Protocols can include oral, intravenous (IV), or a combination of oral and IV administration.

- Although metoprolol tartrate (brand named Lopressor) is probably the most commonly used β-blocker for cardiac CT studies, other options include acebutolol, atenolol, betaxolol, bisoprolol, and esmolol.
- The effects of an oral dose are seen within 1 hour of administration. The peak effect of IV-push metoprolol occurs between 5 and 10 minutes after administration.
- Contraindications are sinus bradycardia, which is defined as a heart rate less than 60 bpm; systolic blood pressure of less than 100 mm Hg; allergy to the medication or its constituents; decompensated cardiac failure; presence of asthma treated with β-agonist inhaler; active bronchospasm; and second- or third-degree atrioventricular block.
- The decision to give β-blockers and about the dosage to be given should be made by a physician and is beyond the scope of the CT technologist.
- A regular heart rate of less than 65 bpm is particularly important when the structures of interest are small, such as the coronary arteries. When imaging larger cardiac structures, heart rate is less of an issue, although a slower, regular heart rate is still preferred.
- Some institutions also give patients nitroglycerin sublingually before coronary CT examinations. The intention is to dilate vessels to improve visualization. In addition, nitroglycerin administration may help to prevent coronary spasm that can mimic stenosis on the CT image and therefore be a potential source of misdiagnosis. If used, short-acting nitroglycerin is given immediately before scan initiation. A dose of 0.3 to 0.4 mg is commonly used.

### ECG Gating

- To minimize cardiac motion artifact, most cardiac CT protocols use images acquired during the point of the cardiac cycle with the lowest cardiac motion.
- Most often, this point is during end-diastole, although different structures may be most still at slightly different phases of the cardiac cycle.
  - The precise point of minimal motion is patient and heart rate dependent. For example, any change in heart rate or rhythm can alter the heart chamber size and subsequently change the location of the target structure in axial or three-dimensional images, even if the individual axial image is not blurred.
- All of these factors should be considered to produce the most diagnostic CT studies.
- The two techniques that attempt to minimize cardiac motion in the study by selecting (or acquiring) images during cardiac segments with relatively

slow cardiac motion are called prospective electrocardiogram (ECG) triggering and retrospective ECG gating.

■ Prospective ECG gating is also known as sequential or cine-mode scanning. This method seeks to identify the areas of lowest cardiac motion and acquire images only in those portions of the cardiac cycle.

■ Retrospective methods acquire images throughout the cardiac cycle while the patient's ECG is recorded. Images are later reconstructed to create image sets at any desired phase of the cardiac cycle.

■ To understand either method of ECG gating, a basic understanding of the ECG tracing is necessary.

● The ECG provides a profile of the heart's electrical activity with time. Each heartbeat in a normally functioning heart exhibits a similar characteristic pattern consisting of five waves referred to as P, Q, R, S, and T (Fig. 20-1).

● The distance between two R waves represents one complete cardiac cycle and is sometimes referred to as the R-R interval. Hence, a scan that covers the entire heartbeat (a continuous acquisition) might be referred to as covering 100% of the R-R interval.

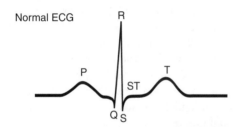

FIGURE 20-1 Each heartbeat in a normally functioning heart exhibits a similar characteristic pattern consisting of five waves referred to as P, Q, R, S, and T, constituting the electrocardiogram (ECG).

■ Prospective ECG gating methods use a signal, usually derived from the R wave of the patient's ECG, to trigger image acquisition. A delay between the R wave and scan initiation can be selected by the technologist. Using this trigger, and the preprogrammed delay, a scan is acquired during a finite portion of the R-R interval (Fig. 20-2). The table then moves to the next position, and the procedure is repeated until the entire area of interest is covered. This is sometimes referred to as a step-and-shoot system to differentiate it from helical CT techniques.

● Because scan acquisition is synchronized with the patient's heart rate, the total time of the examination may vary considerably from one patient to the next.

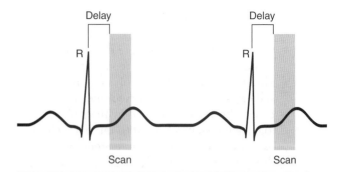

FIGURE 20-2 Prospective electrocardiographic gating methods use a signal, usually derived from the R wave of the patient's electrocardiogram, to trigger image acquisition at a predefined point within the cardiac cycle. Thereafter, the table moves to the next position, and the procedure is repeated until the entire area of interest is covered.

■ The primary advantage of this method over the retrospective method is the dramatic reduction in radiation dose to the patient. This reduction is attributable to the intermittent nature of the scan acquisition.

● Reducing the radiation dose is particularly important if cardiac studies are to be used as a screening examination for patients who have not yet exhibited clear cardiac symptoms but have risks associated with cardiac disease.

■ Disadvantages of prospective methods are that this type of gating is very sensitive to cardiac motion artifacts and image misregistration. This is particularly true in patients with irregular heartbeats.

■ Retrospective ECG-gating methods acquire helical data throughout the cardiac cycle. Using the ECG tracings that are acquired with the scan acquisition, images are reconstructed in specified portions of the cardiac cycle (Fig. 20-3). As a general

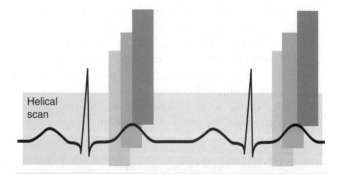

FIGURE 20-3 For retrospective electrocardiographic gating, an MDCT spiral scan is acquired throughout the cardiac cycle (represented by the blue-shaded area). Images are then reconstructed at the portion of the cardiac cycle estimated to have the least motion. Data sets from different segments can be created and evaluated to determine the portion with the least motion. The yellow-shaded area represents the first reconstructed data set, whereas the pink and green areas represent additional reconstructed data sets.

rule, image reconstruction is performed at 60% to 65% of the cardiac cycle. However, reconstructions are often created from other segments of the cardiac cycle and compared to determine which data set demonstrates the least cardiac motion. Some manufacturers have developed software that analyzes the acquired images and automatically selects the best phase with the least cardiac motion for reconstruction.

■ The axial image reconstructions are often referred to as the "source images" because these images are used to create three-dimensional and other image models. Because the retrospective method uses a helical technique, it is possible to combine multiple image sets from different phases in the cardiac cycle to produce a cine loop (i.e., a dynamic image set that resembles a video image).

■ The primary disadvantage of the retrospective ECG-gated method is the relatively high radiation dose to the patient. Although it can be argued that this dose represents an acceptable risk in the symptomatic patient, most researchers worry that it is too high a dose to use the examination as a screening for asymptomatic patients.

● To address this concern, manufacturers have developed methods that automatically decrease the tube current during the systolic phase of the ECG tracing. Hence, the higher tube current is only used during the diastolic phase of the cardiac cycle, the time when images are most likely to be reconstructed. This technique is called ECG-pulsed tube current modulation, or alternatively, ECG pulsing.

● Reducing the kilovoltage setting when scanning slim patients has also been suggested to decrease the radiation dose.

With either gating method, the greatest challenge to obtaining diagnostic images is heart rate variation. Changes in heart rate or rhythm can result in misregistration of the targeted anatomy. In addition, high heart rate variability or the presence of arrhythmia makes the use of ECG-pulsed tube current modulation impossible. Therefore, the advantages of using β-blocker protocols to lower the heart rate not only improve image quality but can reduce the radiation dose to the patient and thus the associated cancer risk.

### Contrast Administration

■ Most cardiac CT protocols require the intravenous administration of iodinated contrast agents.

● Standard screening for contraindications to the contrast agent (e.g., renal impairment, iodine allergy) is necessary.

● An intravenous line is placed using a large-lumen (20-gauge or larger) flexible cannula in a vein of sufficient diameter to accommodate a

relatively high injection rate; typically the antecubital vein is used, preferably on the right side.

● A low-osmolar or isosmolar, nonionic agent with an iodine concentration between 300 and 400 mg/mL is injected, with an injection rate between 3 and 6 mL/s.

● The volume of contrast agent used per examination varies from 70 to 150 mL, depending on the scan protocol, scanner type, and the patient's weight.

■ Techniques for contrast use in cardiac CT continue to evolve. Target enhancement is typically in the range of 200 to 300 HU. However, the target range may vary somewhat depending on the specific indication.

■ Accurate timing of contrast injection and scan initiation is essential. Attempts to use a set time (for instance, 20 seconds when the area of interest is the coronary arteries) for all patients have been unsuccessful. The delay time used must be patient specific.

● The optimal time to start image acquisition can be calculated for each patient using either a timing bolus or bolus tracking.

● The location of the monitoring slices and the placement of the region of interest for either method are dependent on the specific cardiac anatomy being investigated. For instance, the monitoring slice and subsequent ROI is placed in the ascending aorta for studies of the coronary arteries, whereas with pulmonary vein imaging, contrast enhancement is timed to the left atrium.

■ Contrast injection is immediately followed by a saline solution bolus. There are a number of reasons for this practice. One is to make use of the otherwise wasted contrast material present in the IV tubing and in the arm vein of the patient during imaging. In addition, a saline chaser allows for more homogeneous opacification throughout the examination, that is, a more uniform HU from the top of the aorta to the base of the heart. Finally, a saline chaser reduces streak artifacts over the superior vena cava that result from the dense contrast material. A saline chaser can also reduce inhomogeneities that occur, particularly in the superior vena cava and right atrium, when enhanced and nonenhanced blood meet.

### Breath-Hold

■ It is very important that the patient suspend respiration during scan acquisition. Breathing during the scan will result in motion artifact. Careful breath-hold instructions should be given to the patient before the scan begins; moderate inspiration is most frequently used.

### CT Coronary Calcium Screening

- Atherosclerosis is a buildup of fat, plaque, and other substances, including calcium.
- Coronary artery calcification is a marker of coronary artery disease (CAD). Patients with CAD may exhibit no symptoms of the disease; in many patients, myocardial infarction is the first sign of CAD.
- The goal of CT for calcium scoring is to determine the location and extent of calcified plaque in the coronary arteries. This is a helpful diagnostic tool; by measuring the amount of calcium that builds up in the coronary artery, CT can be used to predict the likelihood of subsequent cardiovascular events in people with no symptoms.
- It is frequently performed as a screening study for patients with risk factors for CAD but no clinical symptoms.
- The amount of calcification on cardiac CT is expressed as a calcium score.
  - A negative examination shows no calcification within the coronary arteries and suggests that atherosclerotic plaque is minimal and that the chance of CAD developing during the next 2 to 5 years is low.
  - A positive test means that CAD is present, regardless of whether or not the patient is experiencing any symptoms.
  - Different methods of scoring are used. The Agatston score, the calcium volume score, and the absolute calcium mass measurement are examples of these methods.
- A four-detector-row CT with a 0.5-second gantry rotation time is the minimal equipment requirement for a coronary calcium measurement.
- Because coronary calcium measurement is applied mainly as a screening examination to asymptomatic patients, the radiation dose is of particular concern.
  - Imaging of coronary calcifications is typically performed using a low-dose technique without contrast enhancement.
- The scan time is as short as possible to avoid artifacts from cardiac motion and breathing. Either a prospective or retrospective cardiac gating acquisition technique is used.
- The patient is supine and the scan extends from the midlevel of the left pulmonary artery down to the diaphragm.
- A major criticism of CT coronary calcium scoring is the lack of a standardization regarding image acquisition techniques and with regard to the methods used for quantitative coronary calcification scoring.

### REVIEW QUESTIONS

1. For what study might data be acquired while the patient is lying prone on the CT table?
   a. Routine chest
   b. CT angiography for suspected pulmonary embolism
   c. Cardiac scoring
   d. High-resolution chest CT
2. A volumetric HRCT study refers to a protocol that includes which of the following?
   a. Thin sections, taken at an interval of 20 mm or more between slices, during inspiration, with the patient in a supine position
   b. A sampling technique that is intended to provide representative areas of the lung
   c. Thin sections, in a helical mode, taken contiguously so as to cover the entire lung, during inspiration, with the patient in a supine position
   d. Three series of thin sections, in a helical mode, taken contiguously so as to cover the entire lung; series one is supine inspiratory, series two is supine expiratory, and series three is prone inspiratory
3. Why do many protocols for the evaluation of PE scan in the caudal-to-cranial direction?
   a. To chase the contrast bolus through pulmonary circulation
   b. To reduce radiation exposure
   c. To reduce artifacts attributable to patient motion
   d. To eliminate the need for the patient to hold his or her breath.
4. What must happen to a thrombus for it to be referred to as an embolus?
   a. It must detach from its original site.
   b. It must be formed in the right side of the heart.
   c. It must be formed from clotted blood.
   d. It must lodge in a pulmonary vessel.
5. At a particular institution, the PE protocol includes a second scan series, performed 180 seconds after the IV contrast injection that extends from the iliac crests to the knees. What is the purpose of this second series?
   a. To check for ureteral obstruction.
   b. To check the pelvis and lower extremities for deep vein thrombosis.
   c. To check that the patient is excreting the iodinated contrast.
   d. To assess the patient's cardiac output.
6. What heart valve is located between the right atrium and the right ventricle?
   a. Mitral
   b. Pulmonary
   c. Aortic
   d. Tricuspid
7. β-Blockers are likely to be used as part of a cardiac CT protocol when the
   a. patient has a history of iodine allergy.
   b. patient has asthma and is being treated with an albuterol inhaler.
   c. patient's heart rate is higher than 65 bpm.
   d. patient's heart rate is less than 60 bpm.

8. An imaging technique that attempts to acquire data only during cardiac segments with the lowest cardiac motion is called
    a. a split bolus.
    b. prospective ECG triggering.
    c. retrospective ECG gating.
    d. electron beam CT.

9. A patient who is scheduled for a CT study has an irregular heartbeat with a rate of approximately 85 bpm. For which clinical indication is this the most problematic?
    a. Coronary artery disease
    b. Assessment of ventricular function
    c. Possible thoracic aortic dissection
    d. Evaluation of congenital aortic arch anomaly

10. Why is it recommended that cardiac CT calcium scoring be restricted to patients with risk factors for coronary artery disease, rather than using it as a screening tool for all patients?
    a. It has not proven to be an accurate measure of coronary artery calcification.
    b. A correlation has not been proven between a positive calcium score and a future risk of developing heart disease.
    c. The examination is uncomfortable for the patient.
    d. Risks related to the radiation dose are a concern; for asymptomatic patients with no cardiac risk factors, it is not certain that the benefit of the examination outweighs the risk from the radiation exposure.

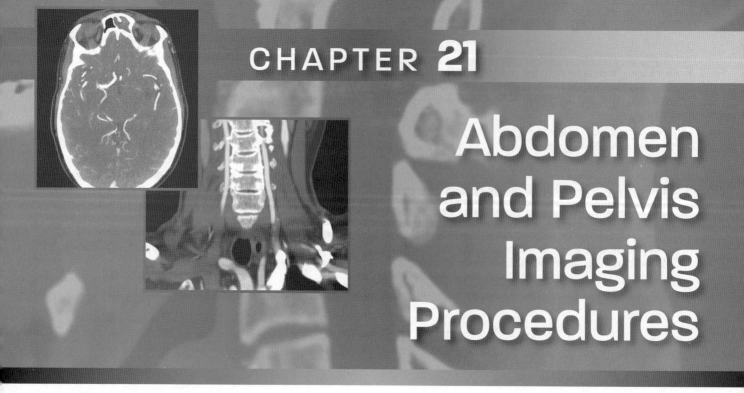

# CHAPTER 21

# Abdomen and Pelvis Imaging Procedures

## GENERAL ABDOMINAL SCANNING METHODS

- CT evaluation of the abdomen and pelvis requires greater attention to patient preparation than does CT evaluation of any other area of the body.
- Most CT scans of the abdomen require the administration of an oral contrast agent to demonstrate the intestinal lumen and to distend the gastrointestinal tract. The use of oral contrast material is imperative to differentiate a fluid-filled loop of bowel from a mass or an abnormal fluid collection.
  - Either a dilute barium suspension or a dilute water-soluble agent may be used with equal effectiveness.
  - In general, the greater the volume of oral contrast material, the better the bowel opacification. Although a volume of at least 600 mL is desired, patient compliance may be a limiting factor.
  - Patients should be given only clear liquids for at least 2 hours before scanning to ensure that food in the stomach is not mistaken for pathologic tissue.
- Air and water are excellent as low-attenuation contrast agents.
  - Air or carbon dioxide is frequently used to insufflate the colon for CT colonography, producing a very high negative contrast.
  - Water or a low-HU oral barium sulfate suspension (e.g., VoLumen, E Z EM) is sometimes used in place of positive contrast agents. These low-HU agents will not obscure mucosal surfaces or superimpose abdominal vessels on postprocessed images. The latter is important in CT angiography (CTA) of the abdomen and pelvis. The use of a low-HU oral contrast has an added advantage in that it does not mask radiopaque stones in the common bile duct or urinary tract.
- Few institutions routinely administer rectal contrast material. When it is used, the most common indication is for colon cancer staging.
- The bladder is best appreciated on CT when filled with urine or contrast agent.
- The vagina is seen in cross section as a flattened ellipse of soft tissue between the bladder and rectum. An inserted tampon will outline the cavity of the vagina with air density and is useful in identification of the vaginal canal.
- Intravenous contrast agents improve the quality of studies of the abdomen and pelvis by opacifying blood vessels, increasing the CT density of vascular abdominal organs, and improving image contrast between lesions and normal structures.
  - The appropriate timing, rate, and dose of the IV contrast agent is essential. For most examinations of the body, image acquisition must be completed before IV contrast medium reaches the equilibrium phase.
  - Modern scanners can accomplish this; as a result, precontrast scans are now seldom obtained for routine abdomen studies, but may be used for specific indications (e.g., diagnosis of fatty infiltration or other alteration of parenchymal attenuation).

- Multiphasic imaging is frequently used for specialized studies of the pancreas, liver, and kidney as well as in many abdominal CTA protocols.
- CT of the abdomen and pelvis is used for the evaluation of virtually all organs and most vessels. Radiologists systematically examine each organ and structure imaged. In any given slice, much more information is present than can be displayed by any single window width and level setting.
  - A routine soft tissue window setting (window width approximately 450; window level approximately 50) will adequately display most abdominal anatomy.
  - The liver may also be examined using "liver windows," which are narrower (window width approximately 150; window level approximately 70) and intended to improve the visibility of subtle liver lesions.
  - The lung bases are contained in slices of the upper abdomen and must be viewed using lung windows (window width approximately 1,500; window level approximately 600).
  - Bone windows (window width approximately 2,000; window level approximately 600) may help to reveal abnormalities of the bones.
- The display field of view (DFOV) should be just large enough to include the skin surface over the key areas of the body. If previous studies are available, it is generally advisable to use the same DFOV, unless a change in patient condition (e.g., large weight gain) necessitates adjustment. Using the same DFOV as the previous study allows easy visual comparison of any changes in size of lesions or structures when both studies are displayed side by side on PACS monitors.
- Although landmarks easily visible on the scout images are often used to guide technologists as to where cross-sectional slices should begin and end, technologists must verify that the anatomy of interest has indeed been scanned. Similarly, scanning should not start or stop in the middle of obvious abnormality.
- Most protocols of the abdomen and pelvis are performed while the patient lies in a supine position on the scan table with the arms elevated above the head. In a few instances, changing the patient position and obtaining additional slices can provide added information.
- Patients are asked to hold their breath during scan acquisition to reduce movement and decrease motion artifacts. Patient movement during scanning will cause anatomic structures to be displaced, distorted, or blurred.
- There is a wide range in the number of protocols used at different institutions for CT of the abdomen and pelvis. Protocols can be of a general nature (e.g., routine abdomen and pelvis), or they can be designed to address a particular clinical question or to evaluate a specific abdominal or pelvic organ (e.g., suspected appendicitis, renal mass).
- At some institutions, scans are routinely checked by a radiologist while the patient is still on the scan table. At others, scans are not reviewed before the patient leaves the department. A third option is that only certain examinations (such as adrenal studies) are checked by the radiologist before the patient leaves the department.
- Technologists are encouraged to carefully review images and call a radiologist whenever they suspect abnormal results could necessitate additional imaging.

## Liver

- The normal CT attenuation of the liver in unenhanced studies varies among individuals and ranges from 38 to 70 HU.
- In healthy subjects, the attenuation of the liver is at least 10 HU greater than that of the spleen.
- Fatty infiltration of the liver is one of the most common abnormalities diagnosed by liver CT and can result from a variety of causes including alcoholism, obesity, diabetes, chemotherapy, corticosteroid therapy, hyperalimentation (i.e., total parental nutrition–intravenous feeding), and malnutrition.
  - Fatty infiltration reduces the CT attenuation of the involved liver. With fatty infiltration, the attenuation of the liver is at least 10 HU lower than that of the spleen.
  - This is most accurately assessed on noncontrast CT.
  - Many operators include a region of interest (ROI) measurement of the liver and spleen. A spleen measurement more than 10 HU higher than that of the liver indicates fatty infiltrate of the liver.
- Another common finding in the liver is that of cavernous hemangiomas. These benign tumors are often discovered incidentally during hepatic imaging by either ultrasonography or CT.
  - Although in the majority of cases hemangiomas are solitary, some patients have multiple lesions.
  - Most hemangiomas have a characteristic appearance on CT. On unenhanced CT, hemangiomas appear as a well-defined hypodense mass of the same density as other blood-filled spaces, such as the inferior vena cava. After IV contrast administration, the lesion shows progressive filling in enhancement from the periphery; eventually, the lesion becomes uniformly enhanced.
- Because the liver derives approximately 25% of its blood supply from the hepatic artery and the

remaining 75% from the portal vein, there are several phases of enhancement after the IV administration of a bolus of contrast material.

- The first is the hepatic arterial phase typically occurring 15 to 25 seconds after the contrast bolus.
- This is followed by the portal venous phase, which begins at 60 to 70 seconds after contrast injection. Based on contrast circulation, the hepatic arterial phase can be further divided.

■ For routine abdominal CT or as part of a chest, abdomen, and pelvic study, the liver is most often scanned just once, during the portal venous phase. However, for some indications (e.g., hypervascular liver lesions or hepatic vascular anatomy), scanning in more than one enhancement phase may improve the examination's sensitivity. In addition to the portal venous phase of the liver, earlier, arterial phase scans are obtained. In some institutions, scans are obtained during three phases of liver enhancement (early arterial, late arterial, and portal venous).

## Pancreas

■ The pancreas differs in size, shape, and location depending on the individual patient. In general, the pancreas is located between the areas of the twelfth thoracic vertebra (superiorly) and the second lumbar vertebra (inferiorly).

■ A technique that includes the use of thin slices and IV contrast enhancement improves the likelihood of visualizing the main pancreatic duct.

■ In a jaundiced patient, noncontrast scans through the area of the common bile duct may allow visualization of common bile duct calculi.

■ Water or low-attenuation oral contrast agents are preferred because dense contrast may obscure small stones.

■ Multiphasic protocols are common for pancreatic indications.

- Most commonly, data acquisition is timed to coincide with the late arterial phase (approximately 35–40 seconds after a bolus injection) and the portal venous phase (approximately 65–70 seconds after a bolus injection).
- Because the exact timing of these phases is patient dependent, bolus-tracking software is often used.

## Kidneys and Ureters

■ Most renal abnormalities are best seen on CT after IV contrast medium administration.

■ Unenhanced CT is generally reserved to demonstrate calcifications and calculi that may be obscured by a contrast agent, or it is used as a baseline for attenuation measurements when enhancement is calculated as a feature of renal mass characterization.

■ When the examination is performed to evaluate a renal mass, scans are typically taken before the contrast bolus and at one or more phases after IV contrast administration. The exact timing of the phases varies depending on patient factors, particularly cardiac output. However, to generalize:

- The corticomedullary phase typically occurs approximately 30 to 70 seconds after the contrast bolus.
- The nephrogram phase is seen from 80 to 120 seconds after the contrast bolus.
- The excretory phase occurs about 3 minutes after injection and can last 15 minutes or longer.

■ 2D and 3D reformations may be helpful in defining certain types of renal abnormalities, such as renal cell carcinoma and ureteropelvic junction (UPJ) obstruction.

■ CTU is an examination optimized for imaging the kidneys, ureters, and bladder. Protocols vary, but all include the use of MDCT with thin-slice imaging, IV administration of contrast medium, and imaging in the excretory phase.

- Protocols may include only the excretory phase, or may contain as many as four phases:
  - Unenhanced
  - Corticomedullary (approximately 60 seconds after injection)
  - Nephrographic (approximately 110 seconds after injection)
  - Excretory (3–16 minutes after injection)

■ Contrast administration is accomplished using one of two different approaches: a single-bolus injection or a split-bolus injection.

- A single-bolus injection administers 100 to 150 mL of LOCM injected at a rate of 2 to 3 mL/s.
- Protocols for split-bolus injections vary somewhat, but all divide the contrast media dose into two bolus injections with a delay of 2 to 15 minutes between injections. The goal of the split bolus is to image a combined nephrographic-excretory phase.

■ Other techniques may be used during CTU to optimize the visualization of the urinary tract, including the use of abdominal compression bands, intravenous saline hydration (approximately 250 mL of 0.9% [normal] saline), and low-dose furosemide injection (Lasix).

■ Multiphase CTU imaging is associated with a relatively high radiation dose. The benefits of the examination must be carefully weighed against the risks on a patient-by-patient basis.

- The split-bolus technique has been gaining in popularity because by combining two phases, the radiation dose is reduced.

# CT of the Adrenal Glands

- CT is the modality of choice in detection and characterization of adrenal masses.
- CT studies are often ordered as a result of unrelated symptoms, and adrenal masses are found incidentally. The term incidentalomas is often used to describe them.
  - The majority of incidentalomas are benign.
  - Although the possibility of malignancy is small, the risk necessitates that each adrenal mass be evaluated further.
- Biopsy can provide a definitive diagnosis, but biopsy is somewhat invasive and is associated with a small but real risk of complications.
- When the appropriate technique is followed, CT can differentiate adrenal adenomas (benign adrenal masses) from metastases.
- The characterization of adrenal masses is accomplished by assessing their attenuation values and by evaluating the degree of iodinated contrast that is washed out of the mass on delayed imaging.
- Because accurate characterization often requires an adjustment in the scan protocol, CT technologists must be familiar with current information. An astute technologist can save a patient the time, money, and radiation exposure of a repeat examination by identifying an incidentaloma and tailoring the study to provide the radiologist with the data necessary to characterize the mass as benign or malignant.
- The adrenal glands are complex endocrine organs named for their location, which is adjacent to the kidneys (thus the name, *ad-renal*). They are also occasionally referred to as suprarenal glands (*supra* means above). Located at the top of each kidney, they are triangular, and a normal gland weighs about 5 g. On a cross-sectional image, adrenal glands have a characteristic Y, V, or T.
- CT imaging protocols attempt to characterize lesions of the adrenal gland. The goals of imaging are to reduce the number of unnecessary biopsies, the number of follow-up studies needed for an accurate diagnosis, and the cost of care.
- There are certain general imaging findings that can help in differentiating benign lesions from malignant ones.
  - Larger lesions have a greater likelihood of being malignant. In particular, lesions greater than 4 cm in diameter are more likely to be either metastasis or a primary adrenal carcinoma than are smaller lesions.
  - Adenomas most often grow slowly, so lesions that change in size may be malignant.
  - The shape of the adrenal mass can also be a helpful indicator of malignancy. Adenomas tend to have smooth margins and a homogeneous density, but metastases are more often heterogeneous and have an irregular shape.
- Unfortunately, although these characteristics are useful indicators in differentiating a benign from a malignant mass, they are not specific enough to be used alone in making a diagnosis.
- Two traits of adenomas, one anatomic and one physiologic, have allowed CT to be used to differentiate adenomas from malignant lesions with a high degree of accuracy.
  - The variance in intracellular lipid (fat) content between adenomas and malignant adrenal masses reflects the anatomic difference.
  - The way each type of mass responds to iodinated contrast enhancement is indicative of the physiologic difference.
- An adrenal mass with an associated attenuation number on CT of less than 10 HU is considered lipid rich and can confidently be identified as an adenoma.
- To rule out malignancy in a mass whose attenuation value is greater than 10 HU, another aspect must be considered, that of contrast washout.
  - This trait is examined by comparing the attenuation value of the mass just after contrast enhancement to the attenuation value of the mass 15 minutes after contrast has been injected.
- The degree of washout can be calculated using either of two simple formulas.
- The first formula assumes that unenhanced, enhanced (at portal venous phase), and 15-minute delayed images are available. If these images are all available, an ROI is placed on the adrenal mass and an HU measurement is taken on each set of images. The washout can then be calculated:

$$\frac{\text{Enhanced} - \text{Delayed}}{\text{Enhanced} - \text{Unenhanced}} \times 100 = \% \text{ washout}$$

To illustrate, an ROI placed on the adrenal mass yields unenhanced = 16 HU, enhanced = 100 HU, and 15-minute delayed = 49 HU. Therefore,

$$\frac{100 - 49}{100 - 16} \times 100 = 62\%$$

- The second formula is designed for situations in which unenhanced images are not available and is called the relative washout. It is calculated:

$$\frac{\text{Enhanced} - \text{Delayed}}{\text{Enhanced}} \times 100 = \% \text{ relative washout}$$

Using the above example:

$$\frac{100-49}{100} \times 100 = 51\% \text{ relative washout}$$

- A washout of greater than 60% is specific for adenoma, and a washout less than 60% indicates malignancy.
- When a relative washout value is used, the threshold is 40%. Hence, a relative washout value that is equal or greater to 40% is specific for adenomas, and when relative washout is less than 40%, malignancy is likely. When washout or relative washout values obtained using CT indicate that an adrenal mass has a high likelihood of malignancy, biopsy is often used to confirm the diagnosis.
- Technologists play an important role in the identification and characterization of adrenal masses, as they are often the first to discover an incidentaloma. A technologist who is aware of the issues surrounding the characterization of adrenal mass can bring an incidentaloma to the attention of the radiologist. Small adjustments such as the addition of delayed images may save the patient the time, the expense, and the additional radiation exposure of a repeat examination.

## CT in the Diagnosis of Acute Appendicitis

- Appendiceal CT has emerged as the dominant imaging method for the evaluation of adults with suspected appendicitis.

### Anatomy and Function of the Appendix

- The appendix is a small, tubelike structure projecting from the cecum.
- Although the base is fixed to the cecum, the tip of the appendix may vary and can be found in the retrocecal, pelvic subcecal, preileal, or right pericolic position.
- The variable position of the appendix contributes to the diverse clinical presentation of acute appendicitis and can make localizing it on cross-sectional images challenging.
- Further complicating identification and diagnosis, the appendix can be naturally absent or duplicated, or easily be mistaken for diverticula.

### Incidence of Acute Appendicitis

- Appendicitis is common, occurring in 7% of the population at some time in their life.
- It can occur at any age but is most common in people between ages 10 and 40.
- The treatment for appendicitis is surgical removal.
- Appendectomies are sometimes done preventatively. These are referred to as incidental appendectomies.

### Prognosis

- The surgical treatment of appendicitis is an effective treatment. Few Americans die from appendicitis.
- The risk of mortality increases if the appendix ruptures before surgical treatment.
- Elderly patients are at an increased risk of mortality and morbidity. This is related, in part, to their increased likelihood of perforation.
- The accurate and timely diagnosis of acute appendicitis is important to minimize poor outcomes.

### Etiology and Pathogenesis

- Fecaliths are the most common cause of appendiceal obstruction.
- Another common cause is the proliferation of normal cells within the appendix; this is typically attributed to viral illnesses such as upper respiratory tract infections, mononucleosis, or gastroenteritis.

### Clinical Presentations

- Diagnosis of acute appendicitis can be problematic for even the most experienced clinicians.
- Patients may present with a wide variety of signs and symptoms. No single clinical finding can effectively rule out or confirm the diagnosis of acute appendicitis.
- Diagnosis is particularly difficult in women of childbearing age because acute gynecologic conditions may mimic signs of appendicitis.
- Abdominal pain, anorexia, nausea, and vomiting are the most common symptoms.
- The position of the appendix will affect the clinical presentation.
  - If the inflamed appendix lies in the typical anterior position, the patient will likely exhibit the classic presentation of right lower quadrant pain, which is most intense at McBurney point, and direct rebound tenderness.
  - If the appendix is in a retrocecal position, the anterior abdominal findings are less pronounced. Instead, tenderness may be more pronounced in the flank.
  - If the appendix is in a posterior position, the patient is likely to exhibit the psoas sign.
  - When the appendix is in the pelvis, abdominal findings may be entirely absent. In this situation, a digital examination of the rectum may aid in diagnosis.

### Differential Diagnosis

- Many other acute processes within or near the peritoneal cavity can present with the same signs and symptoms of acute appendicitis.
- Laboratory tests are helpful but are not specific enough to be used alone to confirm the diagnosis. Many other conditions can produce the identical abnormal laboratory results.

## Imaging Studies

- Plain radiographs of the abdomen may help in ruling out other pathologic processes, but they are rarely helpful in diagnosing acute appendicitis.
- Barium enema is no longer commonly used to diagnose acute appendicitis.
- Ultrasonography is a valuable tool in diagnosis, particularly when there is a concern regarding the radiation dose of CT. Therefore, it is often the primary imaging study in children, and in young or pregnant women. The main disadvantage to ultrasonography is that it is highly operator dependent.
- CT is more precise and reproducible than is ultrasonography.
- Although ultrasonography is recommended as the initial imaging study in children, young women, and pregnant women, CT is most often recommended as the initial study in all other patients.
- CT is also recommended for patients in whom sonographic evaluation is suboptimal, indeterminate, or normal, or for those patients in whom perforation is suspected.

## Common Finding on CT

- The most common CT findings in acute appendicitis are a dilated nonopacified appendix, soft tissue stranding into adjacent periappendiceal fat, and appendicolith.

## Appendiceal CT Protocols

- All current protocols use thin-section images. In all other regards, there are many variations in appendicitis protocols.
- Protocols vary in their use of contrast agents. Protocols may use different combinations of oral, rectal, IV, or noncontrast materials.
- Protocols vary regarding the anatomic area to be included in the scan. Focused appendiceal CT refers to protocols that limit the scan to the lower abdomen and upper pelvis. This is done to reduce the radiation exposure to the patient. Other protocols include the entire abdomen and pelvis. These have the advantage of eliminating the risk for incomplete visualization or nonvisualization of the appendix in an atypical location. In addition, scanning the entire abdomen and pelvis improves the ability to diagnose alternative disease processes when the appendix is found to be normal.
- The most popular CT protocol is to scan the entire abdomen and pelvis with both intravenous and oral contrast materials.

# CT in the Diagnosis of Urinary Tract Calculi

- CT plays an essential role in the diagnosis and initial management of urolithiasis.

## Terminology

- The terms *kidney stones*, *renal stones*, *renal calculi*, *nephrolithiasis*, and *urolithiasis* are often used interchangeably to refer to the gravel-like deposits that may appear in any part of the urinary system, from the kidney to the bladder.
  - These deposits may be small or large and single or multiple. Sometimes they are no bigger than a sugar granule, whereas in other cases, they are so large that they fill the entire renal pelvis.
  - The term *renal calculi* is used to describe stones that are located in the kidney.
  - Ureterolithiasis refers to stones that are in a ureter.
- The passage of renal calculi from the kidney through the urinary tract is frequently accompanied by acute pain that is referred to as renal colic.
- Ureteral stones can sometimes cause ureteral obstruction resulting in dilatation, distention, and enlargement of the collection system in the kidney; these changes are collectively referred to as hydronephrosis.
- However, urinary tract stones are not always painful and sometimes remain undetected for many years. In some cases, stones are discovered as an incidental finding when a patient undergoes imaging studies for unrelated conditions.
- The National Institutes of Health estimates that 10% of people in the United States will have a kidney stone at some point in their lives.
- Kidney stones tend to recur. Approximately 50% of patients with previous urinary calculi have a recurrence within 10 years.
- Sometimes there is no clear precipitating factor identified that can be linked to stone formation. This condition is referred to as idiopathic nephrolithiasis.
- Urinary tract infection and kidney disorders such as polycystic kidney disease are associated with stone formation. A number of metabolic diseases are associated with nephrolithiasis (e.g., hyperparathyroidism, hyperoxaluria).
  - Although certain foods may promote stone formation in people who are susceptible, researchers do not believe that eating any specific food causes stones to form in people who are not susceptible. Therefore, there are no specific dietary recommendations to prevent stone formation. However, once a stone has been analyzed, the patient's diet can be evaluated, and then changes can be recommended that will reduce the likelihood of recurrence.
- There are four basic types of urinary stones: calcium salts, uric acid, magnesium ammonium phosphate (called struvite), or cystine. These four

types of renal calculi are associated with more than 20 different causes. A fifth type of stone is drug induced. A number of medications can precipitate in urine causing stone formation.

- Calcium salt stones are the most common type of stone, accounting for approximately 75% of stone cases.

- It is estimated that 80% to 85% of urinary calculi will pass spontaneously. There are several factors that influence the ability to pass a stone, including the person's size, prior stone passage, prostate enlargement, pregnancy, and the stone's size.
  - A 4-mm stone has an 80% chance of passage, whereas a 5-mm stone has a 20% possibility of passage.

- The classic patient with renal colic is in excruciating unilateral flank or lower abdominal pain, pacing about and unable to lie still. The pain is not related to any precipitating event (such as trauma) and is not relieved by postural changes. This presentation is in contrast to a patient with peritoneal irritation who will typically remain as motionless as possible to minimize discomfort. Some patients with urolithiasis complain of nausea and vomiting that is attributable to stimulation of the celiac plexus. Fever is not part of the presentation of uncomplicated nephrolithiasis.

- The pain of renal colic often begins as vague flank pain and eventually advances into waves of severe pain. It is generally believed that the pain of renal colic is caused by the dilation and spasm of the ureter from transient obstruction as the stone moves through the urinary tract. The symptoms the patient experiences will vary depending on the stone's location.
  - Typically, the pain tends to migrate caudally and medially as the stone works its way down the ureter.
  - It should be noted that the size of the stone does not necessarily predict the severity of the pain; a very tiny crystal with sharp edges can cause intense pain, whereas a larger round stone may not be as problematic.
  - If the stone is too large to pass easily, pain continues as the muscles in the wall of the tiny ureter try to squeeze the stone along into the bladder.
  - As a stone grows or moves, blood may appear in the urine. As the stone moves down the ureter closer to the bladder, the patient may complain of urinary frequency or a burning sensation during urination.

- Many other conditions can cause symptoms similar to those of renal colic.

### Noncontrast Helical CT

- Noncontrast helical CT has become the standard technique for evaluation of suspected renal colic. The advantages of NCHCT compared with all other techniques are as follows:
  - Diagnostic accuracy. More than 99% of stones– including those that are radiolucent on plain film radiography–will be seen on NCHCT. The exceptions are the rarely occurring pure matrix and drug-induced indinavir stones.
  - NCHCT can be rapidly performed and interpreted and does not require the administration of intravenous contrast material.
  - NCHCT provides most of the information required for the management of ureteral calculi, although a KUB is frequently used for follow-up purposes. In addition to demonstrating the size and site of the stone, measurement of stone density can also be useful. Stones of greater than 1,000 HU appear to respond less well to extracorporeal shock wave lithotripsy (ESWL).
  - Through a number of secondary CT signs, the presence of associated urinary tract obstruction can also be inferred from NCHCT.

- Renal stone CT examinations use continuous data acquisition from the top of the kidneys to the base of the bladder. Collimation is typically 2.5 to 3 mm. Thin slices allow identification of small stones that may be overlooked with thicker slices.

- The greatest drawback to the use of NCHCT is that it delivers a relatively high radiation dose, particularly to the gonads. The radiation dose from NCHCT is considerably higher than the dose from a standard intravenous urogram series. This level of radiation exposure is of particular concern because many patients who have stone disease are young and have a tendency to experience repeat stone formation. Therefore, these patients have the potential of undergoing CT of the abdomen and pelvis many times during the course of their lives.

- Because of the concerns regarding the radiation dose, many facilities reduce the tube current for NCHCT, particularly for patients weighing less than 200 pounds.

## REVIEW QUESTIONS

1. Although patient compliance can sometime be a factor, what volume of oral contrast is typically considered the minimum amount needed for a routine CT study of the abdomen and pelvis?
   a. 100 mL
   b. 400 mL
   c. 600 mL
   d. 1,500 mL

2. Which is a window setting used to visualize subtle liver lesions?
   a. 150 ww; 70 wl
   b. 350 ww; 50 wl
   c. 1,500 ww; −600 wl
   d. 2,000 ww; 600 wl
3. A noncontrast CT of the abdomen is ordered on Mr. Smith. The primary indication is a 15-year history of alcoholism. What can the technologist do to help the radiologist determine whether the patient has a fatty liver?
   a. Administer IV contrast and repeat the series.
   b. Administer additional oral contrast and repeat the series.
   c. Continue scanning through the pelvis, even though a pelvic examination was not ordered.
   d. Place a region of interest HU measurement within the liver and spleen.
4. The phase of liver enhancement that occurs 60 to 70 seconds after an IV bolus contrast injection is called the
   a. early arterial phase.
   b. late arterial phase.
   c. portal venous phase.
   d. equilibrium phase.
5. For what clinical indication might a dual-phase (late arterial and portal venous) CT of the abdomen be requested?
   a. To assess possible liver metastasis from a primary thyroid tumor
   b. Detection of suspected liver abscess
   c. Characterization of fatty infiltration of the liver
   d. Acute cholecystitis
6. The nephrogram phase is seen approximately _____ after IV contrast injection.
   a. 30 seconds
   b. 70 seconds
   c. 110 seconds
   d. 5 minutes
7. An adrenal mass that measures less than or equal to 10 HU on unenhanced CT
   a. is an adenoma.
   b. is most likely malignant.
   c. can be either an adenoma or a malignant mass.
   d. is lipid poor.
8. What explains the diversity in clinical presentation of acute appendicitis?
   a. The variable position of the appendix
   b. The skill of the examiner
   c. The varying ability of patients to accurately describe their symptoms
   d. The underlying cause of the obstruction

9. A focused appendiceal CT refers to a scan protocol that
   a. limits the scan area to the lower abdomen and upper pelvis.
   b. uses a rectal contrast agent.
   c. does not include any type of contrast media.
   d. scans the entire abdomen and pelvis with IV and oral contrast material.
10. Select the arrow that points to the appendix in Figure 21-1.
    a. 1
    b. 2
    c. 3
    d. 4

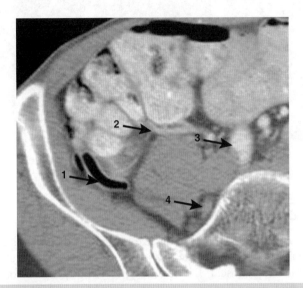

**FIGURE 21-1**

11. What percentage of urinary tract calculi will be seen on noncontrast helical computed tomography?
    a. 40%
    b. 60%
    c. 85%
    d. 99%

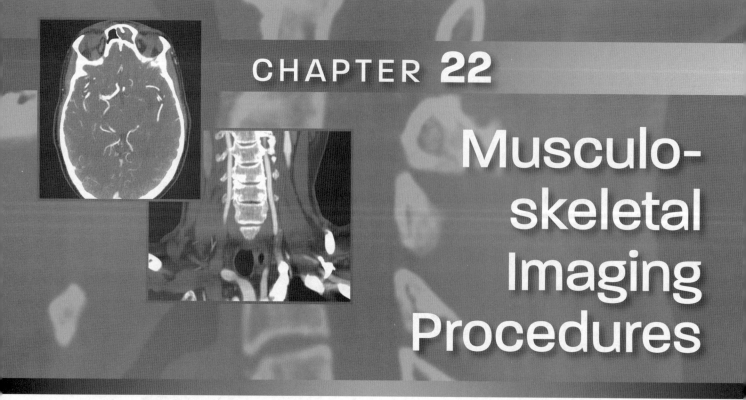

# CHAPTER 22

# Musculo- skeletal Imaging Procedures

## GENERAL MUSCULOSKELETAL SCANNING METHODS

Along with magnetic resonance imaging (MRI), CT is a major method for the evaluation of musculoskeletal anatomy and disease. CT is helpful in providing specific information about bone or other mineralized tissue. It is also a useful method of evaluating bone and soft tissue tumors. It adds details to information obtained with conventional radiography in cases of multiple fractures (e.g., in the pelvis). CT is also used to evaluate joints, especially after air or iodinated contrast material is injected into the joint.

- The development of multidetector row CT (MDCT) has allowed the acquisition of slices as thin as 0.5 mm, resulting in isotropic voxels (Chapter 6). This enables multiplanar reformation (MPR) images to be created in any plane with the same spatial resolution as the original sections.
- In the evaluation of patients with musculoskeletal trauma, scans of the skeleton can be combined with other CT studies. Such is often the case in the evaluation of pelvic trauma, which may include CT angiography (CTA) to look for vascular injury, as well as a CT cystogram to exclude bladder injury.
- The techniques used to scan the musculoskeletal system are tailored to each patient and region being examined.
- Patients should be positioned carefully so that both sides are as symmetric as possible. The lower extremities are usually scanned with the patient supine and placed feet first into the scanner. The upper extremities are often scanned with

the patient supine and placed headfirst into the scanner.
  - Anteroposterior (AP) and lateral scout images are taken to localize the area of interest.
  - In general, the plane of the CT section should be perpendicular to the area of interest.
  - The patient should be made as comfortable as possible with pillows and angle sponges so that inadvertent motion does not degrade the study.
- Intravenous (IV) contrast medium is not routinely administered for musculoskeletal trauma but is often valuable for other indications. IV contrast administration may be helpful in evaluating the vascularity of a tumor or in showing the relationship of major arteries or veins to musculoskeletal masses.
- The reconstruction algorithm selected is based on the clinical application. In cases in which soft tissue or muscle imaging is the primary process, a standard algorithm is used. If bone detail is needed, data are also reconstructed in a high-resolution (bone) algorithm.
- Musculoskeletal images are viewed in both soft tissue (window width approximately 450; window level approximately 50) and bone (window width approximately 2,000; window level approximately 600) window settings.
- The general rules of scanning learned in previous chapters also apply to most musculoskeletal protocols. However, a few specific examinations are worth mentioning for their unique positioning challenges.

## Wrist

- Stable positioning is the key to obtaining good image quality by avoiding motion artifacts. However, patient positioning of the wrist is often awkward and can pose a significant obstacle to the study. Many different approaches are used.
  - Probably the most common is to extend the patient's arm over the head. This can be done with the patient lying either supine or prone.
  - Another approach is to have the patient sit or stand at the far end of the CT scanner with arm resting on the CT table. If direct coronal imaging is desired, the patient's elbow is bent so that the arm is positioned parallel to the gantry. The patient is told to maintain the position while the table moves a short distance and is instructed to move the body along with the table. The patient is asked to look away from the gantry to minimize corneal radiation exposure.
  - If the patient's hand cannot be positioned using one of these approaches, a third method has the patient lying supine on the table with arm resting on the belly. Scans are obtained through both the wrist and the section of the abdomen on which it rests. In this situation, tube current must be increased to at least 300 mAs so that image noise is sufficiently suppressed. Because of the radiation exposure to the patient's abdomen, this method is used only when other approaches have failed.
- Correctly annotating examinations of the hand, wrist, forearm, or elbow can be problematic. Recall that CT systems begin with the assumption that the patient is in the classic anatomic position (Chapter 1). This position is characterized by an individual standing erect, arms down by the sides, with the palms of the hands facing forward. If the technologist inputs directional instructions that the patient is supine and headfirst in the scanner, the scanner assumes the classic anatomic position and annotates images with right/left, superior/inferior, and anterior/posterior accordingly. This annotation system is disrupted when the patient is positioned so that the arm is raised over the head, or is positioned on the far end of the scanner with arm extended.
  - Scanner manufacturers vary in the suggested approach to this dilemma. Technologists should consult the specific scanner's operating instructions or contact the manufacturer's application consultant for the appropriate method of inputting directional instructions on these examinations.
  - Placing a radiopaque marker alongside the anatomy being scanned can help to reduce confusion. For example, an uncoiled, lightweight paper clip (that does not create metallic artifact on the image) can be placed on the right side of the right wrist. The technologist then includes this information in the patient's record for the radiologist interpreting the images.

## Shoulder

- Protocols for shoulder trauma most often include thin slices acquired in the axial plane. Scanning begins at the acromioclavicular joint and terminates a few centimeters below the most inferior fracture line.
- CT arthrography of the shoulder is useful for evaluation of the joint capsule and intracapsular structures and for finding loose bodies within the joint.
  - CT arthrography can be performed with either a single or double contrast technique (0.5–3.0 mL of iodinated contrast material and approximately 10 mL of room air). Thin axial slices begin at just above the acromioclavicular joint and end just below the glenoid fossa.
- For either indication, the patient is positioned supine on the CT table. The arm to be examined is downward, and the opposite arm is extended over the patient's head to reduce the x-ray beam absorption as much as possible.

## Knee

- MRI is the primary modality for the evaluation of the knee. However, CT remains the modality of choice in certain situations, such as tibial plateau fractures.
- The primary indication of knee CT is to assess the degree and alignment of fracture fragments, particularly at the articular surfaces.
- Knee CT is also performed to assess the integrity of the bone around a prosthesis.
- The display field of view (DFOV) is focused on one knee only and must include the patella, both femoral condyles, and the proximal tibia through the fibular head.
- The patient typically lies supine on the scanner table with legs extended and knees side-by-side and enters the scanner feet first.
- CT of the knee is sometimes performed immediately after an arthrogram of the knee in which iodinated contrast or air has been injected directly into the joint space.

## Foot and Ankle

- For CT of the ankle, the DFOV should be large enough to include the hindfoot (talus and calcaneus), the midfoot (navicular, cuboid, and the three cuneiforms), and at least the proximal bases of all five metatarsals. For most patients, it is possible to scan both ankles simultaneously within a 22-cm DFOV, allowing a side-by-side comparison of the symptomatic ankle with the normal ankle.

■ For CT of the foot, the DFOV should be enlarged to include the entire forefoot (metatarsals and phalanges) along with the hindfoot and midfoot.

■ CT data of the foot and ankle can be displayed in a number of different imaging planes. Some of these planes can be obtained directly by positioning the patient in a specific position, whereas other planes are best displayed by reformatting the data. The choice of which plane(s) to display depends on which joint is of primary concern.

● The axial plane is parallel to the plantar surface of the foot. This plane is acquired directly when the patient is positioned so that the toes are pointing straight up.

● Data are collected directly in the oblique coronal plane when the patient is positioned with bent knees so that the feet lie flat on the scanning table. The gantry is then tilted, typically 20° to 30° (top of the gantry away from the patient), so that the scan plane is perpendicular to the subtalar joint.

## REVIEW QUESTIONS

1. Why are isotropic voxels particularly important in images of the musculoskeletal system?
   a. Isotropic voxels will allow good reformations, even if there is motion artifact on the source images.
   b. Isotropic voxels enable MPR images to be created in any plane with the same spatial resolution as the original sections.
   c. Because voxels are isotropic, a wide slice thickness can be used, thereby reducing the data acquisition time.
   d. Isotropic voxels will eliminate streak artifacts from prosthetic devices and other metallic objects.

2. Which of the following clinical indications may result in a musculoskeletal examination being performed with intravenous contrast enhancement?
   a. Trauma
   b. Detection of suspected loose bodies within a joint
   c. Suspected tibial plateau fracture
   d. Suspected infection

3. Why is it recommended to position the patient for a shoulder CT so that the unaffected arm is extended over the patient's head?
   a. To reduce streak artifact
   b. So the IV injection site can be more easily monitored
   c. To make the patient more comfortable
   d. So as not to confuse the unaffected shoulder with that of the symptomatic one

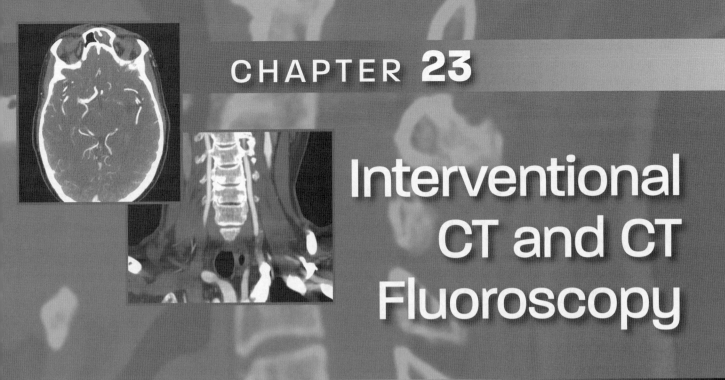

# CHAPTER 23

# Interventional CT and CT Fluoroscopy

CT is a valuable tool for use in interventional procedures such as biopsies and abscess drainage. The use of CT to guide percutaneous procedure offers several advantages.

- High-resolution CT images provide precise three-dimensional localization of lesions.
- CT images permit the clinician to plan an access route to the lesion by showing the relationship of surrounding structures.
- Because the tip of the needle within the structure can be visualized and slice thickness can be as narrow as 0.5 mm, interventions can be performed on small structures.
- Because of the wide latitude of beam attenuation information gathered by CT, an extremely low-density material such as gas can be imaged as well as high-density material such as metal, bone, or synthetic catheters.
- The ability to accurately image high-density material allows the use of any type of instrument (i.e., needle, drainage tube, or other devices).
- Contrast material can be injected when vascularity, an anatomic space, or an abnormal cavity needs further delineation.
- Patients can be placed in a variety of positions to allow easier access to the lesion.

## IMAGING TECHNIQUES FOR CT-GUIDED INTERVENTIONS

- Two different imaging techniques are used for CT-guided interventions: sequential CT and CT fluoroscopy (CTF).

- Sequential CT has all of the advantages listed above, but it does have some drawbacks.
  - The procedure can be lengthy because of the numerous single or helical CT images.
  - More importantly, the intermittent visualization prohibits the clinician from making rapid adjustments that are possible with conventional fluoroscopy.
- CTF allows for the near real-time capabilities of traditional fluoroscopy while maintaining the superior contrast resolution of CT. These benefits expand the ability to perform image-guided interventions in anatomically complex locations.
  - CTF capabilities are not standard on scanners; CTF must be purchased as an addition to a helical scanner.
  - Although there are concerns about the radiation dose delivered from either method, with CTF there is the additional concern for radiation exposure to the CT staff.
- It is not uncommon for a single department to use both approaches, depending on the clinical problem. They can be used separately or in combination.
- Techniques to reduce radiation dose should be used during interventions with either sequential CT or CTF.
  - When sequential CT is used, the mAs should be set as low as possible. One study reported success in both catheter placement and percutaneous biopsy when parameters were reduced to 30 mAs (from the standard setting of 175–250 mAs).

- When CTF is used, it is very important that CTF exposure time and tube current (mA) be kept as low as possible.
  - Dose rates, which can be high with the continuous (i.e., near real time) mode of acquisition, can be minimized by exclusively using intermittent fluoroscopy.
  - Personnel must take care to reduce their own radiation exposure. It is unacceptable to enter the CT beam with the hands. Needle-holding devices have been developed for CTF and have been shown to significantly reduce exposure to the hand.
  - Using a lead drape to cover the nonbiopsy region of the patient can significantly reduce scatter, protecting both the patient and the staff.

## INDICATIONS FOR CT-GUIDED PROCEDURES

- The indications for CT-guided procedures vary from institution to institution, depending on the preference of the radiologists and on the equipment available.
- Some of the most common indications include
  - drainage of abscesses and pneumothoraces
  - punctures of abdominal and thoracic masses and lesion
  - percutaneous diskectomy of herniated disks
  - lumbar spine or pelvic interventions
  - percutaneous administration of chemotherapeutic agents
  - thermoablative or radiofrequency ablative procedures
  - percutaneous vertebroplasty
- The steps to each procedure will vary somewhat. CT-guided biopsies are perhaps the most common interventional procedure; understanding the basic steps involved can provide a framework for other CT-guided procedures.

### CT-Guided Biopsies

- In theory, the risk associated with needle biopsy increases as needle diameter increases. When a cutting needle is used, the risk is even greater. However, the overall complication rate is small, approximately 2%.
  - The primary complication of biopsy procedures is bleeding (often related to undetected coagulopathy).
  - Highly vascularized lesions increase this risk. A bleeding disorder is a contraindication to percutaneous biopsy. However, patients are often treated with blood products or medications to temporarily remedy the disorder so that the biopsy can be performed.

- The most common complication of CT-guided lung biopsy is the occurrence of a pneumothorax during or after the intervention.
- Biopsy (using the sequential CT method) can be performed on any scanner without the purchase of additional computer software, but some supplies, such as specialized needles, are required.
- The purpose of CT-guided biopsy is to document neoplastic disease (primary, metastatic, or recurrent) or to differentiate neoplastic disease from other processes, such as inflammatory disease, postoperative changes, posttherapeutic changes, or normal structures.
- Therefore, the goal in a biopsy procedure is to obtain an adequate sample for laboratory evaluation with minimal trauma to surrounding tissues. The goal is achieved with accurate and expedient placement of the needle.
- CT-guided biopsy can be broken down into several basic steps.
  - The procedure is explained to the patient, and written consent is obtained.
  - Appropriate laboratory values are obtained. Most laboratory evaluations include prothrombin time, partial thromboplastin time, and platelet count.
  - The scan is plotted. This process includes careful review of the patient's previous CT study to determine the optimal patient position, whether oral or intravenous contrast medium is indicated, and the appropriate level for the biopsy.
  - The scan is performed through the selected area. An important consideration in scanning for a biopsy procedure is patient breathing. Clear instructions are essential so that each breath is as similar as possible. The breathing command should be given for each scan sequence. As the needle is placed, the patient is again asked to suspend breathing.
  - The best location for needle entry is selected. Once a location is selected, a metallic marker is placed on the skin with the localizer light on the CT scanner.
  - The scan is repeated to confirm the suitability of the selected entry location.
  - With the distance measurement on the CT system, the distance from the marker on the patient's skin to the lesion is measured. This measure determines the optimal depth and angle for needle placement.
  - The patient's skin is prepared according to aseptic procedure guidelines. A sterile drape is applied, a local anesthetic (lidocaine 1%) is administered, and the biopsy needle is placed.

- The scan is repeated at the needle location as well as one slice above and one slice below the expected needle location until the tip of the needle is visualized.
- If the CT images confirm the correct location of the needle, a tissue sample is taken and prepared according to laboratory protocols.
- A postprocedure scan is taken to identify complications such as pneumothorax or hematoma.

## CT-Guided Abscess Drainage

- The features that make CT an excellent choice for guiding a needle biopsy are also beneficial in performing percutaneous abscess drainage.
- The needle placement technique duplicates that used in percutaneous biopsy.
- In general, the shortest, straightest access route to the collection is favored. However, care should be taken to avoid major vessels, bowel loops, and the pleural space.

- After the needle is placed, a drainage catheter is situated.
- After the catheter is in place, the collection is aspirated as completely as possible. Catheters are usually left to gravity drainage.
- When drainage is complete, the catheter is withdrawn gradually.

## REVIEW QUESTIONS

1. All of the following are methods to reduce radiation dose to the patient and staff from CTF EXCEPT
   a. using intermittent fluoroscopy whenever possible.
   b. using a stand-off needle holder to avoid exposure to the hands.
   c. keeping the tube current as low as possible.
   d. changing the matrix size to 1,024.
2. Which of the following is a contraindication to any CT-guided biopsy?
   a. Infection
   b. Contrast media allergy
   c. Bleeding disorder that does not respond to treatment
   d. Congestive heart failure

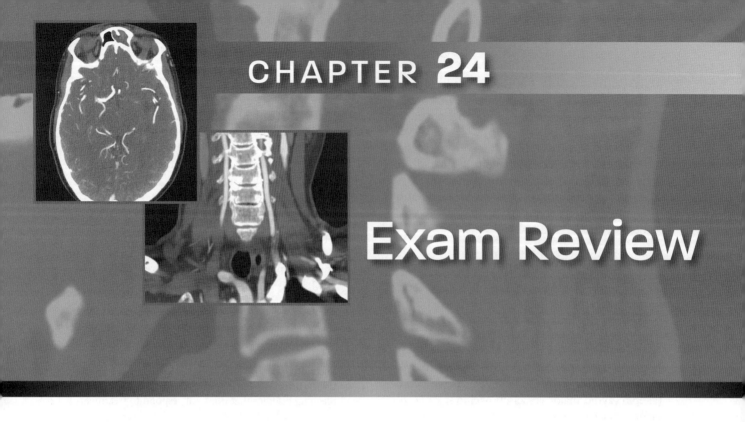

## CHAPTER 24

# Exam Review

## MOCK EXAM

1. In the CT setting, which describes the concept of basic (or simple) consent?
   a. Before the CT examination, the technologist explains the procedure to the patient and asks the patient if he or she agrees.
   b. A written document is given to the patient or guardian (or read to the patient, if necessary). The document lists all of the potential complications of the procedure. The patient must sign the form to acknowledge that he or she understands both the risks and benefits of the examination.
   c. Consent that is inferred from signs or action. For example, if a patient holds out his or her arm so that you can start an intravenous line, it can be implied that he or she gives his or her consent to the procedure.
   d. The requirement that, for minors, one or more parent must consent to the procedure.

2. A patient is being scheduled for a CT examination of the neck. The patient also needs a number of other diagnostic examinations. Which of the following examinations may affect the date scheduled for the CT study?
   a. Upper GI
   b. Nuclear medicine thyroid scan
   c. MR abdomen and pelvis examination
   d. Doppler ultrasound of the lower extremity

3. All of the following are reasons for obtaining a history before a CT examination is performed EXCEPT
   a. to verify that the patient has not exceeded the radiation limit.
   b. to select the appropriate protocol.
   c. to be sure the examination can be performed safely.
   d. to aide the radiologist in his or her interpretation of the CT examination.

4. What is a general rule regarding the administration of intravascular contrast media to patients receiving dialysis?
   a. Patients on dialysis should never be given contrast media.
   b. Patients on dialysis who still have some residual kidney function should not be given contrast media; patients with end-stage renal failure can be given contrast media.
   c. When contrast media is given, dialysis must be scheduled to be performed within 4 hours.
   d. Contrast media poses no risks to patients on dialysis.

5. In many institutions a radiologist is consulted before intravenous contrast medium is administered to patients in whom the eGRF value is less than
   a. 5 mL/min/1.73 m².
   b. 15 mL/min/1.73 m².
   c. 30 mL/min/1.73 m².
   d. 60 mL/min/1.73 m².

6. You complete the CT examination and will remove the intravenous catheter. Which of the following medications may necessitate holding pressure on the puncture site for a longer period?
   a. Coumadin
   b. Benadryl
   c. Tylenol
   d. Synthroid

7. In what circumstances is it acceptable to use a large-bore tunneled dialysis catheter for the injection of iodinated contrast media?
   a. Whenever a standard peripheral IV access is not available.
   b. When the contrast flow rate is 2 mL/s or less.
   c. When the patency of the line has been verified by flushing with saline.
   d. A dialysis catheter should never be used for contrast media administration.

8. Documentation of IV contrast administration is
   a. only necessary when an adverse event occurs.
   b. only necessary when routine injection parameters are modified.
   c. required on all patients and must be cosigned by a radiologist.
   d. required on all patients and should include the name of the agent, the dose, the flow rate, and the injection site.

9. Which is a TRUE statement regarding venipuncture in a peripheral vein for the placement of an IV line for a CT coronary angiogram?
   a. A 22-gauge butterfly infusion set should be used.
   b. An 18-gauge straight needle should be used.
   c. An indwelling catheter set with a flexible plastic cannula should be used, preferably 20 gauge or larger.
   d. A Huber needle should be used.

10. Automated injection triggering methods are used to
    a. simplify the process of contrast injection, so that assistants can perform the task and patient throughput can be increased.
    b. improve patient safety by reducing contrast extravasations.
    c. effectively accommodate for individual differences in circulation time by adjusting the scan delay.
    d. effectively accommodate for individual differences in circulation time by adjusting the contrast flow rate.

11. In what phase of tissue enhancement is the iodinated contrast in Figure 24-1?
    a. Noncontrast
    b. Bolus
    c. Excretory phase
    d. Equilibrium

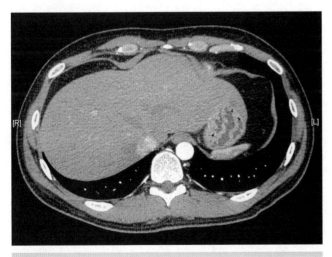

**FIGURE 24-1**

12. What type of heparin is used to flush devices such as PICCs and CVADs?
    a. Concentrated heparin sodium, generally 10,000 units/mL, followed by 5 mL of normal saline.
    b. Concentrated heparin sodium, generally 100 units/mL.
    c. Only a premixed heparin flush solution should be used.
    d. Undiluted, fractionated heparin.

13. What property of intravenous contrast media is responsible for its capacity to increase a structure's ability to attenuate the x-ray beam?
    a. Osmolality
    b. Viscosity
    c. Iodine concentration
    d. Ionic nature

14. Which is a true statement regarding overranging?
    a. Overranging results in streak artifacts on the image.
    b. Overranging only occurs with helical scan sequences.
    c. Overranging is an important technique used to reduce the radiation dose to the patient.
    d. Overranging has been eliminated for scanners with 64, 128, or 256 detectors.

15. A CT of the abdomen and pelvis is ordered for a child weighing 18 kg. Using the standard pediatric formula, what dose of iodinated contrast medium is given?
    a. 9 mL
    b. 18 mL
    c. 36 mL
    d. 54 mL

16. Which is a TRUE statement regarding the risk of iodinated contrast media to the fetus?
    a. At the usual clinical doses, iodinated contrast media does not cross the human placenta and therefore will not enter the fetus.
    b. Many studies have been done on the effects of iodinated contrast media in pregnant women.
    c. Although no definite risk to the fetus has been identified, not enough studies have been done to conclude that there are no risks.
    d. Fetal abnormalities have been reported in pregnant patients who were given iodinated contrast media at the usual clinical doses.

17. Contrast media–induced nephropathy can be defined as
    a. an acute impairment of renal function that occurs within 48 hours following the intravascular administration of contrast material and for which alternative causes have been excluded.
    b. chronic renal failure that is associated with diabetes mellitus.
    c. a short period of mildly reduced kidney function that does not produce symptoms.
    d. any renal impairment, whether mild or severe, that occurs within a month of the intravenous administration of contrast material.

18. Which is an advantage of using higher concentration (≥350 mg iodine/mL) agents?
    a. They possess lower osmolality, so are associated with fewer adverse effects.
    b. They produce fewer high-contrast (streak) artifacts in the injected vein.
    c. They deliver the same amount of iodine at a lower flow rate.
    d. They are of lower viscosity, so are less likely to remain in the venous injection path, and therefore, a saline flush is not necessary.

19. When a mechanical injector is used, a large air embolism can result from
    a. a malfunctioning pressure limit switch.
    b. the incorrect preparation and inadequate connection of the injector syringe and tubing.
    c. the use of butterfly infusion sets or straight needles.
    d. tiny undetected bubbles in the contrast medium.

20. What causes barium peritonitis?
    a. Aspiration of barium into the lungs
    b. The oral administration of a large volume of a barium sulfate solution in patients with an obstructed bowel
    c. The oral administration of a large volume of barium sulfate solution in patients with renal insufficiency
    d. Barium leaking into the peritoneal cavity from a perforation of the gastrointestinal tract

21. When the decision to premedicate using oral medications is made by the radiologist, it is important that the steroids be started
    a. 30 minutes before contrast administration.
    b. at least 2 hours before contrast administration.
    c. at least 6 hours before contrast administration.
    d. 72 hours before contrast administration.

22. Assuming all other factors are held constant, which of the following will increase the radiation dose to the patient for a CT examination of the abdomen?
    a. Widening the window width; increasing the window level
    b. Decreasing the pitch
    c. Using a wider slice
    d. Decreasing the mAs

23. If a single slice of the abdomen delivered a radiation dose of 8 cGy, the entire examination dose from 40 contiguous slices could be estimated as
    a. 0.2 to 0.8 cGy.
    b. 8 cGy.
    c. 10 to 11.2 cGy.
    d. 320 cGy.

24. What type of radiation dose measurement is used when scanner manufacturers report to the Food and Drug Administration and prospective clients the doses typically delivered for their machine?
    a. CTDI
    b. MSAD
    c. DLP
    d. rem

25. How does object size and scan field diameter affect radiation dose to the patient?
    a. Scan field diameter has no effect; it is the display field diameter that has an impact on dose.
    b. Changing from a small scan field, such as that used for a head scan, to a large scan field, such as that used for a body scan, will have a negligible effect on the radiation dose. It could either reduce or increase the dose slightly, depending on the patient factors.
    c. Smaller objects, which are scanned with a small scan field, always absorb a much higher dose than do larger objects, which are scanned with a large scan field.
    d. Smaller objects, which are scanned with a small scan field, always absorb a much lower dose than do larger objects, which are scanned with a large scan field.

26. The relationship between _____ and radiation dose to the patient is linear.
    a. mAs
    b. kVp
    c. display field size
    d. pitch

27. The radiosensitivity of a developing fetus is greatest
    a. from conception to 3 months' gestation.
    b. from 3 to 5 months' gestation.
    c. from 5 to 7 months' gestation.
    d. from 7 to 9 months' gestation.

28. Which of the following is TRUE concerning CT dose uniformity?
    a. Uniformity of dose increases as the scan field of view and patient thickness increase.
    b. The dose in body scans is more uniform than that of head scans.
    c. The peripheral dose, or skin dose, of a body scan can be two to three times higher than the central dose.
    d. Compared with children, adults can be expected to receive a more uniform dose.

29. The lifetime risk of an eventual cancer-related death as a result of pediatric CT is approximately 1 in
    a. 10.
    b. 1,000.
    c. 100,000.
    d. 1,000,000.

30. Why is lead shielding less beneficial in CT than it is in general radiography?
    a. Because of the narrow collimation used in CT, not much radiation is scattered to regions outside the selected scan area.
    b. Because of the high kVp used in CT, photons will penetrate a lead shield.
    c. Scatter radiation is excessive in CT and is not controlled by shielding.
    d. Radiosensitive organs such as the thyroid gland can never be shielded without impairing the scans.

31. Which combination of factors is likely to result in the lowest radiation dose to the patient?
    a. mAs = 180; kVp = 140; pitch = 0.8; 2-mm slice thickness
    b. mAs = 200; kVp = 120; pitch = 1.8; 5-mm slice thickness
    c. mAs = 280; kVp = 120; pitch = 1.5; 2-mm slice thickness
    d. mAs = 300; kVp = 120; pitch = 1.0; 5-mm slice

32. In CT, the uncoupling effect
    a. occurs with digital technology and refers to the fact that the relationship between dose and image quality is less direct than in film-screen radiography.
    b. occurs only in CT and refers to the process of changing pitch.
    c. refers to the process in conventional radiography in which the appropriate dose creates the proper film darkening; that is, too high a dose will create an image that is too dark, whereas too low a dose will result in an image that is too light.
    d. refers to the lack of a relationship, in CT, between patient size and radiation dose.

33. Which of the following is a high-attenuation structure?
    a. Renal cyst
    b. Trachea
    c. Petrous bone
    d. Lung
34. The process of using raw data to create a new image after the initial image has been generated is typically referred to as
    a. prospective reconstruction.
    b. reformatting.
    c. retrospective reconstruction.
    d. step-and-shoot scanning.
35. In a CT system, what is the function of the generator?
    a. It produces an electric current of very high amperage and transmits it to the filament.
    b. It produces high voltage and transmits it to the x-ray tube.
    c. It samples the detectors thousands of times per second.
    d. It dissipates the heat built up during x-ray production.
36. A detector's dynamic range is the
    a. time that is required for the signal from the detector to return to zero.
    b. number of photons absorbed by the detector.
    c. ratio of the maximum signal measured to the minimum signal the detector can measure.
    d. amount of afterglow exhibited.
37. The part of the CT system referred to as the DAS is responsible for
    a. converting the light emitted from the detector to an electric current.
    b. projecting the data from the attenuation profile onto a matrix.
    c. sampling each of the detector cells many times per second.
    d. converting digitized data to shades of gray to be displayed.
38. Increasing the kilovoltage results in an increase in the
    a. speed of the electrons as they travel from filament to anode.
    b. number of electrons that "boil off" of the filament.
    c. speed of electrons as they travel from the anode through the patient.
    d. rate at which the system can rid itself of by-product heat.
39. The configuration of the x-ray tube to the detectors determines a scanner's
    a. heat dissipation rate.
    b. detector efficiency.
    c. generation.
    d. speed.
40. Which are parts of the system's primary memory?
    a. ROM, RAM
    b. SAM, CD-R
    c. MOD, thumb drive
    d. DVD-R, magnetic tape
41. What is an example of a computer output device?
    a. CT detector mechanisms
    b. Microprocessor
    c. Touch-sensitive plasma screen
    d. Monitor

42. What two factors control the slice thickness of an MDCT scanner?
    a. Gantry rotation time and mAs setting
    b. Table speed and kVp setting
    c. Collimation of the x-ray beam and width of the detectors in the $z$ axis
    d. Reconstruction algorithm and detector material
43. What part of the CT system is responsible for converting the digitized data into shades of gray?
    a. Photodiode
    b. Array processor
    c. Display processor
    d. Analog-to-digital converter
44. A hardware component of a CT system that resembles small shutters with an opening that adjusts, dependent on the operator's selection of slice thickness, is a
    a. bow-tie filter.
    b. slip ring.
    c. reference detector.
    d. source collimator.
45. The fraction of a beam of x-rays that is absorbed or scattered per unit thickness of the absorber is referred to as the
    a. attenuation coefficient.
    b. contrast transfer function.
    c. spatial resolution.
    d. modulation transfer function.
46. In the production of x-rays, approximately what percentage of the kinetic energy of the projectile electrons is converted to thermal energy?
    a. 2%
    b. 50%
    c. 75%
    d. 99%
47. The area of the anode where the electrons strike and the x-ray beam is produced is the
    a. filament.
    b. focal spot.
    c. generator.
    d. detector.
48. MDCT systems that contain parallel rows of equal size detectors are called
    a. adaptive arrays.
    b. hybrid arrays.
    c. fourth-generation arrays.
    d. uniform arrays.
49. Which of the following could be retrospectively reconstructed for MDCT data that acquires 64 0.625-mm slices with each gantry rotation?
    a. Slices can be divided to produce one hundred twenty-eight 0.312-mm slices.
    b. Slices can be divided to produce two hundred fifty-six 0.625-mm slices.
    c. Slices can be combined to produce thirty-two 5-mm slices.
    d. Slices can be combined to produce eight 5-mm slices.
50. Computer memory that is imprinted at the factory and is used to store frequently used instructions such as those required for starting the CT system is called
    a. read-only memory (ROM).
    b. serial access memory (SAM).
    c. write-once-read-many times (WORM) memory.
    d. compact disk-recordable (CD-R).

51. Interpolation, as it is used in CT, is
    a. a statistical measure of the spread or dispersion of a set of data; it is the positive square root of the variance.
    b. a mathematical method to estimate a missing value by taking an average of known values at neighboring points.
    c. the method used to convert the electric signal to a digital format.
    d. the method used to convert light levels into an electric current.

52. Image data can be used for
    a. changing the display field size.
    b. changing the reconstruction algorithm.
    c. creating multiplanar reformations.
    d. creating overlapping slices from helical data.

53. Why is it necessary to apply a filter function to an attenuation profile to create a CT image?
    a. To minimize streaks
    b. To increase the signal-to-noise ratio
    c. To eliminate ring artifacts
    d. To reduce radiation exposure to the patient

54. What type of filter accentuates the difference between neighboring pixels to enhance spatial resolution?
    a. A bow-tie filter
    b. A smoothing algorithm
    c. A bone algorithm
    d. A soft tissue algorithm

55. The window width of a specific CT image is set at 120 and the level (or center) is set at 50. How is a structure with a measurement of −40 HU displayed?
    a. It is white.
    b. It is a light shade of gray.
    c. It is a dark shade of gray.
    d. It is black.

56. A narrow window width is best for
    a. displaying the aerated lungs.
    b. displaying the white and gray matter of the brain.
    c. suppressing noise on an image.
    d. reducing the appearance of streak artifact.

57. How is a cursor measurement different than obtaining a region of interest measurement?
    a. A cursor measurement provides only the standard deviation, whereas an ROI provides an HU measurement.
    b. A cursor measurement is the HU measurement for a single pixel, whereas an ROI is the average HU for all pixels within the ROI.
    c. A cursor measurement uses raw data, whereas an ROI uses image data.
    d. A cursor measurement shows what mAs were used to create the image, whereas an ROI obtains both mAs and kVp settings.

58. Using a standard 512 matrix for all studies, which contains the largest pixels?
    a. An image of the pituitary; DFOV = 16; slice thickness = 2 mm
    b. An image of the knee; DFOV = 20; slice thickness = 1 mm
    c. A scan of the neck; DFOV = 30; slice thickness = 3 mm
    d. A scan of the abdomen; DFOV = 44; slice thickness = 5 mm

59. Why is it more common practice to manipulate the mAs, rather than the kVp, for a CT examination?
    a. Changing the mAs does not affect the radiation dose to the patient.
    b. Scanners offer more mA options, and the effect of mAs on image quality is more predictable.
    c. Tube cooling is not affected by adjusting the mAs settings.
    d. Changing the mAs will not affect the quality of the images.

60. What scan parameter determines how the raw data are filtered in the reconstruction process?
    a. Window width
    b. Window level
    c. Reconstruction algorithm
    d. kVp

61. Which of the following is an imaging challenge that depends on spatial resolution?
    a. A liver lesion that is surrounded by healthy liver tissue
    b. Distinguishing between the white matter and gray matter of the brain
    c. A large abdominal abscess
    d. Tiny, contrast-filled arteries that are just 1 mm apart

62. In-plane resolution refers to the resolution
    a. resulting from helical data.
    b. in the $xy$ direction.
    c. in the $z$ direction.
    d. related to the slice thickness.

63. Which of the following parameters will produce near-isotropic voxels?
    a. DFOV = 12; slice thickness = 1 mm
    b. DFOV = 25; slice thickness = 5 mm
    c. DFOV = 35; slice thickness = 0.625 mm
    d. DFOV = 44; slice thickness = 2 mm

64. Temporal resolution refers to
    a. the spatial resolution measurable in images of the temporal bone.
    b. how rapidly the data are acquired by the CT system.
    c. the ability to differentiate between objects with very similar densities as their backgrounds.
    d. the level of noise apparent on an image.

65. What two factors define the quantity of the x-ray energy?
    a. mA and scan time
    b. kVp and heat capacity
    c. Reconstruction algorithm and heat dissipation
    d. DFOV and $x, y$ coordinates

66. Which of the following can be described as possessing high inherent contrast?
    a. Soft tissue
    b. Kidneys
    c. Liver
    d. Lungs

67. What type of 3D display is depicted in Figure 24-2?
    a. Volume rendering
    b. Surface rendering
    c. MIP
    d. MinIP

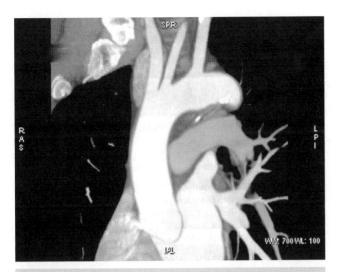

**FIGURE 24-2**

68. In the computing world, _____ is used to describe an arrangement in which two or more components perform the same task—if one element fails, the duplication keeps the system functioning while the failed component is repaired.
    a. redundancy
    b. bandwidth
    c. overlapping
    d. protocol

69. Which is a true statement regarding the linear no-threshold (LNT) model used in radiation physics?
    a. The LNT model has only been accepted as the standard since 2016.
    b. The model assumes that small exposures are harmless and may even be beneficial.
    c. The LNT model assumes that biological damage is directly proportional to the dose of ionizing radiation.
    d. Another name for the LNT model is radiation hormesis model.

70. Spatial resolution can be calculated from the analysis of the spread of information within the system using the modulation transfer function. What is a simpler and more direct way to measure spatial resolution?
    a. Using a line/pairs phantom
    b. Using a water phantom
    c. Using the readout from the scanner's display
    d. Calculating it from the radiation dose delivered

71. Which aspect of the CT quality control program must be performed by a medical physicist?
    a. Spatial resolution measurement
    b. Dosimetric data
    c. Noise and uniformity
    d. All aspects of the CT quality control program must be performed by a medical physicist

72. The process in CT by which different tissue attenuations are averaged to produce one less accurate pixel reading is called
    a. the partial volume effect.
    b. beam hardening.
    c. photon deprivation.
    d. ring artifacts.

73. The primary method of reducing beam-hardening artifacts is
    a. increasing mAs.
    b. decreasing slice thickness.
    c. using a helical technique.
    d. filtering the x-ray beam.

74. Effective slice thickness blooming is
    a. the process in CT by which different tissue attenuations are averaged to produce one less accurate pixel reading.
    b. a disadvantage often associated with the interpolation of helical data.
    c. an improvement to image resolution associated with helical scans.
    d. the trend toward selecting a wider slice thickness to improve spatial resolution.

75. If measurements taken around the perimeter of a water phantom are different from those taken at the center of the phantom, than there is a problem with the system's
    a. linearity.
    b. slice-thickness accuracy.
    c. photon absorption.
    d. cross-field uniformity.

76. Estimate the radiation dose for one CT examination versus the dose for one chest radiograph.
    a. One CT examination is less than or equal to one chest radiograph.
    b. One CT examination is greater than one chest radiograph, but less than 100 chest radiographs.
    c. One CT examination is equal to from 100 to 250 chest radiographs.
    d. One CT examination is equal to or greater than 500 chest radiographs.

77. What postprocessing technique created the image of the heart in Figure 24-3?
    a. MinIP
    b. MIP
    c. Volume rendering
    d. Endoluminal imaging

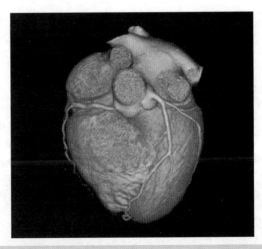

**FIGURE 24-3**

78. The phantom in Figure 24-4 features a series of cylinders with different diameters, all at 0.6% (6 HU) difference from the background material. This phantom is used to measure
    a. slice thickness accuracy.
    b. low-contrast resolution.
    c. high-contrast resolution.
    d. CT number accuracy.

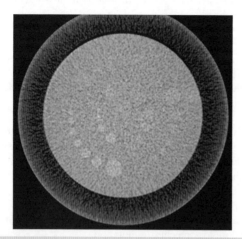

**FIGURE 24-4**

79. Which image artifact can result from an improperly centered patient?
    a. Edge gradient artifact
    b. Undersampling artifact
    c. Tube arc artifact
    d. Out-of-field artifact
80. What is the likely cause of the artifact in Figure 24-5?
    a. Patient motion
    b. Patient arms in the SFOV
    c. Metallic object
    d. Not enough data collected (undersampling)

81. Which type of artifact is only present on images produced from MDCT systems?
    a. Edge gradient
    b. Aliasing
    c. Cone beam
    d. Tube arcing
82. What causes ring artifacts?
    a. Electrical surges (i.e., a "short-circuit") within the x-ray tube
    b. Involuntary patient motion (e.g., heart motion)
    c. Irregularly shaped objects that have a pronounced difference in density from surrounding structures
    d. Imperfect detector elements—either faulty or simply out of calibration
83. The presence of noise on an image degrades its quality, particularly its
    a. low-contrast resolution.
    b. longitudinal resolution.
    c. spatial resolution.
    d. temporal resolution.
84. An image of the abdomen is greatly degraded by quantum mottle. The scan parameters used are as follows: DFOV = 38 cm; slice thickness = 5 mm; mA = 240; tube rotation = 0.5 seconds; kVp = 120. What action will have the best chance of reducing or eliminating the quantum mottle for subsequent scans?
    a. Increase DFOV to 44 cm.
    b. Decrease slice thickness to 2 mm.
    c. Decrease mA to 125, and increase the tube rotation time to 1.0 second.
    d. Increase the mA to 300, and increase the tube rotation time to 0.8 seconds.
85. What plane is the MPR depicted by Figure 24-6?
    a. Sagittal
    b. Coronal
    c. Oblique
    d. Curved

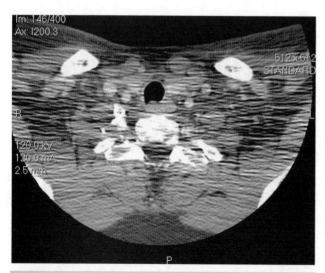

**FIGURE 24-5**

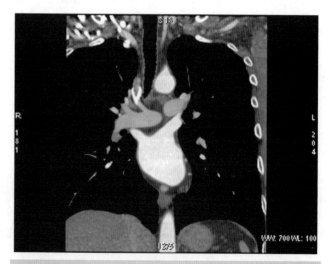

**FIGURE 24-6**

86. A circular ROI is defined and placed on the image, and the resultant measurement is 3 HU. The standard deviation is 0. It can be surmised that
    a. all of the pixels within the region have identical values.
    b. the area measured is composed of a variety of very different tissue types.
    c. the area is likely a calcified nodule.
    d. the patient is obese.

87. 3D printing in CT uses what type of data sets?
    a. MPR
    b. Localizer image
    c. Volume rendered
    d. Surface rendered

88. Comparing the spatial resolution of CT to other modalities:
    a. CT is superior to general radiography, MRI, and ultrasound.
    b. CT is superior to general radiography but is inferior to MRI.
    c. CT is comparable to all other modalities.
    d. CT is inferior to general radiography.

89. Changing the slice incrementation is also referred to as
    a. $z$ axis reconstruction or changing the reconstruction interval.
    b. dynamic or cine scanning.
    c. changing the zoom, target, or display field-of-view.
    d. electron beam or fifth-generation CT.

90. Which of the following is NOT an advantage of using helical CT for the diagnosis of PE?
    a. It is cost-effective.
    b. Quality images are produced even if the patient is uncooperative.
    c. It is often helpful in establishing an alternative diagnosis in the absence of PE.
    d. It is less invasive than pulmonary angiography.

91. High-density contrast agents, such as barium sulfate, are referred to as
    a. positive agents.
    b. negative agents.
    c. neutral agents.
    d. ionic agents.

92. What is the pitch in the following scenario: 64 detector channels used, 0.625-mm slice thickness, table movement of 55 mm per rotation?
    a. 1
    b. 1.375
    c. 1.5
    d. 2

93. When do scan protocols incorporate the use of gapped slices?
    a. When the object of interest is very small (<2 mm)
    b. When metallic objects are present in the area scanned
    c. When the patient is unable to hold still for the duration of the scan
    d. When a survey of an area is needed

94. Pitch is a parameter that is commonly used in helical CT to describe
    a. the number of detectors in the $z$ axis.
    b. tube heat capacity.
    c. table speed.
    d. different types of interpolation methods.

95. Refer to Figure 24-7. Name the structure indicated by arrow #1.
    a. Corpus callosum
    b. Caudate nucleus
    c. Lateral ventricle
    d. External capsule

96. Refer to Figure 24-7. Name the structure indicated by arrows #2 and #5.
    a. Falx cerebri
    b. Pericallosal arteries
    c. Vermis of cerebellum
    d. Central sulcus

97. Refer to Figure 24-7. Name the structure indicated by arrow #3.
    a. Putamen
    b. Caudate nucleus
    c. Thalamus
    d. Pons, medulla oblongata

98. Refer to Figure 24-7. Name the structure indicated by arrow #4.
    a. Basilar artery
    b. Sigmoid sinus
    c. Anterior cerebral artery
    d. Pineal body (calcified)

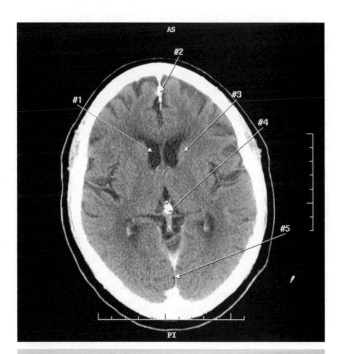

**FIGURE 24-7**

99. Compare 100 mL of Ultravist (iopromide) 300 with 100 mL of Ultravist (iopromide) 370.
    a. Ultravist 370 has a higher viscosity.
    b. Ultravist 370 contains fewer grams of iodine.
    c. Ultravist 370 is a better choice if the IV catheter is a 22 to 24 gauge.
    d. Ultravist 370 has a lower osmolality.

100. In which of the following situations would an LOCM be beneficial when delivered orally?
    a. When a patient is unable to drink the full dose of oral contrast
    b. When oral contrast is needed for neonatal CT examinations
    c. When patients are older than 70 years of age
    d. When patients have a hiatal hernia
101. The difference among the bolus phase, the nonequilibrium phase, and the equilibrium phase of contrast enhancement is primarily determined by the
    a. brand of iodinated contrast agent that is used.
    b. injection rate and scan delay.
    c. type of pathologic disease present.
    d. film processing time.
102. For routine CT of the chest, abdomen, or pelvis, the range of suggested IV contrast flow rates is
    a. 0.2 to 0.5 mL/s.
    b. 1.0 to 2.0 mL/s.
    c. 2.0 to 4.0 mL/s.
    d. 6 to 12 mL/s.
103. Which of the following might be an appropriate protocol for a CT study that is performed for suspected acoustic neuroma?
    a. 10-mm contiguous slices; standard algorithm; with IV contrast; filmed with a narrow window width
    b. 8-mm contiguous slices; bone algorithm; without IV contrast; filmed at two separate window settings
    c. 5-mm slice thickness; 3-mm table increment; without IV contrast; soft (i.e., low contrast) algorithm; filmed with a lung window
    d. 1.0-mm contiguous slices; reconstructed using both a standard and a bone (i.e., high-contrast) algorithm; with IV contrast; filmed in two separate window settings
104. Fresh blood in the brain, as in the case of a recent-onset subdural hematoma, will measure approximately
    a. −80 HU.
    b. 20 HU.
    c. 70 HU.
    d. 150 HU.
105. Patients with metastasis to the brain are at greater risk for _____ after the administration of an IV contrast agent.
    a. seizures
    b. contrast-induced nephropathy
    c. anaphylactoid reaction
    d. pulmonary effects, such as bronchospasm
106. Refer to Figure 24-8. Name the structure indicated by arrow #1.
    a. Mastoid air cells
    b. Incus
    c. Stapes
    d. Cochlea
107. Refer to Figure 24-8. Name the structure indicated by arrow #2.
    a. Malleus
    b. Stapes
    c. Trigeminal nerve branches
    d. Sella turcica

108. Refer to Figure 24-8. Name the structure indicated by arrow #3.
    a. Mastoid antrum
    b. Epitympanic recess
    c. Internal auditory canal
    d. Vestibule

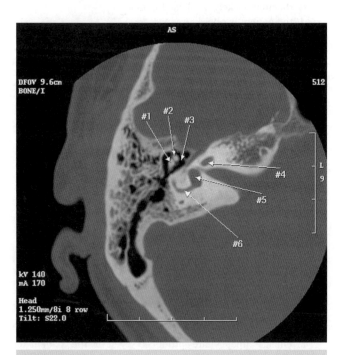

**FIGURE 24-8**

109. Refer to Figure 24-8. Name the structure indicated by arrow #4.
    a. Tympanic sinus
    b. Internal jugular vein
    c. Cochlea
    d. Facial nerve
110. Refer to Figure 24-8. Name the structure indicated by arrow #5.
    a. Vestibule
    b. Facial canal
    c. Cochlea
    d. Internal carotid artery canal
111. Refer to Figure 24-8. Name the structure indicated by arrow #6.
    a. Lateral semicircular canal
    b. Round window
    c. Eustachian tube
    d. Vestibular aqueduct
112. Prospective ECG gating methods for imaging the heart use a signal, usually derived from the _____ of the patient's ECG, to trigger image acquisition.
    a. ST segment
    b. PR segment
    c. R wave
    d. T wave

113. When imaging the heart, particularly when the structures of interest are small, such as the coronary arteries, a regular heart rate of less than _____ is important.
     a. 50 bpm
     b. 70 bpm
     c. 90 bpm
     d. 110 bpm
114. Airway imaging is routinely performed
     a. at both inspiration and expiration.
     b. using a wide slice thickness (≥8 mm).
     c. using a low-contrast (i.e., soft) algorithm.
     d. using a representative technique in which only about 10% of the airway is imaged.
115. In addition to imaging the pulmonary arterial system for patients with suspected PE, CT venography is sometimes performed to assess for venous thrombosis within the pelvis and lower extremities. How is this accomplished?
     a. A single helical scan is obtained in the cranial-to-caudal direction extending from the lung apices to the knees while contrast is in the bolus phase (20–30 seconds after IV contrast injection).
     b. A second scan series is obtained in the nonequilibrium phase (approximately 45 seconds after IV contrast injection) from the iliac crest through the knees.
     c. A second scan series is obtained in a delayed venous phase (approximately 180 seconds after IV contrast injection) from the iliac crest through the knees.
     d. A second scan series is obtained after most of the contrast has washed out of the venous structures (8 to 12 minutes after IV contrast injection) from the iliac crest through the knees.
116. The use of a saline flush after the injection of the iodinated contrast is recommended for CTA pulmonary studies. Why?
     a. To reduce or eliminate beam-hardening artifacts from dense contrast media within the superior vena cava that may obscure small emboli in adjacent vessels
     b. To hydrate the patient and reduce the risk of contrast-induced nephropathy
     c. So that additional images can be acquired with a negative contrast agent
     d. To flush any emboli out of the patient's pulmonary arteries
117. Refer to Figure 24-9. Name the structure indicated by arrow #1.
     a. Left atrium
     b. Aortic arch
     c. Right pulmonary artery
     d. Right brachiocephalic vein
118. Refer to Figure 24-9. Name the structure indicated by arrow #2.
     a. Brachiocephalic artery
     b. Ascending aorta
     c. Right pulmonary vein
     d. Superior vena cava
119. Refer to Figure 24-9. Name the structure indicated by arrow #3.
     a. Right atrium
     b. Ascending aorta
     c. Right ventricle
     d. Superior vena cava

120. Refer to Figure 24-9. Name the structure indicated by arrow #4.
     a. Pulmonary trunk
     b. Descending aorta
     c. Left atrium
     d. Superior vena cava

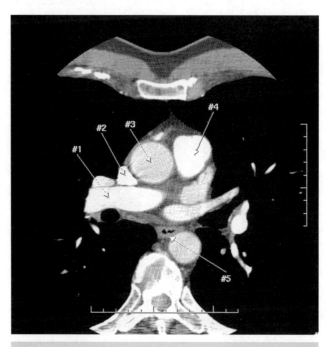

**FIGURE 24-9**

121. Refer to Figure 24-9. Name the structure indicated by arrow #5.
     a. Bronchus intermedius
     b. Azygos vein
     c. Esophagus
     d. Right crus of diaphragm
122. The formation, development, or existence of a clot within the vascular system is referred to as a(an)
     a. embolus.
     b. thrombosis.
     c. ischemic stroke.
     d. myocardial infarction.
123. A CT study done for the screening, detection, or exclusion of pulmonary nodules or infiltrates are typically done
     a. using multiple axial-mode scans, so that the patient must only hold the breath for a few seconds at a time.
     b. using a wide slice thickness (>8 mm) so the scan can be completed quickly, in one breath-hold.
     c. without IV contrast administration.
     d. first without IV contrast administration, followed by a repeat series with IV contrast administration.
124. Refer to Figure 24-10. Name the structure indicated by arrow #1.
     a. Portal vein
     b. Inferior vena cava
     c. Aorta
     d. Left renal artery

125. Refer to Figure 24-10. Name the structure indicated by arrow #2.
    a. Hepatic flexure of the colon
    b. Duodenum
    c. Gastroesophageal junction
    d. Body of the stomach
126. Refer to Figure 24-10. Name the structure indicated by arrow #3.
    a. Portal vein
    b. Inferior vena cava
    c. Superior mesenteric artery
    d. Hepatic artery

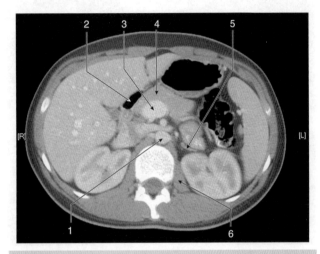

**FIGURE 24-10**

127. Refer to Figure 24-10. Name the structure indicated by arrow #4.
    a. Head of the pancreas
    b. Tail of the pancreas
    c. Duodenum
    d. Left renal artery
128. Refer to Figure 24-10. Name the structure indicated by arrow #5.
    a. Superior mesenteric artery
    b. Superior mesenteric vein
    c. Splenic artery
    d. Left adrenal
129. Refer to Figure 24-10. Name the structure indicated by arrow #6.
    a. Rectus abdominis muscle
    b. Diaphragm
    c. Psoas muscle
    d. Erector spinae muscle
130. A patient is being seen in the emergency department for acute respiratory distress. Pulmonary emboli are suspected and a CT is ordered. A review of the patient's history reveals that he is allergic to shellfish. What action should be taken?
    a. A CT examination using a pulmonary embolism protocol is done.
    b. A CT examination of the chest, without contrast enhancement, is done.
    c. The CT examination is cancelled; most likely it will be replaced by a nuclear medicine V/Q examination.
    d. The patient is given steroids, and the CT examination is delayed for 6 hours.

131. Which is a true statement regarding Figure 24-11?
    a. The gallbladder is absent.
    b. The spleen is absent.
    c. The patient has breast implants.
    d. The patient had a Whipple procedure.

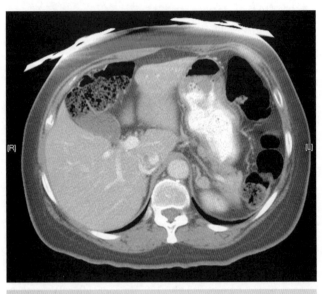

**FIGURE 24-11**

132. Refer to Figure 24-12. Name the structure indicated by arrow #1.
    a. Descending colon
    b. Jejunum/ileum
    c. Inflamed appendix
    d. Ascending colon
133. Refer to Figure 24-12. Name the structure indicated by arrow #2.
    a. Right common iliac vein
    b. Right common iliac artery
    c. Right ovary
    d. Iliacus muscle

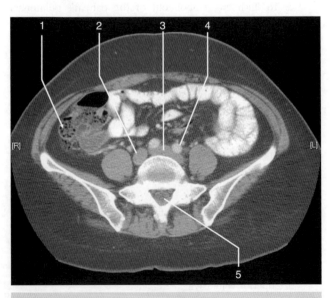

**FIGURE 24-12**

134. Refer to Figure 24-12. Name the structure indicated by arrow #3.
    a. Left common iliac vein
    b. Left common iliac artery
    c. Celiac trunk
    d. Azygos vein

135. Refer to Figure 24-12. Name the structure indicated by arrow #4.
    a. Left common iliac vein
    b. Left common iliac artery
    c. Celiac trunk
    d. Azygos vein

136. Refer to Figure 24-12. Name the structure indicated by arrow #5.
    a. Nucleus pulposus
    b. Vertebral canal with spinal cord
    c. Transverse ligament
    d. Intervertebral foramen

137. A bolus injection of 125 mL of an iodinated contrast media with a concentration of 320 mg of iodine/mL is administered to a 150-pound patient, but because of an unexpected equipment malfunction, scan data could not be acquired. The decision must be made as to whether the patient should be moved to a functioning scanner within the department and the contrast injection repeated. What information will be particularly important for the radiologist making the decision?
    a. The amount of radiation the patient received from the failed attempt
    b. The patient's history of allergy to any food or medication
    c. Evidence of renal impairment or dehydration
    d. The brand of the contrast media being used

138. What can be done to reduce streak artifacts such as those seen in Figure 24-13?
    a. Increase the kVp.
    b. Contrast administration is immediately followed by a saline solution bolus.
    c. Begin scanning 45 seconds after contrast media is seen in the monitoring slice.
    d. Lift the patient's arms over his or her head.

139. On an unenhanced abdominal CT, what is the range of CT attenuation values of a normal liver?
    a. −10 HU to 30 HU
    b. 38 HU to 70 HU
    c. 85 HU to 132 HU
    d. 147 HU to 165 HU

140. In general, the pancreas is located between the areas of the
    a. fifth and eighth thoracic vertebrae.
    b. ninth and eleventh thoracic vertebrae.
    c. twelfth thoracic vertebra and the second lumbar vertebra.
    d. second and fourth lumbar vertebrae.

141. To scan in the nephrographic phase of contrast enhancement, scans should be acquired approximately _____ after a bolus contrast injection.
    a. 15 to 25 seconds
    b. 30 to 70 seconds
    c. 80 to 130 seconds
    d. 3 to 15 minutes

142. The use of flow control mechanical pressure injectors are recommended for CT studies of the chest, abdomen, and pelvis because
    a. there is a reduced risk of extravasation of the contrast media into the soft tissues.
    b. side effects such as heat and nausea are reduced.
    c. contrast media dose and timing can be easily regulated and reproduced in subsequent studies.
    d. the risk of air embolus is eliminated.

143. In scanning the abdomen, what can be done if the patient is unable to take fluids by mouth?
    a. The volume of intravenous contrast material is increased by 25% to compensate for the lack of oral contrast medium.
    b. 600 mL of dilute water-soluble agent is administered by enema.
    c. A nasogastric tube may be inserted for the administration of an oral contrast agent.
    d. A small volume of dilute water-soluble contrast agent can be administered by an inhaler.

144. It is imperative that all scans be completed before the equilibrium phase of contrast enhancement in studies of the
    a. brain.
    b. urinary tract.
    c. liver.
    d. postsurgical lumbar disk.

145. Scanning to the adrenal glands in a CT study of the thorax is sometimes performed because
    a. it ensures that the technologist has scanned the entire lung field.
    b. kidney function can be assessed.
    c. the adrenal glands are part of the respiratory system.
    d. lung cancer may metastasize to the adrenal glands.

146. As a general rule, this is set at a point that has roughly the same value as the average attenuation number of the tissue of interest. What is it?
    a. The x axis in a histogram
    b. Standard deviation
    c. Sampling rate
    d. Window level

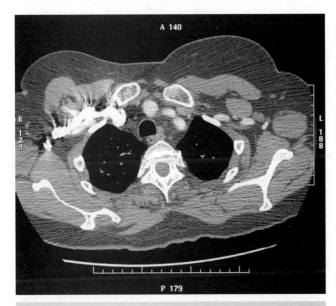

**FIGURE 24-13**

147. The trachea bifurcates at the level of
    a. C6 to C7.
    b. T4 to T5.
    c. T7 to T8.
    d. T10 to T11.
148. An anatomic trait that can help to differentiate an adenoma from a malignant adrenal mass on CT scans is its
    a. intracellular lipid content.
    b. calcium content.
    c. location.
    d. iron content.
149. A set of ROIs, one placed within the liver and one placed within the spleen, is often used to document
    a. splenomegaly.
    b. fatty infiltrate of the liver.
    c. sickle cell disease.
    d. lymphoma.
150. Refer to Figure 24-14. Name the structure indicated by arrow #1.
    a. Sternocleidomastoid muscle
    b. Scalenus muscle
    c. Thyroid gland
    d. Cricoid cartilage
151. Refer to Figure 24-14. Name the structure indicated by arrow #2.
    a. Hyoid bone
    b. Thyroid cartilage
    c. Mandible
    d. Cricoid cartilage
152. Refer to Figure 24-14. Name the structure indicated by arrow #3.
    a. Trachea
    b. Piriform recess
    c. Laryngeal vestibule
    d. Pharynx

153. Refer to Figure 24-14. Name the structure indicated by arrow #4.
    a. Basilar artery
    b. Vertebral artery
    c. Internal jugular vein
    d. Common carotid artery
154. Refer to Figure 24-14. Name the structure indicated by arrow #5.
    a. Pericallosal arteries
    b. Thyroid gland
    c. Jugular vein
    d. Lingual artery
155. For a CT of the foot, the patient is positioned supine, legs flat on the table, toes pointing straight up. There is no gantry tilt. Images acquired are in the direct _____ plane.
    a. sagittal
    b. oblique
    c. coronal
    d. axial
156. In a preliminary scout view of a patient, the abdomen is determined to be 360 mm in length. In this four-slice CT system, the gantry makes a 360° rotation each second. The protocol at this institution calls for a 5-mm slice thickness. To cover the entire abdominal area in a single helical scan, which set of parameters could be selected?
    a. 10-second total acquisition time, 1 pitch
    b. 10-second total acquisition time, 1.2 pitch
    c. 15-second total acquisition time, 1 pitch
    d. 15-second total scan acquisition, 1.2 pitch
157. What technique is often used to differentiate the margins of the pancreas from the duodenum?
    a. Water-soluble contrast medium administered by enema
    b. Acquire scans while the patient is in a right decubitus position
    c. Unenhanced imaging; no oral or intravenous contrast is used
    d. Scan approximately 2 hours after the patient ingests 600 mL of a barium sulfate oral contrast medium
158. Refer to Figure 24-15. Name the structure indicated by arrow #1.
    a. Talus
    b. Calcaneus
    c. Navicular bone
    d. Distal fibula (lateral malleolus)
159. Refer to Figure 24-15. Name the structure indicated by arrow #2.
    a. Talus
    b. Cuneiform (lateral or first)
    c. Cuboid bone
    d. Metatarsal bone
160. Refer to Figure 24-15. Name the structure indicated by arrow #3.
    a. Talus
    b. Cuneiform (interomedial or second)
    c. Navicular bone
    d. Metatarsal bone

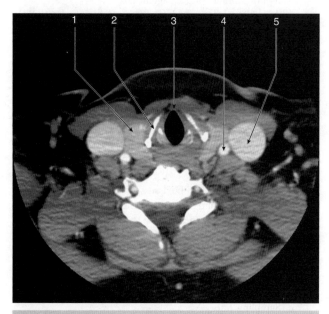

**FIGURE 24-14**

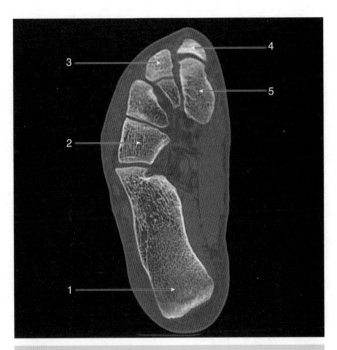

**FIGURE 24-15**

161. Refer to Figure 24-15. Name the structure indicated by arrow #4.
    a. Phalange (proximal)
    b. Distal tibia (medial malleolus)
    c. Navicular bone
    d. Metatarsal bone

162. Refer to Figure 24-15. Name the structure indicated by arrow #5.
    a. Cuneiform bone (medial or first)
    b. Cuboid bone
    c. Calcaneus
    d. Metatarsal bone

163. What is the most superior part of the sternum?
    a. Xiphoid process
    b. Manubrium
    c. Ensiform
    d. Gladiolus

164. Which of the following factors should be adjusted when slice thickness is decreased from 10 to 3 mm?
    a. Increase display field
    b. Decrease matrix size
    c. Lower window level
    d. Increase mAs

165. In scanning the brain, using which one of the following reference lines reduces the radiation exposure to the lens of the eye?
    a. Canthomeatal line
    b. Orbital meatal line
    c. Glabellomeatal line
    d. Infraorbital meatal line

# Appendix

## Answers to Review Questions

### CHAPTER 1: BASIC PRINCIPLES OF CT

1. Answer–d. Manufacturers use different names to describe features in a CT system. Names that have been used to describe the preliminary image include Topogram (Siemens), Scout (GE Healthcare), Scanogram (Toshiba), Pilot (Picker), and CR Image (Shimadzu). The term "spiral scan" is used to describe the method of scanning that includes a continuously rotating x-ray tube and constant table that travel throughout the scan acquisition. (Comprehensive Text Chapter 1; Heading: Terminology)

2. Answer–b. Low-contrast resolution is the ability of the system to display small density differences, such as when an image of the brain clearly shows the difference between the white and gray matter. Choices (a) and (c) are synonyms for a system's ability to define small objects distinctly. Temporal resolution, choice (d), refers to acquisition speed. (Comprehensive Text Chapter 1; Heading: Terminology)

3. Answer–a. (Comprehensive Text Chapter 1; Heading: Computed Tomography Defined)

4. Answer–d. A 1,024 matrix contains 1,024 rows of pixels down and 1,024 columns of pixels across. The total number of pixels in a matrix is the product of the number of rows and the number of columns. (Comprehensive Text Chapter 1; Heading: Computed Tomography Defined)

5. Answer–d. Beam attenuation is a basic radiation principle in which higher-density objects absorb more of the x-ray beam; subsequently fewer photons reach the detectors. The alteration in the beam varies with the density of the structure it passes through. This phenomenon is essential to produce images in which varying shades of gray reflect varying densities within the object. (Comprehensive Text Chapter 1; Heading: Beam Attenuation)

6. Answer–c. A low-attenuation object is one that allows x-rays to pass through relatively unimpeded. Because the trachea contains air, which does not attenuate much of the x-ray beam, it will be repre-sented by a black area on the image. (Comprehensive Text Chapter 1; Heading: Beam Attenuation)

7. Answer–b. In the Hounsfield system, the attenu-ation capacity of water is assigned 0, that of air −1,000, and that of bone 1,000. Objects with a beam attenuation less than that of water have an associated negative number. If an object is slightly less dense than water, an HU of slightly less than 0 can be expected. (Comprehensive Text Chapter 1; Heading: Hounsfield Units)

8. Answer–a. Oral or intravenous iodinated agents fill certain structures with a higher-density material, subsequently raising the structure's ability to attenu-ate the x-ray beam. It is important to note that the contrast agent does not change the body tissues but only resides in them. (Comprehensive Text Chapter 1; Heading: Beam Attenuation)

9. Answer–d. The x-ray beam used in CT contains a vari-ety of x-ray photons, ranging from those that are weak to those that are relatively strong. (Comprehensive Text Chapter 1; Heading: Polychromatic X-ray Beams)

10. Answer–a. Artifacts can be attributed to many different reasons, but they always degrade the image. (Comprehensive Text Chapter 1; Heading: Polychromatic X-ray Beams)

11. Answer–d. Filtering the x-ray beam removes long-wavelength, or "soft," x-rays that do not contribute to the CT image but increase the patient's radiation dose. A second purpose of filtration is to reduce beam-hardening artifacts by creating a more uniform beam intensity. An x-ray beam can only be filtered after it is generated (i.e., leaves the anode); therefore, neither choices (a) nor (c) are possible. (Comprehensive Text Chapter 1; Heading: Polychromatic X-ray Beams)

12. Answer–d. Thinner slices reduce volume averaging by decreasing the amount of patient information included in each voxel. (Comprehensive Text Chapter 1; Heading: Volume Averaging)

13. Answer–a. To accurately image the many small structures of the inner ear, a thin slice is required. It is true that there is a trade-off when it comes to

radiation dose to the patient; thinner slices do result in a higher radiation dose to the patient. However, in the case of the inner ear, the higher dose is justified as only a thin slice will provide the image quality necessary for a diagnosis. As a general rule, if the structures being investigated are very small and the region to be scanned is not extensive, then slice thickness can be quite thin. This type of examination is not done as a screening examination. In addition, when scanning the internal auditory canals, it may be possible to adjust the image plane to reduce radiation exposure to the corneas. (Comprehensive Text Chapter 1; Heading: Volume Averaging)

14. Answer–b. The CT number is the average of all measurements for that pixel. (Comprehensive Text Chapter 1; Heading: Volume Averaging)

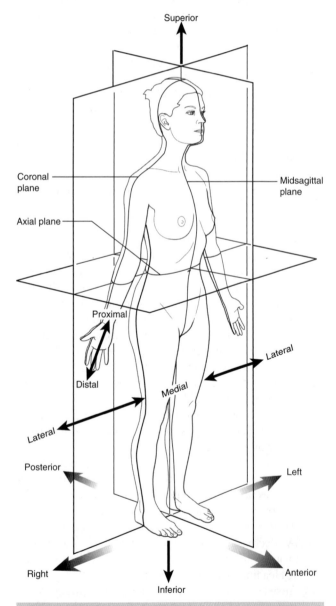

**FIGURE 1-2** The anatomic position.

15. Answer–b. Scan data consist of the information gathered from the detector array but not yet processed to create an image. The other three choices are synonyms for data that have been processed. (Comprehensive Text Chapter 1; Heading: Raw Data Versus Image Data)

16. Answer–c. The anatomic position is characterized by an individual standing erect, with the palms of the hands facing forward (Fig. 1-2). (Comprehensive Text Chapter 1; Heading: Imaging Planes)

17. Answer–a. A coronal plane divides the body into anterior and posterior sections (Comprehensive Text Chapter 1; Heading: Imaging Planes)

## CHAPTER 2: DATA ACQUISITION

1. Answer–a. Three-phase generators are standalone units located near the gantry and require cables. In new CT systems, they have been replaced by smaller, high-frequency generators that are located within the gantry. (Comprehensive Text Chapter 2; Heading: Gantry/Generator)

2. Answer–d. (Comprehensive Text Chapter 2; Heading: Gantry/Generator)

3. Answer–b. Slip rings permit the gantry frame to rotate continuously, making helical scan modes possible. Choice (a) describes the older system of cables, choice (c) describes filtration, and choice (d) describes collimation. (Comprehensive Text Chapter 2; Heading: Gantry/Slip Rings)

4. Answer–d. Although a small tube filament provides better spatial resolution owing to reduced penumbra, a trade-off is necessary because the smaller focal spot cannot tolerate high milliampere (mA) levels. Many systems contain two focal spot sizes, one for lower mA settings and a larger focal spot for settings greater than 300 mA. (Comprehensive Text Chapter 2; Heading: Gantry/X-ray Source)

5. Answer–a. The ability of the tube to withstand the heat resulting from the production of x-rays is called heat capacity and is measured in million heat units (MHU). (Comprehensive Text Chapter 2; Heading: Gantry/X-ray Source)

6. Answer–b. Mechanical filters shape the x-ray beam intensity. Filtering removes soft, or low-energy, x-ray photons and minimizes patient exposure. Bowtie filters are used to reduce the beam intensity at the periphery of the beam, corresponding to the thinner areas of a patient's anatomy. (Comprehensive Text Chapter 2; Heading: Gantry/Filtration)

7. Answer–d. The space occupied by the detector plates relative to the surface area of the detector is an aspect of the geometric efficiency of a detector system. The width and spacing of the detectors affect the amount of scatter that is recorded. (Comprehensive Text Chapter 2; Heading: Gantry/Detectors)

8. Answer–a. Xenon gas must be kept under pressure in an aluminum casing. This casing filters the x-ray beam to a certain extent. Loss of x-ray photons in the casing window and the space taken up by the plates are the major factors hampering detector efficiency. (Comprehensive Text Chapter 2; Heading: Gantry/Detectors/Xenon Gas Detectors)

9. Answer–b. (Comprehensive Text Chapter 2; Heading: Gantry/Scanner Generation)

10. Answer–d. (Comprehensive Text Chapter 2; Heading: Gantry/Detector Electronics)

## CHAPTER 3: IMAGE RECONSTRUCTION

1. Answer–a. (Comprehensive Text Chapter 3; Heading: Reconstruction Terminology/Algorithm)

2. Answer–d. (Comprehensive Text Chapter 3; Heading: Reconstruction Terminology/Interpolation)

3. Answer–c. CT detector mechanisms feed data to the CPU. The microprocessor and primary memory are parts of the CPU. The laser camera is an output device. (Comprehensive Text Chapter 3; Heading: Equipment Components Used for Image Reconstruction/Computer Components)

4. Answer–b. The CPU is sometimes referred to as the brain of the CT system. Using mathematical calculations and data comparisons, it carries out software instructions. (Comprehensive Text Chapter 3; Heading: Equipment Components Used for Image Reconstruction/Central Processing Unit)

5. Answer–c. The raw data include all measurements obtained from the detector array. Typically only a portion of these data is used to create the actual image. (Comprehensive Text Chapter 3; Heading: Data Types/Raw Data)

6. Answer–a. The path the x-ray beam takes from the tube to the detector is referred to as a ray. After the ray reaches the detector and its attenuation accounted for, it is called a ray sum. (Comprehensive Text Chapter 3; Heading: Overview of Image Reconstruction)

7. Answer–d. A view in the CT process can be compared with observing an object from a single angle. It takes many views to obtain a true understanding of the shape of the object. Similarly, it takes many views to create the CT image. (Comprehensive Text Chapter 3; Heading: Overview of Image Reconstruction)

8. Answer–c. The process of taking the information from the attenuation profile and projecting it back onto a matrix is called back projection. The disadvantage of back projection is that it produces streaks in the image. To minimize the streaks, a mathematical filtering process called convolution is applied before the back projection takes place. It can then be referred to as filtered back projection. (Comprehensive Text Chapter 3; Heading: Overview of Image Reconstruction)

9. Answer–b. Different mathematical functions (algorithms) can be used to enhance or suppress parts of the data. Depending on the manufacturer, the filter function used may be called algorithm, convolution filter, or kernel. (Comprehensive Text Chapter 3; Heading: Overview of Image Reconstruction/Filter Functions)

10. Answer–a. The SFOV determines the size of the fan beam, which, in turn, determines the number of detector cells that collect data. (Comprehensive Text Chapter 3; Heading: Overview of Image Reconstruction/Scan Field of View)

11. Answer–b. Changing the DFOV reconstructs the original data differently; therefore, the raw data must be available. In addition, the data selected by the DFOV are a subset of SFOV. Therefore, the display field of view can be equal to or smaller than the SFOV. (Comprehensive Text Chapter 3; Heading: Overview of Image Reconstruction/Digital Field of View)

## CHAPTER 4: IMAGE DISPLAY

1. Answer–b. (Comprehensive Text Chapter 4; Heading: Display Monitors)

2. Answer–c. (Comprehensive Text Chapter 4; Heading: Window Settings)

3. Answer–d. There are more than 2,000 HU, but monitors are unable to display all 2,000 as distinct shades of gray. Even more of a problem is that the human eye can differentiate only a fraction of those shades. Converting the data into shades of gray allows them to be displayed on the monitor or recorded on film. (Comprehensive Text Chapter 4; Heading: Window Settings/Gray Scale)

4. Answer–a. Naturally occurring structures fall in the range of −1,000 (air) to 1,000 (dense bone). Higher HU exist but reflect manmade objects such as dental fillings. (Comprehensive Text Chapter 4; Heading: Window Settings/Gray Scale)

5. Answer–d. A narrow window limits the range of CT numbers displayed to provide greater discrimination between similar densities. A wide window encompasses a wide range of different tissue (e.g., displaying bone and lung) but does so at the expense of subtle density discrimination. Because the window setting is a display function that is set after the image has been acquired, it is impossible for it to affect any scanning parameter such as slice thickness and mAs. The appearance of quantum mottle can be decreased by widening the window width. (Comprehensive Text Chapter 4; Heading: Window Settings/Window Width)

6. Answer–a. The window width selects the range of HU that is to be represented as shades of gray on the image. The window level determines which, of all the

possible HU, are to be included. In this example, the total HU to be represented is 300. Because the center is set at 100, the HU depicted are −50 to 250. This is calculated by dividing 300 in half, then subtracting the quotient from the center (100) to find the lower limit. Add the quotient to 100 to find the upper limit. Everything that falls below these numbers appears black, whereas everything above appears white. Figure 4-2 depicts the process. (Comprehensive Text Chapter 4; Heading: Window Settings/Suggestions for Setting Window Width and Level)

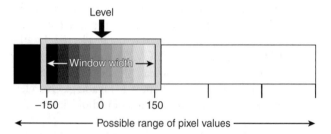

**FIGURE 4-2** The window width selects the range of Hounsfield values displayed. The window level selects the center value.

7. Answer–c. The window level should be set at a point that is roughly the same value as the average attenuation number of the tissue of interest. (Comprehensive Text Chapter 4; Heading: Window Settings/Suggestions for Setting Window Width and Level)

8. Answer–c. The standard deviation indicates the ranges of HU for the pixels within the ROI. Since the standard deviation was 0, this indicates that every pixel within the ROI has the same Hounsfield value. Therefore, the object must be very homogeneous. It is not possible to speculate about the type of structure from the standard deviation alone. The HU reading would help to make that determination. (Comprehensive Text Chapter 4; Heading: Image Display Options/Hounsfield Measurements and Standard Deviation)

9. Answer–b. Changing the display field requires the raw data. In doing this, the pixel size decreases and the spatial resolution increases. (Comprehensive Text Chapter 4; Heading: Image Display Options/Image Magnification)

10. Answer–d. Image magnification is not synonymous with changing the display field size. Because magnification uses only image data and not raw data, pixel size is not affected. A magnified image retains accuracy in all image measurements. (Comprehensive Text Chapter 4; Heading: Image Display Options/Image Magnification)

# CHAPTER 5: METHODS OF DATA ACQUISITION

1. Answer–b. Localizer scans used in CT are very similar to conventional radiographic images in that anatomic structures are superimposed. The radiation dose is typically equivalent to that of conventional radiographs, although the image quality is typically slightly poorer. (Comprehensive Text Chapter 5; Heading: Localizer Scans)

2. Answer–a. In a localizer view, the x-ray tube remains stationary. In this case, the tube is positioned above the patient; the x-ray beam will pass from anterior to posterior creating an AP view, similar to a conventional radiograph known as a flat plate. (Comprehensive Text Chapter 5; Heading: Localizer Scans)

3. Answer–c. The operator incorrectly inputted directional instructions before obtaining the scout in Figure 5-2. The operator indicated the patient position was prone, when in reality, the patient was supine. If the error were to go unnoticed and the scan to proceed, cross-sectional slices would be mislabeled in both the right-left and anterior-posterior aspects. (Comprehensive Text Chapter 5; Heading: Localizer Scans)

4. Answer–a. In an axial sequence, the table moves to the correct position and then stops while the gantry rotates. Each slice is most often created from data acquired during a 360° gantry rotation. Axial scans can be performed with either SDCT or MDCT systems. (Comprehensive Text Chapter 5; Heading: Step-and-Shoot Scanning)

5. Answer–c. Since the table remains stationary during data acquisition, there must be a slight pause between acquisitions while the table moves to the next location. Tube cooling may also contribute to the interscan delay, but only after many slices have been acquired. Detectors are not realigned between data acquisitions, and all current systems perform image reconstruction in a parallel, not a serial, fashion. (Comprehensive Text Chapter 5; Heading: Step-and-Shoot Scanning)

6. Answer–b. The number of scans per cluster is dependent on the speed of the specific scanner used and on how long a patient can reasonably be expected to hold her breath. Although dynamic scans can also consist of groups of axial slices, the technique typically refers to acquiring data for multiple slices at the same table position (most often for the purpose of watching a structure as it fills with iodinated contrast medium). Reformatting refers to the process of using image data to create another image in a different plane. Volumetric scanning refers to the helical method of data acquisition. (Comprehensive Text Chapter 5; Heading: Step-and-Shoot Scanning)

7. Answer–d. The cumulative effect of the pauses between each data acquisition adds to the total examination time. This can be of particular importance when blood vessels, which remain contrast filled for very short periods, are of primary interest. In addition, axial data does not offer as many options for reconstruction as does data acquired in a helical fashion. When motion and timing are not considered (such as when evaluating image quality using phantoms), the image quality of axially acquired data is superior to helical data. Radiation dose is the same and often less, than that of helical scans. (Comprehensive Text Chapter 5; Heading: Step-and-Shoot Scanning/Disadvantages)

8. Answer–a. (Comprehensive Text Chapter 5; Heading: Step-and-Shoot Scanning/Disadvantages/Misregistration)

9. Answer–b. Helical scan systems can contain either a single row of detectors or multiple parallel rows. (Comprehensive Text Chapter 5; Heading: Helical Scanning)

10. Answer–d. Dynamic scanning refers to repeating data acquisitions in the same location. Hence, it is also called nonincremental scanning. This is most frequently done to watch how a structure fills with an iodinated contrast agent. Dynamic scans are most often done using a helical scan method, but they can also be performed with axial scans. (Comprehensive Text Chapter 5; Heading: Helical Scanning)

11. Answer–a. Helical scanners can be of either the third- or fourth-generation design. However, because the fourth-generation design contains so many detectors, it could not be easily adapted to MDCT. Therefore, all scanners made today are of the third-generation design. (Comprehensive Text Chapter 5; Heading: Helical Scanning/Historical Perspective)

12. Answer–b. Helical CT methods create slices that are at a slight tilt. Helical interpolation methods are designed to adjust for that tilt and produce images that are indistinguishable from those acquired with axial methods. (Comprehensive Text Chapter 5; Heading: Helical Scanning/Fundamentals of Helical Technology/Helical Interpolation)

13. Answer–c. $12/(16 \times 0.5) = 12/8 = 1.5$ (Comprehensive Text Chapter 5; Heading: Helical Scanning/Fundamentals of Helical Technology/Pitch/Pitch in MDCT)

14. Answer–d. To calculate scan coverage use the formula: Pitch × total acquisition time × 1/rotation time × (slice thickness × slices per rotation). Therefore, $1.5 \times 15 \times 1/0.5$ s × (2 mm × 4) = 360 mm. (Comprehensive Text Chapter 5; Heading: Helical Scanning/Fundamentals of Helical Technology/Helical Scan Coverage/MDCT Scan Coverage/Distance Covered in an MDCT Helical Scan Sequence)

15. Answer–c. The thinnest images that can be reconstructed for a data set are often predetermined by the slice thickness used for the data acquisition. Images can be added together to create thicker slices for viewing, but in many instances, data cannot be divided to produce thinner slices. It is never possible to create an image that is thinner than the size of the individual detector cell. Any helical data allow the slice incrementation to be changed retrospectively. (Comprehensive Text Chapter 5; Heading: Helical Scanning/Fundamentals of Helical Technology/MDCT: Reconstructed Slice Thickness)

## CHAPTER 6: IMAGE QUALITY

1. Answer–c. Scan parameters are those factors that can be adjusted by the operator. Modern scanners do not allow a choice of matrix. Other scan parameters are DFOV, reconstruction algorithm, and kVp. (Comprehensive Text Chapter 6; Heading: Scanning Parameters)

2. Answer–d. Choice (a) is 150 mAs. Choice (b) is 400 mAs. Both choices (c) and (d) equal 350 mAs; however, choice (d) is preferable because the shortest possible scan time should be used for cardiac imaging to reduce the effect of cardiac motion. (Comprehensive Text Chapter 6; Heading: Scanning Parameters/Milliampere-Second Setting)

3. Answer–a. Many technologists are not aware that with digital technology the image quality is largely uncoupled from the dose, so even when an mAs or kVp setting that is too high is used, a good image results. This effect can make it difficult to identify when a dose that is higher than necessary is used, so that adjustment can be made to future scans. (Comprehensive Text Chapter 6; Heading: Scanning Parameters/The Uncoupling Effect)

4. Answer–d. Bone filters accentuate the difference between neighboring pixels to optimize spatial resolution but must make sacrifices in low-contrast resolution. Although this type of filter is best when the interest is fine bone detail, the trade-off is reduced visibility of the soft tissue structures where the high-contrast filter produces a noisy effect. (Comprehensive Text Chapter 6; Heading: Spatial Resolution/Factors Affecting Spatial Resolution/Reconstruction Algorithm)

5. Answer–d. Although they are inferior to full scans, a partial scan can be created from less than a 360° tube arc. Although these scans are slightly more than a half circle, they are often referred to as half-scan. (Comprehensive Text Chapter 6; Heading: Scan Geometry)

6. Answer–a. Although many objective measures of image quality exist, the true test of an image is whether it is useful in providing an accurate diagnosis. For example, an image of an infant using a very low technique may appear quite noisy, and by measurable standards, the quality may be quite low, but it may still

be adequate if the image is taken to follow up a large abnormality, such as an abscess. (Comprehensive Text Chapter 6; Heading: Image Quality Defined)

7. Answer–b. Many factors affect the main features of spatial and contrast resolution. Pixel size, slice thickness, focal spot size, reconstruction algorithm, and pitch have an effect on spatial resolution. Pixel size and slice thickness also affect contrast resolution, but for different reasons. In addition, mAs, patient size, subject contrast, and the inherent contrast of the object scanned contribute to the degree of contrast resolution present in the image. (Comprehensive Text Chapter 6; Heading: Image Quality Defined)

8. Answer–d. The ability to differentiate on an image a structure that varies only slightly in density from its surrounding is its contrast resolution. Brain imaging requires good low-contrast resolution because of the small density difference between white matter and gray matter. The ability to resolve (as separate objects) small, high-contrast structures, such as contrast-filled vessels, tiny bones, or a calcified nodule, is a system's spatial resolution. (Comprehensive Text Chapter 6; Heading: Contrast Resolution)

9. Answer–a. How *frequently* an object will fit into a given *space* is its spatial frequency. Therefore, large objects will have low spatial frequency and small objects will have high spatial frequency. (Comprehensive Text Chapter 6; Heading: Spatial Resolution/Direct Measurement of Spatial Resolution/Spatial Frequency)

10. Answer–b. The modulation transfer function (MTF) is a measure of the capability of the scanner to produce an image that accurately reflects the object scanned. It offers information on the resolution capability of the scanner as a function of spatial resolution. The MTF is often represented by a graph such as the one in Figure 6-1. (Comprehensive Text Chapter 6; Heading: Spatial Resolution/Evaluating Spatial Resolution Using the MTF)

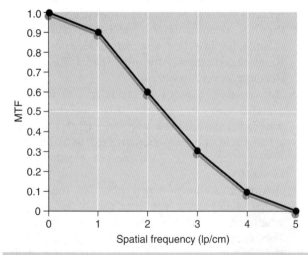

**FIGURE 6-1** A typical MTF graph. The *x* axis corresponds to the spatial frequency of the object.

11. Answer–a. Pixel size can be calculated by dividing the DFOV by the matrix size. Therefore, the pixel size of choice (a) is 0.31 mm; choice (b) is 0.49 mm, choice (c) is 0.68 mm, and choice (d) is 0.82 mm. The smaller the pixel size, the higher the spatial resolution of the image (holding all other factors constant). (Comprehensive Text Chapter 6; Heading: Spatial Resolution/Factors Affecting Spatial Resolution/ Matrix Size, Display Field of View, Pixel Size)

12. Answer–c. An isotropic voxel is a cube, measuring the same in the *x*, *y*, and *z* directions. (Comprehensive Text Chapter 6; Heading: Spatial Resolution/Factors Affecting Spatial Resolution/Slice Thickness)

13. Answer–d. Choices (a), (b), and (c) refer to the level of detail that is visible on the image. For example, if two thin wires lie close together in an object, will they be seen as two distinct lines on the image? (Comprehensive Text Chapter 6; Heading: Contrast Resolution)

14. Answer–b. Image noise is the undesirable fluctuation of pixel values in an image of a homogeneous material (such as water). Noise is most often caused by an mAs setting that is too low (an mAs setting that is too high will not affect the image quality). Using a wider slice thickness can help to reduce image noise as it results in a greater number of detected photons. (Comprehensive Text Chapter 6; Heading: Contrast Resolution/Noise)

15. Answer–c. Although in medicine the word temporal often refers to being near the temple of the head, in discussion of image quality, temporal refers to the characteristic of being limited by time. Therefore, temporal resolution refers to the speed that a scanner acquires data. This is an important consideration in imaging moving structures, such as the heart. (Comprehensive Text Chapter 6; Heading: Temporal Resolution)

## CHAPTER 7: QUALITY ASSURANCE

1. Answer–b. Performing the tests in a quality assurance program is most often a responsibility shared by technologists and medical physicists. (Comprehensive Text Chapter 7; Heading: Quality Assurance Methods)

2. Answer–a. A line pairs phantom is used to measure spatial resolution. (Comprehensive Text Chapter 7; Heading: Quality Assurance Methods/Spatial Resolution)

3. Answer–d. (Comprehensive Text Chapter 7; Heading: Quality Assurance Methods/Slice Thickness Accuracy)

4. Answer–b. (Comprehensive Text Chapter 7; Heading: Quality Assurance Methods/Noise and Uniformity)

5. Answer–a. A water phantom is expected to be uniform in density throughout. Standard deviation measurements indicate fluctuation in the individual pixel measurement with the ROI. An image is noisy if the standard deviation exceeds 10. Noise can be reduced on subsequent images by increasing the mAs or kVp setting. It can also be reduced by using a wider slice

thickness. (Comprehensive Text Chapter 7; Heading: Quality Assurance Methods/Noise and Uniformity)

6. Answer–a. With time, a system's linearity can be degraded by small changes in detector channel variation and responses. Daily calibration helps to avoid fluctuation in linearity by compensating for these tiny changes. (Comprehensive Text Chapter 7; Heading: Quality Assurance Methods/Linearity)

7. Answer–c. Dose measurement must be performed for each of a facility's CT scanners and must be performed by a medical physicist. (Comprehensive Text Chapter 7; Heading: Quality Assurance Methods/Radiation Dose)

8. Answer–a. The beam is hardened more by dense objects. Increasing the kVp will increase the average photon energy of the beam, reducing beam hardening to some extent. The best strategy to minimize beam-hardening artifacts is to select the appropriate SFOV. (Comprehensive Text Chapter 7; Heading: Image Artifacts/Beam Hardening)

9. Answer–d. Insufficient projection data can result in aliasing artifacts. This can occur when the helical pitch is greatly extended, or when a partial scan is used rather than a full 360° tube rotation. (Comprehensive Text Chapter 7; Heading: Image Artifacts/Aliasing)

10. Answer–b. Streaks or shading (both light and dark) may arise from irregularly shaped objects that have a pronounced difference in density from surrounding structures. In this case, the artifacts are caused from air in the stomach. (Comprehensive Text Chapter 7; Heading: Image Artifacts/Edge Gradient Effect)

# CHAPTER 8: POSTPROCESSING

1. Answer–b. Any process that reuses the raw data is called reconstruction. Reformation, whether it is multiplanar or 3D, uses only image data. (Comprehensive Text Chapter 8; Heading: Retrospective Reconstruction/Retrospectively Changing Image Thickness)

2. Answer–a. When the voxels from the source data are isotropic, or near isotropic, overlapping reconstructions provide little benefit and are not generally worth the inconvenience. To determine whether a voxel is isotropic, first calculate pixel size (DFOV in mm/512), then compare the pixel size to the slice thickness. When slice thickness is considerably greater than the pixel size, overlapping reconstructions are likely to be beneficial. In choice (a), the pixel size is 0.48–nearly the same as the slice thickness. (Comprehensive Text Chapter 8; Heading: Retrospective Reconstruction/Overlapping Reconstructions)

3. Answer–b. To create a reformation, source images must possess the same DFOV, image center, and gantry tilt, and they must be contiguous. If the raw data are available, new source images can be created that possess the same center (choice c) and DFOV (choice d).

Reformations can be made from images with variable slice thicknesses. However, nothing can be done retrospectively that will change the gantry angle of the original acquisition. (Comprehensive Text Chapter 8; Heading: Retrospective Reconstruction)

4. Answer–b. Review Chapter 1 for an explanation of the various body planes. (Comprehensive Text Chapter 1; Heading: Imaging Planes)

5. Answer–d. An MPR uses only image data, and it is 2D in nature (meaning it displays the original CT attenuation values). The image quality of an MPR matches that of the source image only when the source data contains isotropic voxels. Modern software allows MPRs to be created quickly and easily from either the operator's console or a workstation. (Comprehensive Text Chapter 8; Heading: Image Reformation/Multiplanar Reformation)

6. Answer–c. On most scanners, if oblique or curved reformations are needed, the technologist must create them manually. (Comprehensive Text Chapter 8; Heading: Image Reformation/Multiplanar Reformation/Scanner-Created MPR)

7. Answer–b. In many institutions, MDCT data are combined to create thicker slices for viewing. These slices tend to be better for radiologist interpretation and easier to transmit via the PACS, and consume less computer memory to store. However, to create the highest quality reformations on the workstation, the thinnest possible slices must be available. Data sets from MDCT are frequently huge, potentially slowing down the PACS network. Only image data are used to create MPRs, not raw data. (Comprehensive Text Chapter 8; Heading: Image Reformation/Multiplanar Reformation/Workstation-Created MPR)

8. Answer–d. (Comprehensive Text Chapter 8; Heading: Image Reformation/Three-Dimensional Reformation/Surface Rendering)

9. Answer–a. Setting the appropriate threshold CT values for surface rendering is critical. Setting the threshold too high will include unwanted structures that may obscure the area of interest; setting the threshold too low may cause important structures to be omitted from the display. (Comprehensive Text Chapter 8; Heading: Image Reformation/Three-Dimensional Reformation/Surface Rendering)

10. Answer–d. MIPs are best used for higher-attenuation structures such as bone, calcifications, and contrast-filled structures. Lower-attenuation structures, such as the bronchial tree, are not well visualized. (Comprehensive Text Chapter 8; Heading: Image Reformation/Three-Dimensional Reformation/Projection Displays)

11. Answer–d. MinIP involves selecting voxels with the minimum values for display. These are useful for displaying low-attenuation structures such as the bronchial tree. Image 8-2 is a sagittal MinIP

demonstrating the trachea and portions of the nasopharynx. (Comprehensive Text Chapter 8; Heading: Image Reformation/Three-Dimensional Reformation/Projection Displays)

12. Answer–a. An advantage of VR over other 3D techniques is that all voxels contribute to the image. This allows VR images to display multiple tissues and show their relationship to one another. (Comprehensive Text Chapter 8; Heading: Image Reformation/Three-Dimensional Reformation/Volume Rendering)

13. Answer–b. VR displays are built by collecting and manipulating data along an imaginary line from the viewer's eye through the data set. VR techniques assign each voxel an opacity value based on its Hounsfield unit, then they use this value to determine how much the voxel will contribute (along with other voxels along the same line) to the final image. (Comprehensive Text Chapter 8; Heading: Image Reformation/Three-Dimensional Reformation/Volume Rendering)

14. Answer–c. Segmentation is done to remove obscuring structures from the 3D image. (Comprehensive Text Chapter 8; Heading: Image Reformation/Region-of-Interest Editing)

15. Answer–c. Metallic artifacts from the patient's dental fillings degrade this coronal MPR. (Comprehensive Text Chapter 8; Heading: Image Reformation/Factors That Degrade Reformatted Images/Artifact)

## CHAPTER 9: DATA MANAGEMENT

1. Answer–d. Computerized physician order entry (CPOE) systems are designed to allow physicians to electronically order tests, procedures, and medications. Electronic ordering improves patient safety because it eliminates the risks associated with handwritten orders and multiple "hand offs" from one person to the next (such as when a doctor writes an order and a clerk must transcribe it). (Comprehensive Text Chapter 9; Heading: Introduction to Informatics)

2. Answer–a. The RIS is typically used for scheduling patients, storing reports, patient tracking, protocoling examinations, and billing. The PACS manages the storage, retrieval, distribution, and display of images. (Comprehensive Text Chapter 9; Heading: Introduction to Informatics)

3. Answer–d. A necessary component of any PACS is a skilled team of IT personnel to keep the PACS running smoothly. (Comprehensive Text Chapter 9; Heading: PACS Fundamentals)

4. Answer–c. A server is a computer that facilitates communication between, and delivers information to, other computers. Servers are passive, that is, they wait for requests from client computers. (Comprehensive Text Chapter 9; Heading: PACS Fundamentals/Networking)

5. Answer–b. The functions of core servers include DICOM gateway, examination import and export, image storage, RIS interfacing, and image distribution services. (Comprehensive Text Chapter 9; Heading: PACS Fundamentals/Networking)

6. Answer–a. Bandwidth represents the capacity of the network connection. (Comprehensive Text Chapter 9; Heading: PACS Fundamentals/Networking)

7. Answer–d. Lossy compression methods (such as fractional coding and scalar and vector quantization) are known to introduce some level of artifacts to the image. In many cases, the artifacts are imperceptible, but because it is difficult to know how much lossy compression can be applied to a radiographic image without affecting its clinical usefulness, many PACS use only lossless compression methods. (Comprehensive Text Chapter 9; Heading: PACS Fundamentals/Networking)

8. Answer–b. The DICOM standard has made it possible to send images over a network from one electronic system to another. (Comprehensive Text Chapter 9; Heading: PACS Fundamentals/Electronic Standards/DICOM)

9. Answer–a. Although the purchase price of the LCD monitor can be two to three times higher than the price of a CRT monitor, this cost is offset by the longer life span of the new monitors. (Comprehensive Text Chapter 9; Heading: PACS Fundamentals/Workstation Monitors)

10. Answer–d. Optical jukeboxes are also called optical disc libraries, robotic drives, or autochangers. (Comprehensive Text Chapter 9; Heading: PACS Fundamentals/Data Storage/Optical Storage)

## CHAPTER 10: PATIENT COMMUNICATION

1. Answer–c. Often there is no good response when a patient expresses concerns about their medical condition. It is unwise to offer false hope or to attempt to advise the patient on legal matters. Although choice (b) is true, this is not the best time to lecture the patient about the habits that may have contributed to his symptoms. The best response is an empathic one that reassures the patient that everything possible is being done to provide him with quality health care. (Comprehensive Text Chapter 10; Heading: Practical Advice/Communication Habits to Avoid)

2. Answer–b. Reflective speech is a technique that can help clarify a patient's message. To use this technique, the technologist tries to paraphrase what he or she thinks the speaker means and allows the speaker to correct any misunderstanding. In this example, it may be necessary for the technologist to follow up with more questions, such as, "Mr. Smith, can you explain what you mean when you say they 'kick started' your kidneys?" (Comprehensive Text

Chapter 10; Heading: Practical Advice/Communication Habits to Adopt)

# CHAPTER 11: PATIENT PREPARATION

1. Answer–a. In addition to physicians, clinicians who may order diagnostic tests include nurse practitioners (NP) and physician assistants. (Comprehensive Text Chapter 11; Heading: Examination Initiation)

2. Answer–d. At least two methods of verifying a patient's identity before performing any care are necessary. A sign on the door of a patient's hospital room is not a reliable method of verification. (Comprehensive Text Chapter 11; Heading: Medical History)

3. Answer–b. In patients with a history of hyperthyroidism, iodinated contrast media administered intravascularly can intensify thyroid toxicosis (excessive thyroid hormone). In rare cases, iodinated contrast media can precipitate a thyroid storm, which is a severe, life-threatening condition resulting when thyroid hormone reaches a dangerously high level. (Comprehensive Text Chapter 11; Heading: Medical History/Patient Safety)

4. Answer–b. BUN, creatinine, and eGFR are important indicators of renal function. This is important because patients with impaired renal function who receive an injection of an iodinated contrast agent are at risk of developing contrast-induced nephropathy. (Comprehensive Text Chapter 11; Heading: Medical History/Laboratory Values)

5. Answer–c. Examinations such as biopsies carry the risk of excessive bleeding. PT, PTT, and platelet count are laboratory tests that can indicate problems with the blood's ability to form clots. (Comprehensive Text Chapter 11; Heading: Medical History/Laboratory Values)

6. Answer–c. In most facilities, a signed consent is not necessary for routine CT studies. However, studies of a more invasive nature, such as CT-guided fluid aspirations, require that a consent form be signed. Before signing the form, the relevant facts regarding the examination and any associated risk must be explained to the patient. The patient must be in possession of his or her reasoning faculties. The consent form must be signed before the patient is given any medication that could affect the mental status. (Comprehensive Text Chapter 11; Heading: Patient Education and Informed Consent)

7. Answer–b. Restraints should be used to protect a patient from falling or to immobilize a part to improve image quality. Whenever possible, the patient should consent to the use of the restraining device. Technically, a clinician's order is required to use a restraining device for a patient who cannot provide consent. Strict safety rules must be adhered to whenever restraining devices are used. These include the rule that if leg immobilizers are necessary, wrist immobilizers must also be applied to prevent the patient from either unfastening the device or unintentionally hanging themselves in an attempt to leave the table or gurney. (Comprehensive Text Chapter 11; Heading: Immobilization and Patient Restraint Devices)

8. Answer–d. Throughout the CT examination, the patient should be monitored visually and spoken to frequently using the scanner's intercom system. This reassures the patient and allows the technologist to intervene quickly should problems arise. (Comprehensive Text Chapter 11; Heading: Assessment and Monitoring Vital Signs)

9. Answer–a. The vital signs are body temperature, pulse, respirations, and blood pressure. (Comprehensive Text Chapter 11; Heading: Assessment and Monitoring Vital Signs)

10. Answer–d. (Comprehensive Text Chapter 11; Heading: Assessment and Monitoring Vital Signs/Pulse)

11. Answer–a. (Comprehensive Text Chapter 11; Heading: Assessment and Monitoring Vital Signs/Respirations)

12. Answer–a. (Comprehensive Text Chapter 11; Heading: Assessment and Monitoring Vital Signs/Blood Pressure)

# CHAPTER 12: CONTRAST AGENTS

1. Answer–a. A density difference between adjacent structures will result in different beam attenuation, ultimately producing an image that clearly displays the different tissue types. (Comprehensive Text Chapter 12; Introduction)

2. Answer–b. All contrast agents that contain iodine, and most agents that contain barium, are considered positive agents. That is, their density is higher than the structure that it fills. (Comprehensive Text Chapter 12; Introduction)

3. Answer–b. Most brands of iodinated contrast medium have a greater osmolality than plasma. The osmolality of blood plasma is approximately 290 mOsm/kg. The osmolality of HOCM range from approximately 1,300 to 2,140 mOsm/kg. The osmolality of LOCM range from about 600 to 850 mOsm/kg. (Comprehensive Text Chapter 12; Heading: Intravascular Contrast Agents/Properties of Iodinated Agents/Osmolality)

4. Answer–c. Dehydration may result from HOCM contrast media administration because the significant difference in osmolality between the agent and body fluids causes a shift of fluids from the cellular spaces into the plasma. (Comprehensive Text Chapter 12; Heading: Intravascular Contrast Agents/Adverse Effects of Iodinated Contrast Medium/Chemotoxic Reactions/Contrast Media-Induced Nephropathy/Prevention of CIN/Hydration)

5. Answer–c. Viscosity can be described as the thickness or friction of the fluid as it flows. In the case of intravenous iodinated contrast agents, a higher concentration of iodine results in a more viscous solution. Heating the agent from room temperature to body temperature significantly decreases the solution's viscosity. Molecular structure also affects viscosity; therefore, different brands of iodinated contrast media will possess varying viscosities. (Comprehensive Text Chapter 12; Heading: Intravascular Contrast Agents/Properties of Iodinated Agents/Viscosity)

6. Answer–d. To compare the dose of iodine from different concentrations of contrast media, it is useful to calculate the total grams of iodine delivered. This is done by multiplying the dose times the concentration. The protocol calls for 32 g of iodine (100 mL × 320 mgI/mL = 32 g). Therefore, for each of the doses given, (a) 84 mL × 240 mgI/mL = 20 g, (b) 100 mL × 240 mgI/mL = 24 g, (c) 125 mL × 240 mgI/mL = 30 g, and (d) 133 mL × 240 mgI/mL = 32 g. It is not necessary to match the grams of iodine exactly. In actual practice, the dose of the lower concentration agent would likely be rounded off to 130 or 140 mL. (Comprehensive Text Chapter 12; Heading: Intravascular Contrast Agents/Dose)

7. Answer–a. There is no agreed-on standard used to describe adverse reactions to contrast media. In some instances, the term is used to describe all undesired effects, such as the feeling of heat that often follows an intravenous injection. In other instances, it is used exclusively to describe the less common, more serious side effects that may require treatment or even be life threatening. (Comprehensive Text Chapter 12; Heading: Intravascular Contrast Agents/Adverse Effects of Iodinated Contrast Medium/Mechanism of Adverse Reactions)

8. Answer–b. All hemodynamic disturbances and injuries to organs (such as the kidneys) or vessels perfused by the contrast medium are considered chemotoxic reactions. Allergic-like reactions, such as hives and nasal stuffiness, are considered idiosyncratic reactions. (Comprehensive Text Chapter 12; Heading: Intravascular Contrast Agents/Adverse Effects of Iodinated Contrast Medium/Mechanism of Adverse Reactions)

9. Answer–c. Acute idiosyncratic reaction are usually classified as mild, moderate, or severe. Moderate reactions are not immediately life threatening, although they may progress to be so. Symptoms of a moderate reaction require treatment. (Comprehensive Text Chapter 12; Heading: Intravascular Contrast Agents/Adverse Effects of Iodinated Contrast Medium/Idiosyncratic Reactions/Classifications of Idiosyncratic Reactions)

10. Answer–b. The reported rate of both idiosyncratic and chemotoxic reactions is much lower with LOCM. Some data suggest that there is also a lower mortality rate with LOCM. (Comprehensive Text Chapter 12; Heading: Intravascular Contrast Agents/Adverse Effects of Iodinated Contrast Medium/Idiosyncratic Reactions/Incidence and Risk Factors for Idiosyncratic Reactions)

11. Answer–a. Although a previous contrast reaction is considered to be the most important relative risk factor, the incidence is still relatively low. It is estimated to be from 16% to 35% when an HOCM is given, but just 5% when an LOCM is given. (Comprehensive Text Chapter 12; Heading: Intravascular Contrast Agents/Adverse Effects of Iodinated Contrast Medium/Idiosyncratic Reactions/Incidence and Risk Factors for Idiosyncratic Reactions/Previous Contrast Medium Reaction)

12. Answer–b. Idiosyncratic reactions are not dose dependent; reactions have resulted from very small volumes of iodinated contrast media. Therefore, test injections are of no predictive value. Although pretreating high-risk patients with steroids is generally believed to reduce the rate of idiosyncratic reactions, the degree to which that risk is reduced is unknown. The single best method of reducing reactions is to use LOCM. The risk associated with these agents is four to five times lower than that of HOCM. However, it is not uncommon to use both strategies when dealing with high-risk patients–both steroid pretreatment and the use of LOCM. (Comprehensive Text Chapter 12; Heading: ntravascular Contrast Agents/Adverse Effects of Iodinated Contrast Medium/Idiosyncratic Reactions/Prevention of Acute Idiosyncratic Reactions)

13. Answer–b. Each kidney contains from one to two million nephrons. The nephron produces urine by filtering out from the blood small molecules and ions and then reclaiming the needed amounts of useful materials. Surplus or waste molecules and ions are discarded as urine. (Comprehensive Text Chapter 12; Heading: Intravascular Contrast Agents/Adverse Effects of Iodinated Contrast Medium/Chemotoxic Reactions/Contrast Media-Induced Nephropathy/Renal Anatomy and Physiology)

14. Answer–c. There are significant limitations in using SeCr as an absolute measure of renal function. Many factors can affect the SeCr value including sex, age, race, and nutritional status. Despite its drawbacks, SeCr is a good reflection of any major drug-induced fluctuation in GFR and remains a useful clinical tool in assessing kidney function. (Comprehensive Text Chapter 12; Heading: Intravascular Contrast Agents/Adverse Effects of Iodinated Contrast Medium/Chemotoxic Reactions/Contrast Media-Induced

Nephropathy/Renal Function/Serum Creatinine as an Index of GFR)

15. Answer–c. Multiple risk factors have a cumulative effect in increasing the risk of CIN. Risk factors for CIN include preexisting renal insufficiency, diabetes mellitus (particularly when combined with renal impairment), and studies that use a high volume of contrast material. (Comprehensive Text Chapter 12; Heading: Intravascular Contrast Agents/Adverse Effects of Iodinated Contrast Medium/Chemotoxic Reactions/Contrast Media-Induced Nephropathy/ CIN Incidence and Risk Factors)

16. Answer–d. Although metformin-associated lactic acidosis is rare, when it does occur, it is fatal in about half of patients. It can occur after CIN, because the reduced renal function can allow metformin to accumulate in the body. (Comprehensive Text Chapter 12; Heading: Intravascular Contrast Agents/Adverse Effects of Iodinated Contrast Medium/Chemotoxic Reactions/Contrast Media-Induced Nephropathy/ Metformin Therapy)

17. Answer–a. Patients who have conditions that disrupt the blood-brain barrier are at increased risk of seizures after contrast administration. (Comprehensive Text Chapter 12; Heading: Intravascular Contrast Agents/Adverse Effects of Iodinated Contrast Medium/Chemotoxic Reactions/Other Organ or System-Specific Adverse Effects/Central Nervous System)

18. Answer–c. Patients report many symptoms of late reactions after a CT examination, including headache, skin rash, itching, nausea, dizziness, urticaria, fever, arm pain, and gastrointestinal disturbances. However, when investigated, all but the skin reactions appeared equally in the group that had only undergone an unenhanced CT. (Comprehensive Text Chapter 12; Heading: Intravascular Contrast Agents/ Adverse Effects of Iodinated Contrast Medium/ Delayed Reactions)

19. Answer–a. Barium peritonitis is associated with a significant mortality rate. A water-soluble iodinated oral contrast should be substituted whenever perforation is possible, such as in cases of ulcerative colitis. (Comprehensive Text Chapter 12; Heading: Gastrointestinal Contrast Medium/Barium Sulfate Solutions)

20. Answer–d. Research with pediatric patients has concluded that LOCM offers a significant reduction in complications compared with either barium sulfate or HOCM. LOCM are indicated when the possibility of entry of the contrast agent into the lung exists or when the possibility of leakage of contrast agent from the gastrointestinal tract exists. (Comprehensive Text Chapter 12; Heading: Gastrointestinal Contrast Medium/Iodinated Agents)

# CHAPTER 13: INJECTION TECHNIQUES

1. Answer–c. Because of the increased risk of contrast media extravasation, the use of metal needles should be avoided, particularly when a mechanical injector will be used for contrast media injection. (Comprehensive Text Chapter 13; Heading: Vascular Access/Starting a Peripheral Intravenous Line)

2. Answer–a. Open-ended catheters must be clamped when not in used. Most manufacturers recommend that between uses they be flushed with a heparinized saline flush to maintain the catheter's patency. A popular method is the SASH method: saline flush, administer medication or draw blood, saline flush, heparinized saline flush. (Comprehensive Text Chapter 13; Heading: Vascular Access/Managing Patients With Existing Vascular Access/Using a Central Venous Access Device)

3. Answer–b. Implanted ports are typically used for long-term intermittent access such as that required for chemotherapy. The port is accessed by use of a special needle, called a Huber needle. Placing the needle requires special training; improper placement of the access needle could result in the extravasation of injected fluid into the subcutaneous tissues of the chest. (Comprehensive Text Chapter 13; Heading: Vascular Access/Managing Patients With Existing Vascular Access/Using a Central Venous Access Device/Nontunneled and Tunneled Central Venous Catheters)

4. Answer–b. The difference between the three general phases is predominantly determined by the rate at which the contrast material is delivered and the time that elapses from the start of the injection and when scanning is initiated. (Comprehensive Text Chapter 13; Heading: Basic Principles of Intravenous Contrast Administration/General Phases of Tissue Enhancement)

5. Answer–c. The AVID indicates the point in the circulatory process the injected contrast media is at a given time. This is done by comparing the degree of contrast enhancement in the arteries (specifically, the aorta) to that contained in the venous structures (specifically, the inferior vena cava). (Comprehensive Text Chapter 13; Heading: Basic Principles of Intravenous Contrast Administration/General Phases of Tissue Enhancement)

6. Answer–a. This phase immediately follows an IV bolus injection. The arterial structures are filled with contrast medium; contrast medium has not yet reached venous structures. (Comprehensive Text Chapter 13; Heading: Basic Principles of Intravenous Contrast Administration/General Phases of Tissue Enhancement)

7. Answer–b. Scanning of the liver must take place before the equilibrium phase, which can begin as early as 2 minutes after the contrast bolus. This is

particularly important when the clinical indication is to evaluate for metastatic lesion. The impact of an unanticipated delay can only be estimated, because factors such as the speed of the particular scanner and how soon after the start of injection the delay occurs affect the timing window. For purposes of illustration, let us assume the scanner at this facility will acquire the scans through the liver in 20 seconds. Although the routine scan protocol at this facility calls for a delay of 60 seconds between the start of injection and the start of scanning, the scan could be delayed an additional 40 seconds and still acquire all of the scans before 2 minutes has elapsed. Because the scan delay is so critical for many studies, it is best to prepare the patient for any potential effects of the contrast injection before beginning the injection. The patient should be given clear instructions on what effects will be transient (i.e., warm feeling, metallic taste) and what warrant interrupting the study (i.e., pain at or near the injection site). (Comprehensive Text Chapter 13; Heading: Basic Principles of Intravenous Contrast Administration/General Phases of Tissue Enhancement)

8. Answer–a. The injection rate is not important for routine scans of the brain. The scan delay is only important in that it is long enough to allow contrast to leak across a disrupted blood-brain barrier. The scan delay for other studies is typically measured in seconds, whereas the scan delay for routine brain studies is most often several minutes. (Comprehensive Text Chapter 13; Heading: Basic Principles of Intravenous Contrast Administration/General Phases of Tissue Enhancement)

9. Answer–c. The drip infusion method does not allow scans of the body to be acquired before the equilibrium phase of contrast enhancement. It cannot produce peak enhancement of sufficient magnitude for CT angiography. However, it can be used for routine brain studies because precise flow rates and scan delays are not critical. (Comprehensive Text Chapter 13; Heading: Basic Principles of Intravenous Contrast Administration/Methods of Contrast Media Delivery/Drip Infusion)

10. Answer–d. If a standard PICC line is the only option available for contrast injection, most manufacturers recommend contrast be administered using the hand bolus technique. (Comprehensive Text Chapter 13; Heading: Basic Principles of Intravenous Contrast Administration/Methods of Contrast Media Delivery/Bolus Technique/Hand Bolus Technique)

11. Answer–c. If the flow rate remains the same, it will take longer to inject a higher volume of contrast material. If the same flow rate is used, the contrast will reach a specific enhancement point at the same time regardless of the total volume; however, increas-

ing the volume means that the magnitude of the enhancement will continue to climb. (Comprehensive Text Chapter 13; Heading: Basic Principles of Intravenous Contrast Administration/Factors Affecting Contrast Enhancement/Pharmacokinetic Factors/Contrast Media Volume, Flow Duration, Flow Rate)

12. Answer–a. When the flow rate is reduced, it takes longer for contrast to reach peak enhancement, so the scan delay must be increased. In most cases, the total volume of contrast remains unchanged. (Comprehensive Text Chapter 13; Heading: Basic Principles of Intravenous Contrast Administration/Factors Affecting Contrast Enhancement/Pharmacokinetic Factors/Contrast Media Volume, Flow Duration, Flow Rate)

13. Answer–b. For most clinical application, a single injection rate and a set scan delay can be used. CT angiography and other specialized studies often use more complex injection techniques. (Comprehensive Text Chapter 13; Heading: Basic Principles of Intravenous Contrast Administration/Factors Affecting Contrast Enhancement/Pharmacokinetic Factors/Contrast Media Volume, Flow Duration, Flow Rate)

14. Answer–c. A reduction in a patient's cardiac output will not reduce the magnitude of the peak enhancement, only the time it takes to achieve it. When the patient's heart pumps less efficiently, the contrast will take longer to reach the various vessels and organs. This requires the scan delay to be extended in proportion to the degree of cardiac impairment. (Comprehensive Text Chapter 13; Heading: Basic Principles of Intravenous Contrast Administration/Factors Affecting Contrast Enhancement/Patient Factors Affecting Contrast Enhancement)

15. Answer–b. The optimal scan delay time is equal to the time that elapsed from the start of the test injection to that of the imaging showing maximum enhancement. Therefore, 12 (trial scan delay) + 2 (interval between trial scans) × 4 (image showing maximum enhancement) = 20 seconds. Experience has shown that the best results are achieved by adding 3 seconds to this calculated delay; the adjusted value is 23 seconds. (Comprehensive Text Chapter 13; Heading: Basic Principles of Intravenous Contrast Administration/Factors Affecting Contrast Enhancement/Equipment Factors Affecting Contrast Enhancement/Automated Injection Triggering/Test Bolus)

## CHAPTER 14: RADIATION DOSIMETRY IN CT

1. Answer–d. Although appropriate patient selection is critical, it is primarily the radiologist's responsibility to enforce ACR guidelines. It is primarily

the responsibility of the technologist to ensure that adequate image quality is achieved using the lowest possible dose. (Comprehensive Text Chapter 14; Heading: Basic Dose Concepts)

2. Answer–d. Comparisons of reported radiation dose can be difficult because it is reported in many different units. (Comprehensive Text Chapter 14; Heading: Basic Dose Concepts/Measurement Terminology)

3. Answer–a. (Comprehensive Text Chapter 14; Heading: Basic Dose Concepts/Measurement Terminology)

4. Answer–b. The gray (Gy) is the SI unit for absorbed dose. The rad is the older unit for absorbed dose that is now obsolete. (Comprehensive Text Chapter 14; Heading: Basic Dose Concepts/Measurement Terminology)

5. Answer–d. (Comprehensive Text Chapter 14; Heading: Basic Dose Concepts/Measurement Terminology)

6. Answer–a. The quality factor or the radiation weighting factor must be applied to the absorbed dose to account for the different degree of biologic damage caused by different types of radiation. (Comprehensive Text Chapter 14; Heading: Basic Dose Concepts/Measurement Terminology)

7. Answer–b. Effective dose is difficult to calculate because it depends on an accurate estimate of the dose to radiosensitive organs from the CT procedure. (Comprehensive Text Chapter 14; Heading: Basic Dose Concepts/Measurement Terminology)

8. Answer–a. The area of scatter into adjacent tissue, or tails, explains why the total dose will be higher when multiple scans are performed. (Comprehensive Text Chapter 14; Heading: Basic Dose Concepts/Dose Geometry/$Z$ Axis Variations)

9. Answer–a. Because most CT applications involve multiple slices, dose is usually calculated from multiple scans. Both MSAD and CTDI measurements calculate the dose for multiple scans. (Comprehensive Text Chapter 14; Heading: Basic Dose Concepts/Dose Geometry/$Z$ Axis Variations)

10. Answer–b. The $CTDI_{vol}$ accounts for the nonuniformity of dose both within a single slice (i.e., the difference between the dose at the periphery and the dose at the central portion) and the variation of exposure in the $z$ direction. This measurement is particularly useful for evaluating the dose from helical scan sequences. (Comprehensive Text Chapter 14; Heading: Basic Dose Concepts/Dose Geometry/$Z$ Axis Variations)

11. Answer–b. The relationship between mAs and dose is linear. That is, if the mAs setting is doubled, the dose will be doubled. Likewise, if the mAs setting is halved, the dose is halved. (Comprehensive Text Chapter 14; Heading: Basic Dose Concepts/Factors Affecting Dose/Radiographic Technique)

12. Answer–c. CT examinations carry a higher radiation dose than do most other radiographic procedures; therefore, they contribute disproportionately to the overall radiation dose. (Comprehensive Text Chapter 14; Heading: Why the Growing Concern?/Commonly Used and Relatively High Radiation Doses)

13. Answer–b. The risk associated with a single CT procedure is much lower–it has been estimated that one child per thousand exposed may eventually develop a fatal cancer that is attributable to the CT examination. Many variables affect cancer risk so that it is impossible to predict with any certainty which specific child will be affected. However, parents should be informed that although there is a small risk associated with the examination, everything possible is being done to minimize that risk. In addition, parents can be assured that the CT examination is the appropriate choice to answer the diagnostic question posed. (Comprehensive Text Chapter 14; Heading: Perception of Risk)

14. Answer–c. (Comprehensive Text Chapter 14; Heading: Special Considerations for the Pediatric Population/Increased Sensitivity)

15. Answer–b. (Comprehensive Text Chapter 14; Heading: Special Considerations for the Pediatric Population/Increased Sensitivity)

16. Answer–d. Technologists can play an important role in ensuring that all of the strategies listed are used to reduce the radiation dose to the patient. (Comprehensive Text Chapter 14; Heading: Strategies for Reducing Dose/General Strategies)

# CHAPTER 19: NEUROLOGIC IMAGING PROCEDURES

1. Answer–c. The slice angle is determined by the position of the patient's head and the tilt of the gantry. Having the patient tuck his chin down may allow a slice angle that avoids scanning through the eye, thereby reducing radiation exposure to the lens. The lens of the eye is known to be more sensitive to radiation; exposure increases the risk of developing cataracts later in life. On all scanners, the gantry can be tilted in the axial mode. However, on many MDCT scanners, the gantry cannot be angled in the helical mode. (Comprehensive Text Chapter 19; Heading: General Imaging Methods for the Head)

2. Answer–b. The ventricles of the brain are filled with cerebrospinal fluid that typically measures from 4 to 8 HU. (Comprehensive Text Chapter 19; Heading: General Imaging Methods for the Head)

3. Answer–a. The injection protocol for a routine brain scan must allow time for contrast to leak across a disrupted blood-brain barrier. Choice (b) does not have a long enough scan delay. Choice (c) is an injection protocol typical for a neck; the split bolus allows for the opacification of both vessels

and slower-to-enhance tissue, such as lymph nodes. (Comprehensive Text Chapter 13; Heading: Basic Principles of Intravenous Contrast Administration/ General Phases of Tissue Enhancement)

4. Answer–b. CT venography (CTV) is used for the depiction of venous anatomy. Scan parameters are quite similar to CTA, except images are acquired while contrast is in the venous enhancement phase. (Comprehensive Text Chapter 19; Heading: CTA of the Head and Neck)

5. Answer–c. A CT scan of the head is done to determine the presence of blood. Thrombolytic therapy is contraindicated for hemorrhagic stroke. A CT scan must be performed soon after the patient arrives in emergency department because t-PA must be administered within 3 hours of the first signs of stroke. (Comprehensive Text Chapter 19; Heading: Specific Neurologic Protocols/A Profile of Stroke/Diagnosis and Treatment of Stroke)

6. Answer–d. CT perfusion techniques measure cerebral blood flow, which can be used to distinguish infacted tissue from penumbra. An unenhanced CT scan of the head is done to rule out intracranial bleeding. The time of stroke onset is determined by interviewing the patient or the patient's family. The patient is not a candidate for t-PA if the onset time cannot be determined. CTA with three-dimensional reformation is done to depict the spatial relationship of vascular lesions to the surrounding structures. (Comprehensive Text Chapter 19; Heading: Specific Neurologic Protocols/CT Brain Perfusion Scans)

## CHAPTER 20: THORACIC IMAGING PROCEDURES

1. Answer–d. For high-resolution chest studies, prone images can help to differentiate disease from the effects of gravity that can mimic disease on the CT images. (Comprehensive Text Chapter 20; Heading: High-Resolution CT)

2. Answer–c. Volumetric HRCT protocols use a helical mode scan to cover the entire lung, rather than representative slices, for the supine inspiratory series. The other two series (supine expiratory and prone inspiratory) are done in representative slices (thin slice but wide interval) so as to limit the radiation exposure to the patient. (Comprehensive Text Chapter 20; Heading: High-Resolution CT)

3. Answer–c. Respiratory motion is greatest at the lung bases. Scanning in a caudal-to-cranial direction may help to minimize respiratory artifact because scans through the lung bases are acquired when the patient is most likely able to hold his or her breath. (Comprehensive Text Chapter 20; Heading: Thoracic CTA/CTA of Pulmonary Embolism/CTA/ Disadvantages)

4. Answer–a. An embolus can be formed from a number of different materials and can originate from many different sites in the body. A thrombus is called an embolus when it detaches from its original site. If it detaches and lodges in a pulmonary vessel, it is called a pulmonary embolism. If it detaches and lodges in a cerebral vessel, it causes an ischemic stroke. (Comprehensive Text Chapter 20; Heading: Thoracic CTA/CTA of Pulmonary Embolism/ Anatomy and Terminology Review)

5. Answer–b. Many pulmonary emboli are caused from thrombi originating in the lower extremities. A delayed scan, sometimes called CT venography, can help to identify these clots. (Comprehensive Text Chapter 20; Heading: Thoracic CTA/CTA of Pulmonary Embolism/CTA)

6. Answer–d. The appropriately name tricuspid valve has threefolds and is in the right side of the heart, between the right atrium and the right ventricle. The mitral valve is in the left side of the heart, between the left atrium and left ventricle. The pulmonary valve is in the right side of the heart, between the right ventricle and the entrance to the pulmonary artery. The aortic valve is in the left side of the heart, between the left ventricle and the entrance to the aorta. (Comprehensive Text Chapter 20; Heading: Cardiac CT/ Cardiac Anatomy/Valves and Openings)

7. Answer–c. A rapid heart rate increases the chance that motion artifact will degrade cardiac CT images. β-Blockers are used to lower the heart rate to less than 65 beats per minute and to make the rhythm more regular. (Comprehensive Text Chapter 20; Heading: Cardiac CT/Technique/Pharmacologic Heart Rate Control)

8. Answer–b. The prospective ECG gating method attempts to synchronize the data acquisition with the quietest phase of the heart cycle (usually diastole). This method reduces the radiation dose to the patient (compared to the retrospective ECG gating method) since the exposure is intermittent. However, in patients with irregular heartbeats, it can be difficult to accurately time data acquisition with a specific cardiac cycle–motion artifact and misregistration can result. (Comprehensive Text Chapter 20; Heading: Cardiac CT/Technique/ECG Gating)

9. Answer–a. Visualization of the coronary arteries, because they are of relatively small caliber and are often tortuous in shape, is more sensitive to cardiac motion artifacts and image misregistration than larger structures, such as the aorta. (Comprehensive Text Chapter 20; Heading: Cardiac CT/Technique/ Pharmacologic Heart Rate Control)

10. Answer–d. Cardiac CT calcium scoring studies are generally not recommended for asymptomatic patients with no coronary risk factors because of the radiation dose delivered. In addition, many

insurance companies do not pay for the study. However, for patients with risk factors, CT calcium scoring examinations offer a convenient and noninvasive way of evaluating the coronary arteries. The examination takes little time and causes no pain; it does not require a contrast agent and therefore avoids possible side effects. Results from the study can suggest the presence of coronary artery disease, even when the coronary arteries are less than 50% narrowed. Standard cardiac tests will not reliably detect this level of blockage, and more than half of all heart attacks occur with less than 50% narrowing [http://www.radiologyinfo.org/en/info.cfm?pg=ct_calscoring&bhcp=1#part_nine]. (Comprehensive Text Chapter 20; Heading: Cardiac CT/CT Coronary Calcium Screening)

# CHAPTER 21: ABDOMEN AND PELVIS IMAGING PROCEDURES

1. Answer–c. (Comprehensive Text Chapter 21; Heading: General Abdominopelvic Scanning Methods)

2. Answer–a. When narrower window widths are used, the number of HU values distributed over a set number of shades of gray is reduced. Therefore, fewer HU are included in each shade of gray, making subtle density differences more discernible (Chapter 4). (Comprehensive Text Chapter 21; Heading: General Abdominopelvic Scanning Methods)

3. Answer–d. Fatty infiltration reduces the CT attenuation of the involved liver. This can be confirmed by including an HU measurement of the liver and spleen before filming. A spleen measurement that is more than 10 HU higher than that of the liver indicates fatty infiltrate of the liver. Fatty infiltration of the liver is most accurately assessed on noncontrast CT, so IV contrast is not necessary for the diagnosis. (Comprehensive Text Chapter 21; Heading: Organ-Specific Considerations/Liver)

4. Answer–c. The portal venous phase occurs from 60 to 70 seconds after IV injection. This phase is also sometimes referred to as the redistribution phase. The early arterial phase typically occurs within the first 20 seconds after an IV bolus injection, whereas the late arterial phase typically occurs between 30 and 35 seconds after injection. The equilibrium phase, sometimes called the late or delayed phase, occurs several minutes after injection. (Comprehensive Text Chapter 21; Heading: Organ-Specific Considerations/Liver)

5. Answer–a. Some tumors are supplied by an abnormal number of blood vessels (i.e., hypervascular tumors). Because of this increased blood supply, these tumors will display more intense enhancement after an IV contrast injection; these are often described as hyper-

attenuating. Tumors that are hyperattenuating relative to the surrounding liver tissue are best detected during the late arterial phase. Liver metastases tend to be hypervascular in cases of primary tumors of the thyroid or pancreatic islet cells, carcinoid tumors, renal cell carcinoma, some breast tumors, and melanoma. When these are suspected, dual-phase imaging is often beneficial. However, the majority of liver metastases are hypovascular and develop from primary tumors of the colon and rectum, pancreas, lung, urothelium, prostate, and most gynecologic malignancies. When these conditions are suspected, images are typically acquired in a single (portal venous) phase.(1) (Comprehensive Text Chapter 21; Heading: Organ-Specific Considerations/Liver)

6. Answer–c. (Comprehensive Text Chapter 21; Heading: Organ-Specific Considerations/Kidneys and Ureters)

7. Answer–a. An adrenal mass that measures less than 10 HU is high in fat (lipid-rich). This is useful because malignant adrenal masses contain very little fat. Therefore, an adrenal mass that measures less than 10 HU on a noncontrast CT image is benign. Unfortunately, the converse assumption cannot be made. That is, lesions measuring greater than 10 HU on unenhanced CT cannot automatically be assumed to be malignant. To determine whether these masses are benign or malignant, the scan protocol must be adjusted so that additional images are acquired, through the adrenal glands, from 5 to 15 minutes after the contrast injection. The delayed images will allow the radiologist to assess the degree of contrast media washout and determine whether the adrenal mass is malignant. It is important that the technologist recognize an adrenal mass so that the appropriate adjustment can be made to the examination (i.e., delayed images can be obtained). (Comprehensive Text Chapter 21; Heading: Protocol Development for Specific Abdominopelvic Applications/CT of the Adrenal Glands/Characterization of Adrenal Masses/Intracellular Lipid Content)

8. Answer–a. The appendix's variable location is an important reason why patients with appendicitis describe a wide variety of symptoms. This variation in location also makes the appendix more challenging to locate on cross-sectional images. (Comprehensive Text Chapter 21; Heading: Protocol Development for Specific Abdominopelvic Applications/CT in the Diagnosis of Acute Appendicitis/Anatomy and Function of Appendix)

9. Answer–a. A focused appendiceal CT limits the scan area to the lower abdomen and upper pelvis, thereby reducing the radiation dose to the patient. However, disadvantages to this technique are that if the appendix is in an atypical position (i.e., one that resides in the pelvis), it might not be scanned

and it may reduce the ability to provide alternative diagnoses when the appendix is found to be normal. (Comprehensive Text Chapter 21; Heading: Protocol Development for Specific Abdominopelvic Applications/CT in the Diagnosis of Acute Appendicitis/Imaging Studies/Appendiceal CT Protocols)

10. Answer–a. Appearance of a normal appendix (arrow marked as 1) on a scan done with IV and oral contrast. (Comprehensive Text Chapter 21; Heading: Protocol Development for Specific Abdominopelvic Applications/CT in the Diagnosis of Acute Appendicitis/Anatomy and Function of Appendix)

11. Answer–d. More than 99% of urinary tract stones–including those that are radiolucent on plain film radiography–will be seen on noncontrast helical CT. Interestingly, this is not true of stones located elsewhere. For example, gallstones are only detected by CT about 85% of the time, which is much less than that of ultrasonography or oral cholecystography (which is why CT is not the primary modality for imaging the gallbladder). (2) (Comprehensive Text Chapter 21; Heading: Protocol Development for Specific Abdominopelvic Applications/CT in the Diagnosis of Urinary Tract Calculi/Diagnosis/Diagnostic Imaging/Noncontrast Helical CT)

## REFERENCES

1. Valette PJ, Pilleul F, Crombe-Ternamian A. Imaging benign and metastatic liver tumors with MDCT. In: Marchal G, Vogl TJ, Heiken JP, Rubin GD, eds. *Multidetector-Row Computed Tomography, Scanning and Contrast Protocols*. Milan, Italy: Springer, 2005:32.
2. Brant WE. Biliary tree and gallbladder. In: Webb WR, Brant WE, Major NM, eds. *Fundamentals of Body CT*. 3rd Ed. Philadelphia: Saunders, 2006:241.

## CHAPTER 22: MUSCULOSKELETAL IMAGING PROCEDURES

1. Answer–b. MPR images are a particularly important aspect of musculoskeletal protocols. When MPR images are created from isotropic voxels, the image quality of the reformations remains as high as that of the source images. A thin slice is necessary to produce isotropic voxels. Unfortunately, isotropic voxels will have no effect on image artifacts. (Comprehensive Text Chapter 22; Heading: General Musculoskeletal Scanning Methods)

2. Answer–d. Clinical indications such as tumor, infection, or abscess may require the examination be done with IV contrast. The detection of loose bodies within the joint may be improved by intra-articular contrast administration (i.e., CT arthrography). (Comprehensive Text Chapter 22; Heading: General Musculoskeletal Scanning Methods)

3. Answer–a. The dense bone of the shoulder girdle often absorbs a high percentage of the x-ray beam, resulting in streak artifacts owing to beam hardening. (Comprehensive Text Chapter 22; Heading: Examinations With Unique Challenges/Shoulder)

## CHAPTER 23: INTERVENTIONAL CT AND CT FLUOROSCOPY

1. Answer–d. To limit the radiation dose to patients and personnel, it is very important that CTF exposure time and mA be kept as low as possible and that the near real-time mode of image acquisition be avoided as much as possible. Another suggested technique is to reduce scatter radiation by draping nonbiopsy areas with lead shielding. (Comprehensive Text Chapter 23; Heading: Imaging Techniques for CT-Guided Interventions)

2. Answer–c. The most likely potential risk during any biopsy procedure is the occurrence of bleeding. The vascularity of the lesion being biopsied as well as the specific organ of interest affects the level of risk. For example, liver hemangiomas are associated with high potential bleeding risk. To avoid complications, it is important to ensure that the patient's laboratory values are within acceptable ranges. (Comprehensive Text Chapter 23; Heading: Indications for CT-Guided Procedures/CT-Guided Biopsies)

## CHAPTER 24: EXAM REVIEW

1. Answer–a. Basic consent is appropriate for most types of radiologic procedures. Choice (b) describes informed consent, which is required for procedures of a more invasive nature, such as image-guided biopsies. Choice (c) describes implied consent. Choice (d) describes parental consent. (Comprehensive Text Chapter 11; Heading: Patient Education and Informed Consent)

2. Answer–b. The iodinated contrast material used for the CT examination of the neck can interfere with the results of a radioactive thyroid uptake study. Therefore, CT studies that use iodinated contrast material should not be scheduled sooner than 2 weeks before the nuclear medicine thyroid study. (Comprehensive Text Chapter 12; Heading: Effects on Thyroid Function)

3. Answer–a. There is no established radiation limit for patients receiving diagnostic tests. A medical history can discover risk factors for contrast media administration, determine pregnancy status in women of childbearing age, verify that the appropriate examination protocol is selected, and provide the radiologist with diagnostic information that can help when

interpreting the CT images. (Comprehensive Text Chapter 11; Heading: Medical History)

4. Answer–b. If the intention is that the dialysis is short-term therapy, with the hope that the kidney will recover, the patient should not be given intravascular contrast media. The aim is to avoid any risk of further renal insult that could diminish residual renal function and result in the renal failure becoming chronic with the need for ongoing hemodialysis. (Comprehensive Text Chapter 12; Heading: Dialysis and Contrast Media)

5. Answer–c. In general, the normal range for estimated glomerular filtration rate is 60 mL/min/1.73 m² or higher. Radiologists are typically consulted whenever the eGFR is less than 30 mL/min/1.73 m². (Comprehensive Text Chapter 11; Heading: Laboratory Values)

6. Answer–a. Coumadin (or warfarin) belongs to the class of medications called anticoagulants. These drugs, used to treat a variety of health conditions including stroke, inhibit coagulation. (Comprehensive Text Chapter 11; Heading: Laboratory Values)

7. Answer–d. (Comprehensive Text Chapter 13; Heading: Nontunneled and Tunneled Central Venous Catheters)

8. Answer–d. Documentation of IV contrast administration is a legal necessity and should include all injection parameters. It should also include the date, the time of the injection, and the person administering it. Accurate documentation allows the study to be reproduced, should follow-up examinations be necessary. (Comprehensive Text Chapter 13; Heading: Basic Principles of Intravenous Contrast Administration)

9. Answer–c. CT coronary angiograms require the use of mechanical injectors. Whenever these injectors are used, both straight needles and butterfly infusion sets should be avoided to reduce the risk of contrast extravasation. A Huber needle is a noncoring hooked needle used for accessing implantable ports. (Comprehensive Text Chapter 13; Heading: Vascular Access)

10. Answer–c. Both the test bolus method and the bolus triggering method allow the scan delay to be individualized to the patient. Unfortunately, they do not improve patient safety. In fact, the major disadvantage of bolus triggering is that the technologist is no longer able to monitor the injection site during the initial seconds of the contrast injection. Although the software is not particularly complicated, both methods require the technologist to understand the programs and correctly input information. Because a timing bolus requires an additional series of scans to calculate the delay, it increases the total examination time (compared with using a standard flow rate and scan delay) rather than decreasing it. (Comprehensive Text Chapter 13; Heading: Bolus Triggering)

11. Answer–b. The bolus phase is the earliest phase, which occurs following an IV bolus injection. It is characterized by a dramatic attenuation difference between the aorta and the inferior vena cava. (Comprehensive Text Chapter 13; Heading: General Phases of Tissue Enhancement)

12. Answer–c. Technologists must be sure that they are administering a premixed heparin flush solution. Concentrated heparin sodium could result in serious bleeding complications for the patient. Fatalities from accidental overdose have been documented, such as when infants accidentally received 1,000 times more heparin than intended when vials containing 10,000 units/mL instead of 10 units/mL were used to flush the infants' vascular access lines. (Comprehensive Text Chapter 13; Heading: Peripherally Inserted Central Catheters)

13. Answer–c. The iodine atoms in the contrast material are exclusively responsible for an enhanced structure's increased beam attenuation capacity. The degree to which this occurs is directly related to the concentration of iodine in the contrast material. (Comprehensive Text Chapter 12; Heading: Dose)

14. Answer–b. Overranging occurs with helical scanning and refers to the extra data acquired above and below the designated area of interest. It adds to the patient dose and is more pronounced with 64, 128, or 256 detector scanners. (Comprehensive Text Chapter 14; Heading: Overranging)

15. Answer–c. The most common formula for calculating the dose of contrast material for pediatric studies is 2 mL/kg. (Comprehensive Text Chapter 12; Heading: Dose)

16. Answer–c. Although no definite risk to the fetus has been identified, there is insufficient evidence to conclude contrast agents pose no risk. Therefore, it is recommended that if a patient is known to be pregnant, both the potential radiation risk and the potential added risks of contrast media should be considered before proceeding with the study. The radiologist should confer with the patient's referring physician. (Comprehensive Text Chapter 12; Heading: Iodinated Contrast Media During Pregnancy and Lactation)

17. Answer–a. Although a functional definition varies in the literature, the common measure is a reported rise in serum creatinine of greater than 25% above baseline or an absolute rise of 0.5 mg/dL within 48 hours of receiving an iodinated contrast agent. (Comprehensive Text Chapter 12; Heading: Contrast Media-Induced Nephropathy)

18. Answer–c. Higher concentration agents are particularly well suited when multislice scanners are used and the scan duration is quite short. (Comprehensive Text Chapter 13; Heading: Contrast Medium Characteristics)

19. Answer–b. Large air embolism after contrast administration by means of a mechanical injector can only occur as a result of human error. Although butterfly infusion sets and straight needles are not recommended when using a mechanical injector, this is because of the increased risk of contrast extravasation (not air embolism). Although technologists should make every attempt to remove air bubbles from the syringe and tubing, small quantities of air can be absorbed by the body without harm. (Comprehensive Text Chapter 13; Heading: Mechanical Injection Systems)

20. Answer–d. The mortality rate from barium peritonitis is significant. To prevent this condition, a water-soluble solution is recommended whenever there is suspicion of a gastrointestinal tract perforation. (Comprehensive Text Chapter 12; Heading: Barium Sulfate Solutions)

21. Answer–c. Oral steroids must be given a minimum of 6 hours (but preferably 12 hours) before the examination. Probably the most common premedication regimen for adult patients calls for three 50-mg doses of prednisone, beginning 12 hours before the scheduled examination and given every 6 hours. Often a single 50-mg dose of diphenhydramine is also given shortly before the examination. Intravenous steroid administration can provide the same risk reduction in a shorter time (5 hours) and is sometimes used for inpatient or emergency department patients. (Comprehensive Text Chapter 12; Heading: Role of Premedication)

22. Answer–b. A change in window settings has no effect on radiation dose, as it is done after the data acquisition. Using a wider slice for an examination that contains multiple slices will reduce the radiation dose, as will decreasing the mAs. Decreasing the pitch will increase the radiation dose to the patient. For example, it is estimated that decreasing the pitch from 1.5 to 1.0 will result in a dose increase of approximately 33% (assuming all other factors are held constant). (Comprehensive Text Chapter 14; Heading: Factors Affecting Dose)

23. Answer–c. In general, radiation that spills over from adjacent slices (or "tails") will contribute approximately 25% to 40% additional dose, as compared with the dose from a single slice. Therefore, if a single slice delivered 8 cGy, then the entire dose from a contiguous slice study would range from 10 cGy (i.e., 8 cGy + 2 cGy) to 11.2 cGy (i.e., 8 cGy + 3.2 cGy). (Comprehensive Text Chapter 14; Heading: $Z$ Axis Variation)

24. Answer–a. The computed tomography dose index, or CTDI, can only be calculated if slices are contiguous, that is, there are no overlapping or gapped slices. The multiple scan average dose (MSAD) will allow for gapped or overlapping slice protocols. Although the dose-length product (DLP) more closely reflects the radiation dose for a specific CT examination, its value is affected by variances in patient anatomy. Therefore, CTDI is a more useful measurement for comparing radiation doses among different scanners and different protocols. (Comprehensive Text Chapter 14; Heading: Measurement Terminology)

25. Answer–c. Holding all technical factors constant, smaller objects always absorb a higher dose by a factor of at least two. This effect is primarily attributed to the fact that total exposure is made up of both entrance radiation and exit radiation. For smaller patients, the patient has less tissue to attenuate the beam, which results in a much more uniform dose distribution. Conversely, for a larger patient, the exit radiation is much less intense owing to its attenuation through more tissue. (Comprehensive Text Chapter 14; Heading: Dose Geometry)

26. Answer–a. All other factors held constant, if the mAs setting is doubled, the radiation dose is also doubled. Likewise, if the mAs setting is halved, the dose to the patient is also halved. Although kVp does affect the radiation dose, the effect is not linear. With all other factors held constant, changing from 120 to 140 kVp increases the radiation dose about 30% to 45%. Pitch also affects the radiation dose to the patient, but the effect is not linear. (Comprehensive Text Chapter 14; Heading: Factors Affecting Dose)

27. Answer–a. From conception to 3 months' gestation, the fetus is most sensitive to the effects of radiation because this is the time of organ and neural crest development. (Comprehensive Text Chapter 14; Heading: Radiation Dose to the Fetus)

28. Answer–c. As the scan field and patient size increase, the x-ray beam must travel a greater distance and penetrate more tissue to arrive at the center. The greater distance and increased thickness of the absorber provide more opportunity for the beam to be attenuated. Hence, the uniformity of the dose decreases as the scan field of view and patient thickness increase. Therefore, body scans are less uniform than head scans. (Comprehensive Text Chapter 14; Heading: Dose Geometry)

29. Answer–b. The latency time for cancer induction at the dose ranges used in CT is 10 to 30 years. However, because of their younger age, children have more time to express a cancer, and more time to undergo more CT examinations, than do adults. In addition, because of their youth, they have more rapidly dividing cells, which are more radiosensitive. It is worth noting that controversy does exists regarding methods of estimating the risk of cancer induction by low-dose radiation that put estimates such at this into question and suggest that the risk may be much lower. (Comprehensive Text Chapter 14; Heading: Increased Sensitivity)

30. Answer–a. Because the x-ray beam does not typically scatter great distances in CT, shielding in not

nearly as effective in reducing the radiation dose to the patient as it is in general radiography. However, shielding in CT is not without benefit and is particularly useful in demonstrating to the patient (or the patient's family) that everything possible is being done to minimize the risks from radiation exposure. (Comprehensive Text Chapter 14; Heading: Patient Shielding)

31. Answer–b. In general, increasing radiation dose results from increasing mAs, increasing kVp, decreasing pitch, and decreasing slice thickness. Although choice (a) includes the lowest mAs, it is more than offset by the increased kVp and decreases in pitch and slice thickness. (Comprehensive Text Chapter 14; Heading: Factors Affecting Dose)

32. Answer–a. With digital technology, the image is uncoupled from the dose, so even when an mA or kVp setting that is too high is used, a good image results. Many technologists currently working in the field were trained before the routine use of digital radiography and may be unfamiliar with this characteristic. (Comprehensive Text Chapter 6; Heading: The Uncoupling Effect)

33. Answer–c. A high-attenuation object is one that absorbs or scatters a high percentage of the x-ray beam. The trachea and lung are composed mostly of air, which does not attenuate much of the x-ray beam. A renal cyst is fluid-filled and is, therefore, relatively low-attenuation (approximately 0 HU). The petrous bone is dense, consisting of calcium and other dense minerals, and will attenuate much of the x-ray beam; it will be represented as a white area on the CT image. (Comprehensive Text Chapter 1; Heading: Beam Attenuation)

34. Answer–c. Prospective reconstruction is that which occurs automatically with scanning. Reformatting includes only image data. Step-and-shoot scanning is also called axial scanning and refers to a nonhelical scan process in which the table movement is stopped during each scan acquisition. (Comprehensive Text Chapter 1; Heading: Raw Data Versus Image Data)

35. Answer–b. The generator produces high voltage and transmits it to the x-ray tube. This high voltage propels the electrons from the x-ray tube filament to the anode. High amperage is not necessary for the production of x-rays. (Comprehensive Text Chapter 2; Heading: Generator)

36. Answer–c. Choice (a) is the response time of the detector. Choice (b) is the detector absorption efficiency. Choice (d) refers to the brief, persistent flash of scintillation that occurred with older detector materials. (Comprehensive Text Chapter 2; Heading: Detector)

37. Answer–c. (Comprehensive Text Chapter 2; Heading: Detector Electronics)

38. Answer–a. Electrons "boil off" of the heated filament and are propelled across to strike the anode, where they disarrange the target material to produce x-ray photons. The x-ray photons (not electrons) then travel from the anode to the patient. Increasing the kilovoltage, increases the speed at which they travel. Ultimately, this results in a higher photon energy of the resultant x-ray beams. (Comprehensive Text Chapter 6; Heading: Milliampere-Second Setting)

39. Answer–c. (Comprehensive Text Chapter 2; Heading: Detector Electronics)

40. Answer–a. Primary storage refers to the computer's input/output channels. Primary memory is used to store data that are likely to be in active use. (Comprehensive Text Chapter 3; Heading: Computer Memory)

41. Answer–d. Output devices accept processed data from the computer. Other examples of output devices are laser cameras, printers, and archiving equipment such as optical disks or magnetic tape. CT detector mechanisms and touch-sensitive plasma screens are examples of input devices that feed data into the computer. The microprocessor is part of the CPU. (Comprehensive Text Chapter 3; Heading: Computer Components)

42. Answer–c. MDCT systems modify many of the rules established with SDCT. MDCT contains multiple parallel rows of detector elements that can be combined in various ways to yield slices with different section thicknesses. In SDCT, slice thickness was controlled exclusively by the degree of physical collimation. But in MDCT, slice thickness is also affected by the width of the detectors in the $z$ axis. (Comprehensive Text Chapter 5; Heading: Multidetector Row Systems)

43. Answer–c. The digitized data are sent from the reconstruction processor to the display processor, which then converts it to shades of gray. (Comprehensive Text Chapter 4; Heading: Gray Scale)

44. Answer–d. The source collimator is located near the x-ray source and limits the amount of x-ray emerging to thin ribbons. Because it acts on the x-ray beam before it passes through the patient, it is sometimes referred to as prepatient collimation. (Comprehensive Text Chapter 2; Heading: Collimation)

45. Answer–a. The attenuation coefficient is a number derived from a specific strength beam as it travels through a specific substance. For example, with a CT scanner that is operating in the typical range of 120 kVp, the linear attenuation coefficient for water is approximately 0.18 cm$^{-1}$. This means that when the beam passes through 1.0 cm of water, about 18% of the photons are either absorbed or scattered. (Comprehensive Text Chapter 1; Heading: Beam Attenuation)

46. Answer–d. Dissipating the by-product heat generated in the production of x-rays is an important

aspect of the CT system design. (Comprehensive Text Chapter 2; Heading: X-ray Source)

47. Answer–b. The focal spot is also called the anode target. (Comprehensive Text Chapter 2; Heading: X-ray Source)

48. Answer–d. MDCT systems with detectors that contain thinner rows centrally are called adaptive arrays, nonuniform arrays, or hybrid arrays. Fourth-generation scanners (in which detectors are situated in a complete ring) are not used in MDCT systems because too many detector elements would be required. (Comprehensive Text Chapter 5; Heading: Multidetector Row Systems)

49. Answer–d. The thinnest that images can be reconstructed for a data set is predetermined by the slice thickness used for data acquisition. Images can be added together to create thicker slices for viewing, but in many cases, data cannot be divided to produce thinner slices. On systems that will allow data to be divided, the slice can never be thinner than the smallest detector element. In this example, 40 mm of data are acquired with each data acquisition. Slice thickness can be reconstructed in multiples of 0.625. For example, 32 slices that are each 1.25 mm, 16 slices that are each 2.5 mm, or 8 slices that are each 5 mm (Comprehensive Text Chapter 5; Heading: MDCT: Reconstructed Slice Thickness)

50. Answer–a. ROM is a type of solid-state memory. It is part of the system's primary memory. Primary storage refers to the computer's internal memory. It is accessible to the CPU without the use of the computer's input/output channels. (Comprehensive Text Chapter 2; Heading: Computer Memory)

51. Answer–b. This method is used in helical scanning. The system takes the slanted helical data and estimates what its appearance would be if the slices were taken axially, with each slice parallel to the plane of the table. The greater the slant (i.e., the higher the pitch), the more interpolation is required. Choice (a) is the definition for standard deviation. (Comprehensive Text Chapter 5; Heading: Helical Interpolation)

52. Answer–c. Multiplanar reformation software stack up images, and then slice the stacked whole in a plane specified by the operator. These can be created from image data, providing the images possess the same display field size, center, and gantry tilt and the slices are contiguous. Changes to the display field size, the reconstruction algorithm, or the slice increment must be done using raw data. (Comprehensive Text Chapter 8; Heading: Multiplanar Reformation)

53. Answer–a. Streaks are inherent in the back-projection process; therefore, it is essential to apply a mathematical filtering process before back projection. (Comprehensive Text Chapter 3; Heading: Filter Functions)

54. Answer–c. This type of filtering is applied to scan data before back projection occurs. Many different filters are available that use different algorithms depending on which part of the data must be enhanced or suppressed. Bone (or high-contrast algorithms) accentuate the difference between neighboring pixels to optimize spatial resolution but must make sacrifices in low-contrast resolution. These filters are most often used when there are great extremes of tissue density and when optimal low-contrast resolution is not necessary. (Comprehensive Text Chapter 6; Heading: Reconstruction Algorithms)

55. Answer–d. The window width selects the range of HU that is to be represented as shades of gray on the image. The window level determines which, of all the possible HU, are to be included. In this example, the total HU to be represented is 120. Because the center is set at 50, the HU depicted are −10 to 110. This is calculated by dividing 120 in half, then subtracting the quotient from the center (50) to find the lower limit. Add the quotient to 50 to find the upper limit. Everything that falls below this range appears black, whereas everything above this range appears white. (Comprehensive Text Chapter 4; Heading: Window Settings)

56. Answer–b. Tissues types with similar densities, such as the white and gray matter of the brain, should be displayed in a narrow window width. Wider window settings are used to suppress image noise and to reduce the appearance of streak artifact. Wider window widths encompass greater anatomic diversity (such as aerated lung), but subtle density discrimination is lost. (Comprehensive Text Chapter 4; Heading: Window Settings)

57. Answer–b. Both a cursor measurement and an ROI obtain an HU measurement. Because the ROI is the average HU for all the pixels within the region, the standard deviation can also be calculated. Both a cursor measurement and an ROI use image data. Neither indicates what scan parameters were used for data acquisition. (Comprehensive Text Chapter 4; Heading: Region of Interest)

58. Answer–d. The slice thickness is irrelevant in determining pixel size. Pixel size can be calculated by dividing the DFOV by the matrix size. Therefore, the pixel size of choice (a) is 0.31 mm; choice (b) is 0.39 mm; choice (c) is 0.59 mm; and choice (d) is 0.86 mm. (Slice thickness does not impact pixel size, only voxel size.) (Comprehensive Text Chapter 6; Heading: Matrix Size, Display Field of View, Pixel Size)

59. Answer–b. (Comprehensive Text Chapter 6; Heading: Impact of mAs and kVp Settings on Radiation Dose)

60. Answer–c. It is important to differentiate reconstruction algorithms from setting a window width and level. Changing the window setting merely changes

how the image is viewed. Changing the reconstruction algorithm will change the way the raw data are manipulated to reconstruct the image. (Comprehensive Text Chapter 6; Heading: Reconstruction Algorithms)

61. Answer–d. Spatial resolution is also called detail resolution. Spatial resolution is the system's ability to resolve, as separate forms, small objects that are very close together. (Comprehensive Text Chapter 6; Heading: Spatial Resolution)

62. Answer–b. Resolution in the $xy$ direction is called in-plane resolution. The in-plane resolution is affected by pixel size, which is affected by the DFOV. Resolution in the $z$ direction is called longitudinal resolution. This is affected largely by slice thickness and (in helical scans) pitch. (Comprehensive Text Chapter 6; Heading: In-Plane Versus Longitudinal Resolution)

63. Answer–c. An isotropic voxel is a cube, measuring the same in the $x$, $y$, and $z$ directions. The pixel size is the $xy$ size (because pixels are square). The pixel size for the four choices are (a) 0.23, (b) 0.49, (c) 0.68, and (d) 0.86. For the voxel to be near-isotropic, the pixel size must be close to that of the slice thickness (the $z$ direction). (Comprehensive Text Chapter 6; Headings: Spatial Resolution, Slice Thickness)

64. Answer–b. In the context of image quality, the word "temporal" refers to the characteristic of being limited by time and relates to a scanner's data acquisition speed. The temporal resolution of a system is typically reported in milliseconds. (Comprehensive Text Chapter 6; Heading: Temporal Resolution)

65. Answer–a. The product of the mA and scan time is known as mAs, or tube current. It determines the amount of x-ray photons. The kVp determines the quality (or average photon energy) of the x-ray beam. Neither DFOV nor reconstruction algorithm has any affect on the x-ray beam; rather they control how the raw data are back projected to create an image. (Comprehensive Text Chapter 6; Heading: Scanning Parameters)

66. Answer–d. The lungs are considered to have high inherent contrast because they are primarily composed of air and provide a background that makes nearly any object contained within the lung easy to see. On the contrary, the physical properties of the body's soft tissues and many other organs possess low inherent contrast, often making it difficult to differentiate adjacent structures; to increase the inherent contrast in these organs, iodinated contrast medium is often administered. (Comprehensive Text Chapter 6; Heading: Other Contrast Resolution Considerations)

67. Answer–c. The MIP (maximum-intensity projection) examines each voxel along a line from the viewer's eye through the data set and selects only the voxel with the highest value for inclusion in the displayed image. This method tends to display bone and contrast-filled structures; lower-attenuation structures are not well visualized. (Comprehensive Text Chapter 8; Heading: Projection Displays)

68. Answer–a. Redundancy can also refer to the duplication of data to provide an alternative in case of failure of one part of the process. Planning for redundancy is an important part of any radiology information system. (Comprehensive Text Chapter 9; Heading: Networking)

69. Answer–c. The LNT model assumes that the long-term, biological damage caused by ionizing radiation is directly proportional to the dose–that is, it is linear. In addition, the model assumes that any radiation is considered harmful with no safety threshold. It has been the accepted standard for many years and has been used to set radiation protection standards. The radiation hormesis model asserts that radiation at very small doses can be beneficial. (Comprehensive Text Chapter 14; Heading: Information Concerning the Effects of Low-Dose Radiation)

70. Answer–a. A typical line/pairs phantom contains groups of lead strips having different strip width and spacing. In each group, the lead width is equal to the lead spacing. The spatial resolution is given as the maximum number of visible line pairs (lead strip and space) per millimeter. (Comprehensive Text Chapter 6; Heading: Direct Measurement of Spatial Resolution)

71. Answer–b. Responsibility for performing and documenting quality control tests is often shared between CT technologists and medical physicists. However, a medical physicist must perform dose measurements. (Comprehensive Text Chapter 7; Heading: Quality Assurance Methods)

72. Answer–a. The partial volume effect occurs when more than one type of tissue is contained within a voxel. (Comprehensive Text Chapter 7; Heading: Partial Volume Artifact)

73. Answer–d. As x-ray beams pass through an object, lower-energy photons are preferentially absorbed, creating a "harder" beam. Individual rays are hardened to differing degrees, and this variation cannot be adjusted for by the reconstruction algorithm. CT systems use three features to minimize beam hardening: filtration, calibration correction, and beam-hardening correction software. Filtering the beam with a material such as aluminum filters out the lower-energy components of the beam before they pass through the patient. (Comprehensive Text Chapter 7; Heading: Beam Hardening)

74. Answer–b. Interpolation methods used with helical data can result in a scan that is wider than that selected by the operator. This is referred to as slice thickness blooming or degradation of the slice sensitivity profile. (Comprehensive Text Chapter 5; Heading: Effective Slice Thickness)

75. Answer–d. Cross-field uniformity refers to the ability of the scanner to yield the same CT number in a homogeneous object (i.e., water phantom) regardless of the location of the region of interest. (Comprehensive Text Chapter 7; Heading: Noise and Uniformity)

76. Answer–c. In a 2004 study, researchers asked patients, ED physicians, and radiologists to estimate the radiation dose for one CT examination versus the dose for one chest radiograph. The results from that study demonstrated the lack of awareness regarding the radiation dose associated with CT examinations. None of the estimates given by the patients were in the accurate range. Twenty-two percent of ED physicians surveyed reported dose estimates in the accurate range. Most surprising, only 13% of radiologists surveyed reported dose estimates in the accurate range. In all groups, the majority of participants underestimated the dose from CT examinations. (Comprehensive Text Chapter 14; Heading: Why the Growing Concern?/Lack of Awareness)

77. Answer–c. VR is a 3D semitransparent representation of the imaged structure. It has become the favored 3D image technique because all voxels contribute to the image. (Comprehensive Text Chapter 8; Heading: Volume Rendering)

78. Answer–b. (Comprehensive Text Chapter 6; Heading: Contrast Resolution; and Chapter 7; Heading: Contrast Resolution [Low-Contrast Resolution])

79. Answer–d. Out-of-field artifacts occur when portions of the patient lie outside the selected scan field of view. (Comprehensive Text Chapter 7; Heading: Out-of-Field Artifacts)

80. Answer–b. The most likely cause of the streak artifact is from the patient's arms positioned down by his or her sides for scanning. This can be inferred, even without the scout image to confirm, by examining the streaks, which appear to have their origins outside, on either side, of the displayed image. This type of artifact is broadly categorized as out-of-field artifacts. (Comprehensive Text Chapter 7; Heading: Out-of-Field Artifacts)

81. Answer–c. As the number of detector channels increases, a wider collimation is required and the x-ray beam becomes cone-shaped, rather than fan-shaped. This can result in cone beam artifacts, which are more pronounced for the outer detector rows. The larger the cone beam (i.e., more detector channels), the more pronounced the effect. (Comprehensive Text Chapter 7; Heading: Spiral and Cone Beam Effect)

82. Answer–d. Sometimes ring artifacts can be eliminated simply by recalibrating the scanner. If that fails, a service engineer must be called to repair the defective detector. (Comprehensive Text Chapter 7; Heading: Ring Artifacts)

83. Answer–a. We can recognize noise as the grainy appearance or "salt-and-pepper" look on an image. Contrast resolution involves differentiating an object from its very similar density background. Because the difference between object and background is small, noise plays an important role in low-contrast resolution. (Comprehensive Text Chapter 6; Heading: Noise)

84. Answer–d. Quantum mottle occurs when there are an insufficient number of photons detected and results in image noise. Doubling the mAs of the study increases the number of photons detected per pixel by approximately 40%. (Comprehensive Text Chapter 6; Heading: mAs/Dose)

85. Answer–b. (Comprehensive Text Chapter 8; Heading: Multiplanar Reformation)

86. Answer–a. The standard deviation indicates the amount of CT number variance within the ROI. (Comprehensive Text Chapter 4; Heading: Hounsfield Measurements and Standard Deviation)

87. Answer–c. 3D printing uses VR data sets to produce models that will accurately portray the detail of both surface and interior structures. (Comprehensive Text Chapter 8; Heading: 3D Modeling)

88. Answer–d. The spatial resolution of a CT image does not compare favorably with other modalities. Where CT excels is in its low-contrast resolution, for which it is superior to all other clinical modalities. (Comprehensive Text Chapter 6; Heading: Evaluating Spatial Resolution Using the MTF)

89. Answer–a. Changing the slice incrementation is only possible with helical CT data. (Comprehensive Text Chapter 5; Heading: Changing Slice Incrementation Retrospectively; and Chapter 8; Heading: Retrospective Reconstruction)

90. Answer–b. Overt patient motion will create artifacts that can greatly degrade image quality. It is unlikely that a diagnostic examination can be produced in a patient unable to lie still for the length of time required to complete the test. Although newer scanners can often complete the arterial phase acquisition in just seconds, the patient must be able to lie still for that short time. (Comprehensive Text Chapter 20; Heading: CTA of Pulmonary Embolism)

91. Answer–a. A positive agent creates image contrast because it has a higher density than surrounding tissues. Iodine and barium sulfate are examples of positive agents. (Comprehensive Text Chapter 12; introductory text)

92. Answer–b. $55/(64 \times 0.625) = 55/40 = 1.375$ (Comprehensive Text Chapter 5; Heading: Pitch in MDCT Systems)

93. Answer–d. Gapped images are taken when representative slices are sufficient and imaging every part of the region is not required. Because some areas are not exposed, studies comprising gapped slices will reduce the radiation dose to the patient.

(Comprehensive Text Chapter 14; Heading: Slice Width and Spacing)

94. Answer–c. Pitch is most commonly defined as the travel distance of the CT scan table per 360° rotation of the x-ray tube, divided by the x-ray beam width. In the case of MDCT, the beam width can be determined by multiplying the number of slices by slice thickness. (Comprehensive Text Chapter 5; Heading: Pitch)

95. Answer–c. Lateral ventricle. (Comprehensive Text Chapter 15; Heading: Brain)

96. Answer–a. Falx cerebri. (Comprehensive Text Chapter 15; Heading: Brain)

97. Answer–b. Caudate nucleus. (Comprehensive Text Chapter 15; Heading: Brain)

98. Answer–d. Calcified pineal body. (Comprehensive Text Chapter 15; Heading: Brain)

99. Answer–a. Both the viscosities and the osmolalities of contrast agents classified as nonionic/low osmolality will rise slightly with the concentration. Because higher concentration agents are more viscous, they may not flow through small-gauge IV catheters as easily as lower concentration agents. One hundred milliliters of a 300 concentration agent will contain 30 g of iodine, whereas 100 mL of a 370 concentration agent will contain 37 g of iodine. (Comprehensive Text Chapter 12; Heading: Properties of Iodinated Agents)

100. Answer–b. In most situations, HOCM (e.g., Hypaque) is used for oral administration because it is less expensive than LOCM (e.g., Omnipaque) and provides equivalent gastrointestinal opacification. However, in some cases, LOCM has advantages. If aspirated, LOCM causes less pulmonary edema than HOCM. In newborns, researchers have noted a reduction in complications when LOCM is used compared with barium sulfate or HOCM. Barium sulfate is preferred when a patient is unable to drink the full dose of oral contrast. This is because in small amounts barium sulfate tends to cling to the intestinal wall, providing at least a small amount of visible contrast. In comparison, the bowel usually absorbs a small quantity of water-soluble oral contrast. (Comprehensive Text Chapter 12; Heading: Comparison of Positive Oral Contrast Agents)

101. Answer–b. (Comprehensive Text Chapter 13; Heading: General Phases of Tissue Enhancement)

102. Answer–c. (Comprehensive Text Chapter 20; Heading: Thoracic Protocols; and Chapter 21; Heading: Abdomen and Pelvis Protocols)

103. Answer–d. Acoustic neuromas, or more properly vestibular schwannoma, originate in the internal auditory canal (IAC). Although medium and large acoustic neuromas extend outside the IAC and into the brain cavity, many of these tumors are quite small and are confined to the IAC. Contrast-enhanced CT using a narrow slice thickness is typically needed to detect small acoustic neuromas. (Comprehensive Text Chapter 19; Heading: Neurologic Protocols)

104. Answer–c. The appearance of an intracranial hemorrhage (ICH) will change with the passage of time, as red blood cells begin to deteriorate outside the vasculature. As a general rule, ICH will appear hyperdense to normal brain tissue for approximately 3 days, after which it will gradually decrease in density. (Comprehensive Text Chapter 19; Heading: General Imaging Methods for the Head)

105. Answer–a. The use of iodinated contrast media has been shown to provoke seizures in patients who have diseases that disrupt the blood-brain barrier. In these patients, the risk of seizure can be reduced by a one-time oral dose of diazepam, 30 minutes before contrast administration. Seizures that occur can also be controlled with diazepam. (Comprehensive Text Chapter 12; Heading: Central Nervous System)

106. Answer–b. Incus. (Comprehensive Text Chapter 15; Heading: Temporal Bone)

107. Answer–a. Malleus. (Comprehensive Text Chapter 15; Heading: Temporal Bone)

108. Answer–b. Epitympanic recess. (Comprehensive Text Chapter 15; Heading: Temporal Bone)

109. Answer–c. Cochlea. (Comprehensive Text Chapter 15; Heading: Temporal Bone)

110. Answer–a. Vestibule. (Comprehensive Text Chapter 15; Heading: Temporal Bone)

111. Answer–a. Lateral semicircular canal. (Comprehensive Text Chapter 15; Heading: Temporal Bone)

112. Answer–c. (Comprehensive Text Chapter 20; Heading: ECG Gating)

113. Answer–b. Motion artifact can be a problem when the patient's heart rate is greater than 70 bpm or if the heart rate is irregular. When imaging larger cardiac structures, heart rate is less of an issue, although a slower, regular heart rate is still preferred. (Comprehensive Text Chapter 20; Heading: ECG Gating)

114. Answer–a. CT imaging of the airways is most often performed in a helical mode, using thin sections and an overlapping z axis image reconstruction of 50% so that images can be postprocessed. Airway imaging is routinely performed at both inspiration and expiration. (Comprehensive Text Chapter 20; Heading: CT of the Airways)

115. Answer–c. (Comprehensive Text Chapter 20; Heading: CTA)

116. Answer–a. (Comprehensive Text Chapter 20; Heading: Important Considerations)

117. Answer–c. Right pulmonary artery. (Comprehensive Text Chapter 16; Heading: Chest)

118. Answer–d. Superior vena cava. (Comprehensive Text Chapter 16; Heading: Chest)

119. Answer–b. Ascending aorta. (Comprehensive Text Chapter 16; Heading: Chest)

120. Answer–a. Pulmonary trunk. (Comprehensive Text Chapter 16; Heading: Chest)
121. Answer–c. Esophagus. (Comprehensive Text Chapter 16; Heading: Chest)
122. Answer–b. A thrombosis is a blood clot. If the thrombus detaches from its original site, it is referred to as an embolus. If the embolus occludes a vessel in the brain and disrupts the blood supply, it results in an ischemic stroke. A myocardial infarction (i.e., heart attack) occurs when the heart does not receive an adequate blood supply. (Comprehensive Text Chapter 19; Heading: Types of Stroke; and Chapter 20; Heading: Anatomy/Terminology Review)
123. Answer–c. IV contrast administration is not necessary for all thoracic indications because the structures of the thorax possess high intrinsic natural contrast. (Comprehensive Text Chapter 20; Heading: General Thoracic Scanning Methods)
124. Answer–c. Aorta. (Comprehensive Text Chapter 17; Heading: Abdomen)
125. Answer–b. Duodenum. (Comprehensive Text Chapter 17; Heading: Abdomen)
126. Answer–a. Portal vein. (Comprehensive Text Chapter 17; Heading: Abdomen)
127. Answer–a. Head of the pancreas. (Comprehensive Text Chapter 17; Heading: Abdomen)
128. Answer–d. Left adrenal gland. (Comprehensive Text Chapter 17; Heading: Abdomen)
129. Answer–c. Psoas muscle. (Comprehensive Text Chapter 17; Heading: Abdomen)
130. Answer–a. Allergy to foods that contain iodine (e.g., seafood) does not increase the risk of intravenous contrast medium reactions. Seafood allergy results from hypersensitivity to a protein within the seafood and has no association with iodine. Assuming the history does not reveal any contraindications to iodine, the examination should proceed as ordered. (Comprehensive Text Chapter 12; Heading: Allergies)
131. Answer–b. The gallbladder is present in the expected location adjacent to the liver. A Whipple procedure consists of removal of the gallbladder (along with the distal portion of the stomach, the distal portion of the common bile duct, the head of the pancreas, the duodenum, and the proximal jejunum). The high-density objects on the anterior chest wall are breast shields, intended to reduce radiation to the breast. (Comprehensive Text Chapter 17; Heading: Abdomen)
132. Answer–d. Ascending colon (cecum). (Comprehensive Text Chapter 17; Heading: Abdomen)
133. Answer–a. Right common iliac vein. (Comprehensive Text Chapter 17; Heading: Pelvis)
134. Answer–a. Left common iliac vein. (Comprehensive Text Chapter 17; Heading: Pelvis)
135. Answer–b. Left common iliac artery. (Comprehensive Text Chapter 17; Heading: Pelvis)
136. Answer–b. Vertebral canal with spinal cord. (Comprehensive Text Chapter 17; Heading: Pelvis)

137. Answer–c. Most institutions set guidelines as to the upper limit of contrast media that can routinely be given (typically 64 g of iodine). However, the guidelines are typically quite cautious, and specific circumstances (such as equipment malfunction) may necessitate exceeding the limit. A radiologist will determine whether the guidelines can safely be exceeded by considering individual factors, such as a patient's level of hydration and renal function. Several studies have shown a direct correlation between the volume of contrast administered and the risk of contrast-induced nephropathy. (Comprehensive Text Chapter 12; Heading: Chemotoxic Reactions)
138. Answer–b. A "saline chaser" reduces streak artifacts over the superior vena cava that result from dense contrast material. Although increasing the scan delay (choice c) would reduce the streak artifact by allowing the contrast to dilute, the examination would be degraded. (Comprehensive Text Chapter 20; Heading: Contrast Administration)
139. Answer–b. The normal CT attenuation of the liver in unenhanced studies varies among individuals and ranges from 38 to 70 HU. (Comprehensive Text Chapter 21; Heading: Liver)
140. Answer–c. (Comprehensive Text Chapter 21; Heading: Pancreas)
141. Answer–c. The nephrogram phase occurs when the contrast media reaches the kidneys. (Comprehensive Text Chapter 21; Heading: Kidneys)
142. Answer–c. The use of mechanical injection systems in CT produces the best results. However, precautions must be taken to prevent contrast media extravasation and care must be taken in the preparation and connection of the injector and cannula to avoid the risk of large air emboli. (Comprehensive Text Chapter 13; Heading: Mechanical Injection Systems)
143. Answer–c. (Comprehensive Text Chapter 12; Heading: Gastrointestinal Contrast Medium)
144. Answer–c. (Comprehensive Text Chapter 13; Heading: General Phases of Tissue Enhancement; and Chapter 21; Heading: Liver)
145. Answer–d. In many institutions, the protocol for a thoracic CT extends to the adrenal glands when patients have a history of lung cancer. (Comprehensive Text Chapter 20; Heading: Thoracic Protocols)
146. Answer–d. (Comprehensive Text Chapter 4; Heading: Suggestions for Setting the Window Width and Level)
147. Answer–b. (Comprehensive Text Chapter 16; Heading: Chest)
148. Answer–a. Although both adenomas and metastatic lesions enhance rapidly, because of differences in their intracellular lipid content, metastatic lesions retain the contrast longer. (Comprehensive Text Chapter 21; Heading: Contrast Washout)
149. Answer–b. Fatty infiltration reduces the CT attenuation of the involved liver. With fatty infiltration, the

liver is at least 10 HU lower than that of the spleen. (Comprehensive Text Chapter 21; Heading: Liver)

150. Answer–c. Thyroid gland. (Comprehensive Text Chapter 15; Heading: Neck)

151. Answer–b. Thyroid cartilage. (Comprehensive Text Chapter 15; Heading: Neck)

152. Answer–a. Trachea. (Comprehensive Text Chapter 15; Heading: Neck)

153. Answer–d. Common carotid artery. (Comprehensive Text Chapter 15; Heading: Neck)

154. Answer–c. Jugular vein. (Comprehensive Text Chapter 15; Heading: Neck)

155. Answer–d. The axial plane is parallel to the plantar surface of the foot. (Comprehensive Text Chapter 22; Heading: Foot and Ankle)

156. Answer–d. The distance covered in an MDCT helical scan sequence can be calculated using the following formula: Pitch × total acquisition time × 1/rotation time × (slice thickness × slices per rotation). Therefore, (a) $1 \times 10 \times 1 \times (5 \text{ mm} \times 4) = 200$ mm; (b) $1.2 \times 10 \times 1 \times (5 \text{ mm} \times 4) = 240$ mm; (c) $1 \times 15 \times 1 \times (5 \text{ mm} \times 4) = 300$ mm; (d) $1.2 \times 15 \times 1 \times (5 \text{ mm} \times 4) = 360$ mm. (Comprehensive Text Chapter 5; Heading: Helical Scan Coverage)

157. Answer–b. When initial scans fail to differentiate the margins of the pancreas from the duodenum, the patient is often given additional oral contrast material and additional slices are obtained with the patient lying in a right decubitus position. (Comprehensive Text Chapter 21; Heading: Pancreas)

158. Answer–b. Calcaneus. (Comprehensive Text Chapter 18; Heading: Foot)

159. Answer–c. Cuboid bone. (Comprehensive Text Chapter 18; Heading: Foot)

160. Answer–b. Cuneiform (interomedial or second). (Comprehensive Text Chapter 18; Heading: Foot)

161. Answer–d. Metatarsal bone. (Comprehensive Text Chapter 18; Heading: Foot)

162. Answer–a. Cuneiform bone (medial or first). (Comprehensive Text Chapter 18; Heading: Foot)

163. Answer–b. (Comprehensive Text Chapter 16; Heading: Chest)

164. Answer–d. Because of the increased collimation, a narrower slice results in fewer x-ray photons. To compensate, mAs must be increased. (Comprehensive Text Chapter 6; Heading: Factors Affecting Contrast Resolution/Slice Thickness)

165. Answer–c. The glabellomeatal line is the imaginary reference line that runs approximately 15° cephalad from the orbital meatal line. The glabella is the surface of the frontal bone lying between the eyebrows. (Comprehensive Text Chapter 19; Heading: General Imaging Methods for the Head)

# Index

*(Note*: Page numbers followed by "*f* " denote figures; those followed by "*t* " denote tables.)